Lives Interrupted

Psychoanalytic Studies: Clinical, Social, and Cultural Contexts

Series Editor
Michael O'Loughlin, Adelphi University

Mission Statement

Psychoanalytic Studies seeks psychoanalytically informed works addressing the implications of the location of the individual in clinical, social, cultural, historical, and ideological contexts. Innovative theoretical and clinical works within psychoanalytic theory and in fields such as anthropology, education, and history are welcome. Projects addressing conflict, migrations, difference, ideology, subjectivity, memory, psychiatric suffering, physical and symbolic violence, power, and the future of psychoanalysis itself are welcome, as are works illustrating critical and activist applications of clinical work.

See https://rowman.com/Action/SERIES/LEX/LEXPS for a list of advisory board members.

Titles in the Series

Lives Interrupted: Psychiatric Narratives of Struggle and Resilience, edited by Michael O'Loughlin, Secil Arac-Orhun, and Montana Queler
Women and the Psychosocial Construction of Madness, edited by Marie Brown and Marilyn Charles
Revisioning War Trauma in Cinema: Uncoming Communities, by Jessica Datema and Manya Steinkoler
Women & Psychosis: Multidisciplinary Perspectives, edited by Marie Brown and Marilyn Charles
Psychoanalysis from the Indian Terroir: Emerging Themes in Culture, Family, and Childhood in India, edited by Manasi Kumar, Anup Dhar, and Anurag Mishra
A Three-Factor Model of Couples Psychotherapy: Projective Identification, Level of Couple Object Relations, and Omnipotent Control, by Robert Mendelsohn

Lives Interrupted

Psychiatric Narratives of Struggles and Resilience

Edited by Michael O'Loughlin,
Secil Arac-Orhun,
and Montana Queler

LEXINGTON BOOKS
Lanham • Boulder • New York • London

Published by Lexington Books
An imprint of The Rowman & Littlefield Publishing Group, Inc.
4501 Forbes Boulevard, Suite 200, Lanham, Maryland 20706
www.rowman.com

6 Tinworth Street, London SE11 5AL

British Library Cataloguing in Publication Information Available

Library of Congress Cataloging-in-Publication Data

ISBN: 978-1-4985-6833-3 (cloth)
ISBN: 978-1-4985-6834-0 (electronic)

This book is dedicated to the memory of Tod Sloan (1952–2018),
professor, humanitarian, social justice activist, and friend.

Contents

Foreword

Listen In

Erin Soros

When I was in the psychiatry ward, someone stole my diary and returned it with new entries. I remember the violation I felt on noticing its absence—what else did I have in that institution but my words? And I remember the surprising joy when I found it on the common room table and opened it to discover handwriting other than my own. Another patient had felt compelled to write—to herself? to me? to us both?—in what was now an oddly shared private space. Her longing on one page, mine on the other: side by side our entries formed an intersubjective madness. We were still speaking to ourselves, in our own worlds, but here was that fold connecting us.

Madness is supposed to be kept private. In fact it is often kept locked. We were both held captive within that ward, unable even to go for a stroll on the grounds without timed supervision, and involuntarily medicated so that our minds would quiet, no one willing to listen to our words and their secrets—but now I held this journal returned with its new daring permissions.

I recalled these written intimacies—those taken and those offered—when I first encountered the pages of this book, which contains both the words of those who experience severe psychic struggle and those who have learned from them: reflections, insights and critiques that are sometimes on the same page, as when commentary addresses issues and themes within the interviews, and sometimes in separate sections, as with the introduction and afterword, but all bound here together nevertheless. I wonder how readers will approach these voices with their divergent titles and roles. Which ones will possess authority and how will that authority be shaped? Who is the knower and who is the known? Will the words of those who experience madness in fact ultimately trouble the words of those we think do not? We may assume we can distinguish easily between the authorial positions of those people recorded here who survive psychic distress and those who listen to them, but I am curious if we might find an intersubjective madness on *these* pages too, something shared through language—shared in the sense of being understood, and in the sense of being transmitted. Given how rarely the insight of those who experience severe psychic distress is actually elicited—how unusual is this collection of voices—one could well assume that the act of valuing and elevating this input amounts to a form of madness itself. For what is the fold between sanity and insanity when we begin to attend with respect and humility to those who have been institutionally silenced? Do we indeed risk becoming mad when involved in such transgressive and attuned listening? Is that fear not in some sense gripping us in those moments when we refuse to hear? What will happen to your own words, then, to your companion notes, when you write them down in response to this reading? When you close this book, how will it enter the maps of your dreams?

I have never met the people who are recorded here. I do not know their real names. After sitting with both the delicacy and force of their recollections, I experienced a daunting reluctance to join my own voice to this collection, my contribution seeming somehow as presumptuous as stealing another's journal and adding my own thoughts. The stories articulated in the interviews are powerful and poignant, immediate and intimate: revealing not just suffering, and not just struggle, but startling and challenging insight from the very cusp of the human mind. We are taken on an intricate journey, encountering desire and talent, unexpected humor and found kinship, testimony of individual and collective trauma, rage against societal injustices and grief after repeated violation—madness not as wound, but rather a way to communicate its location.

Here too is trust. Here is the private emerging as public. Here is freedom and the risks it brings. When we say the word "I" to another and we are heard, even for a fleeting moment, we can experience a pivotal release. In these pages you can hear hesitancy, and also the pleasure of disclosure. What could not be expressed, what was supposed to be kept hidden, has a witness. And the stories are given time on the page: while readers are provided significant and helpful clinical framing and theoretical context, the excerpts of each personal tale also find their own rhythms and express their own illuminating and often troubling sense. People are not reduced to symptom and diagnosis: instead we hear the nuance and specificity of what they choose to tell. And the connections we encounter on these pages were developed over months before any formal interview took place. So there is vulnerability on both sides of this listening, with the requirement and opportunity that clinicians join a therapeutic community beyond their designated roles. Yet a book such as this one does have its enclosures. The dialogue has been edited and then shaped by commentary. The names published on the cover do not direct us to those interviewed, those who have so much to teach. These people instead required the protections offered by anonymity, their words existing independent of their identities, like a written confession found in a common room. Listening becomes both gift and theft.

You were not originally there to listen within those white walls holding both pain and beauty, but now you can listen in: you grasp stories in your hands, interior landscapes, words originally trusted to someone other than yourself. How will you now honor what has been left open for you to read?

Acknowledgments

One of the pleasures of writing an academic book is acknowledging the genealogical traces and ancestral wisdom from which our ideas are born. The list of works cited pays homage to some of that genealogical continuity. The book you hold in your hands, or the virtual book in which these words are inscribed, is also a powerful testament to the workings of community. Our ancestors came together to offer communal labor for purposes such as barn raising. The Amish people in the United States still maintain this beautiful tradition. Creating a book of this scope also entails the collaborative effort of many people—not all of them compensated—to collaborate on a shared production. It is a privilege for us, as editors, to be the beneficiaries of such largesse, and we would like to acknowledge here some of the more than fifty people who have joined communally to create the book you are about to read.

Our debt to the participants in this study is indescribable. We are deeply grateful to the people who entrusted us with their stories, and who spoke with grace, compassion, and heartfelt sincerity about privileged aspects of their life histories. The only form of recompense that we can imagine doing justice to their participation is the hope that this book contributes to humanizing and complexifying our understanding of severe psychic distress. We are also deeply grateful to Fountain House. Kenneth Dudek, President, Elliott Madison, Program Director, and Andrew Schonebaum, Chief Financial Officer, put their moral weight and financial support from Fountain House behind this project, and offered wisdom and guidance at crucial moments. We are also deeply grateful to members of the Fountain House Research Board for approving the project and providing oversight over a lengthy period of time. We are grateful to: Nancy L. Farrell, Dr. Howard Fillit, Alexandra Herzan, Dr. Howard Owens, Charles J. Marsden, Stephen B. Rice, and Guy Szeto. In addition, Yusselffy Denize, Betty Eastland, and Cyrus Napolitano of Fountain House provided invaluable feedback after viewing videotaped sessions.

At Adelphi University, Jay Crosby, a graduate of Derner School of Psychology doctoral program, helped us gain entrée to Fountain House, and we are grateful for his assistance. A cohort of graduate assistants, funded by Derner School of Psychology, provided an invaluable service in faithfully transcribing thirty-nine hours of interviews. We are deeply grateful to Rachel Ether, Meredith Friedson, Jacqueline Hrzich, Julia Krebs, Caitlin Lapine, Bri McMahan, Dolores Paul, and Melodie Piciullo for their painstaking work. Sigi Gradwohl also contributed to transcription, and Janani Sundaram assisted with preparation of the index.

The idea for this project took shape while Michael O'Loughlin was working on a psychosis research project at Austen Riggs Center in collaboration with Marilyn Charles. While Marilyn's work in this book speaks for itself, her understanding of the experience of persons with severe distress, and her humanitarian approach to therapeutic work has deeply infused our thinking. Lucy Newlyn, whose beautiful poem opens the introduction, is a model for how a person who has suffered significant psychic suffering pursues her life with grace, dignity, and creativity, and we thank her for allowing us to use her work. We are also deeply grateful to Erin Soros who authored the foreword. Her work serves as a beautiful invitations to readers to engage with the book. We are honored that Robin Taylor from Fountain House Gallery has granted us permission to use her evocative *Ghost Jenny* on the cover.

Kasey Beduhn, Associate Acquisitions Editor at Lexington Books, and Assistant Editors Alison Keener and Megan Murray handled the coordination and production process with grace and efficiency. Kasey is the editor for both of Michael O'Loughlin's book series and she combines talent and receptivity with a deep commitment to publishing the highest quality academic books.

On a personal level, Michael O'Loughlin wishes to express thanks to Margaret Healy, who has provided the continuing emotional support and forbearance that makes this kind of long-term work possible. Michael is enormously grateful to Daniel Griffin, MD, who managed his care during a serious illness in Summer 2018. Secil Arac-Orhun wishes to express gratitude to Eren Orhun, who has been an amazing source of support through all aspects of this project, from start to finish. She also wishes to thank Nilgun and Sukru for providing the emotional support needed to complete this work. Montana Queler would like to thank Victor Bonilla, who has provided enduring kindness, love, and boundless support; and Michael O'Loughlin, for his dedication to creating a work of integrity, and for approaching the task of mentorship with the same spirit of humanity and respect.

Introduction

Narrating the Prose of Severe Psychic Suffering

Michael O'Loughlin,
Secil Arac-Orhun, and Montana Queler

The self now seeing
They hide behind their shiny screens
to muse, and gloze, and pry—
a little clan of medicine men
whose hospital's hard by.

I see them in my nightmares
In suits and serried rows.
They trap me with their lures and snares—
Until the black mood goes.

My stock of little poison-pills
Tucked in their plastic sheet
And covered in thin metal foil—
It tempts me, "Come and eat!"

I'm stupefied by medicine
My numbed brain put on hold.
My limbs are like a mannequin's—
I wander, dull and cold.

Five months go past; there is a wall
That grows with time more wide,
Till February comes—and still
No warmth can get inside.

But now the poison-pills are done—
I'll have no more of them.
The serried rows of suits are gone—
Dismissed, upon a whim

Prescribe me nothing, I am free
To flout this world of men—
And spring is here to welcome me
Back to my blues again.

Lucy Newlyn [1]

In her frank and moving autobiography, poet and Oxford professor Lucy Newlyn (2018) charts the course of a significant psychiatric disturbance that she first experienced in her forties, while she kept vigil as her father lay dying. Newlyn offers a harrowing account of the fifteen years since she first experienced psychosis, was sectioned, and was forcibly taken to the emergency room (known in U.K. as Casualty or A & E) in a state of frightened confusion, exacerbated, perhaps, by the precipitous manner in which she was inducted into the psychiatric system:

> Arriving in Casualty I thought I had been put prison. When a psychiatrist interviewed me I didn't know who I was or even what time of day it was. I had turned into a strange thing I couldn't recognize as myself. I sat on a seat which was also a toilet in a large white empty room on my own where a strong bright light shone on me perpetually. I shouted for a long, long time. When I was let out of the observation room I saw the A & E area, where people were lying on stretchers or trolleys. I was sure they were war-victims; there was one whose face was bloated—her whole body was swollen and it seemed to be in a sack. She looked like my mum. There were other people whose heads I could see over the tops of screens, and I thought two of them were my sisters. I kept hearing their voices and they seemed to be lying about me—their accounts of me were a tissue of lies, designed to show that I was no carer. They wanted me punished. I kept screaming at the top of my voice: "LISTEN." (pp. 22–23)

Newlyn's narrative charts unsparingly the many ups and downs of her condition; her struggles with socially sanctioned stigma and institutional anomie in her workplace; her battle with medications that flattened her symptoms but at the cost of also flattening out the creative spikes that were so vital to her poetry-making; and, of course, the monkey wrench that her psychic struggles threw into the personal and professional relationships she was seeking to stabilize and maintain. Newlyn lifts the veil on the complex and often downright perplexing nature of psychic suffering. Benefiting from her experiences in counseling and from her struggles to articulate self-understanding in her poetry, Newlyn offers a deeply reflective, nuanced account that serves as a counter-narrative to simplistic, reductionist diagnoses and classifications, as well as to the idea that there is any single, simple "magic bullet" or single pill to "cure" severe psychic suffering. It says a lot about Western societies' attitudes to mental distress that a distinguished author such as Newlyn, struck by a form of madness that is just a whisper away from being triggered for any one of us, given straitened circumstances, must frame her work as a coming-out story—with all the connotations of overcoming shame and stigma that this implies. Mad Pride still has a long way to go in creating a space that renders madness nameable and speakable.[2] Is madness still a condition that, to borrow from Lord Douglas, "dare not speak its name"?[3]

The narrative tone of Newlyn's work is also worthy of note. Modern, industrialized, corporatized medicine, with its constant pressure for automation, for cost-cutting, and for the generation of putatively "evidence-based," cost-conscious treatment protocols and the completion of time-consuming records, places enormous billing pressures on medical providers to see as many patients as possible. Too often there is neither time nor interest in listening to the patient—in *getting the story* of human suffering. The patient narrative that frames the origin and meaning of a medical or psychological/spiritual crisis is at risk of disappearing from general medical practice and, indeed, from psychiatry. Even strictly medical conditions come with attendant spiritual and existential crises that merit attention and anxieties that should be recognized so they might be assuaged. With the notable exception of her general practitioner, Newlyn noted that despite the essential help her carers offered, for the most part there was little interest in the total circumstances of her distress, in the meaning of her experience, or in the effects these aberrant and terrifying intrusions were having on her daily living. About her family physician, she remarked: "In the day to day management of mental illness I've found GPs to be more helpful than psychiatrists, since they are not committed to any particular methodology: one just talks to them as to another human being." (pp. 4–5). In a review of Alison Vaspe's (2017) book on the U.K.'s National Health Service [NHS], Michael O'Loughlin summarized the increasing shift away from listening and from the provision of psychosocial support in healthcare:

> What family physicians and mental health workers have offered historically, as many of the writers here note, is *continuity of care* through deep immersion in patient narratives across lifespans and even generations. In mental health care, the capacity for hospitals to provide for *communality of care* through creation of supportive mental health communities, of the kind that Barbara Taylor (2015) has described as so beneficial to her recovery in the now extinct asylum system, has also disappeared. The model that is emerging in the NHS is of time-limited physician visits (i.e., 10 minute, single-issue consultation with whatever physician happens to be on duty). (O'Loughlin, 2018a, p. 446)

In Vaspe's book, Clare Gerada, former chairperson of the Council of the Royal College of General Practitioners, states that now the emphasis in the NHS is too often on conformity rather than delivery of care:

> This, together with an extremely onerous regulatory burden—here captured in the rubric of endless *box ticking* and the conversion of general practitioners into factory workers, leads to the kind of depersonalized, atomized, and commodified health care delivery that is marketed as consumer choice. As Marilyn Miller notes, "the production line model, with its focus on time, activity, and money—squeezing more out of each GP—also means that patients are being looked at as things rather than people. . . . It is part of an archaic industrial model of Taylorism" (p. 196). Referring specifically to mental health, Gerada explores how manualized, scripted therapies, outcomes-based therapies, rationed treatments, time-limited therapies, and a system where performance is judged by computerized feedback sheets reflects exactly the same thinking.
>
> Where, in all of this, is there a place for relationship or narrative? Where is there room for the physician, nurse, or therapist to keep the patient in mind? Who keeps the physician, nurse, or therapist in mind when, inevitably, they are overwhelmed by the schizoid anxieties the system is continually manufacturing? In the current NHS, as Tim Darlington (Chapter 10) notes, care is denigrated and insight is regulated, all in the interest of what Gerada calls "machine-marked care indices" (p. 204). Gerada tells us that her physician head "is full of patient stories," (p. 204) but all she can see around her is pervasive grief as altruistic, dedicated professionals are driven to alienation. (O'Loughlin, 2018a, p. 461)

ETHICAL LONELINESS

We are not naïve enough to believe that the neoliberal ideology behind the money-driven, pharmaceutical/medical model of healthcare will be easily reversed. However, with this book, we hope to make one important, if humble, contribution. Our goal is to illustrate the complexity of human psychic, existential, and spiritual suffering and the need for medical and community-based solutions that provide spaces where people can gain the psychological containment and psychosocial support to facilitate recovery. This book, then, is a book of life stories. The beauty of these stories—and the many other survivor stories that have been published[4]—is that they resist the kind of simplification and reductionism that essentialize and objectify persons with psychiatric struggles, atomize their experiences, and all too often lead to simplistic, and sometimes even coercive, "treatment" plans. We hope that readers will use these stories to complexify the conversation and expand their thinking about psychic suffering. Most important, we hope that readers of this work will double down on the value of getting the story rather than checking off boxes and formulating diagnoses and treatment plans that then lead to supposedly cost-effective—and all too often exclusively pharmaceutical—and ultimately unhelpful short-term revolving-door interventions for what are, after all, very complex forms of human suffering. This suffering has arisen in the course of living a life and will be exacerbated or alleviated by the provision or absence of appropriate familial and psychosocial supports. This observation would be fairly mundane, were it not that it is often strikingly absent from neoliberal health care.

The shift towards term-limited, manualized, or didactic therapies, as well as the increasing use of medication as an exclusive treatment for severe psychic distress, is antithetical to narrative approaches to healing. Music therapies (cf., Ready, 2016), expressive art therapies (Attard & Larkin, 2016), progressive mirror drawing (cf., Peciccia & DiBenedetto, 1998), social justice–oriented therapies (Martin Baró, 1996; Watkins & Shulman, 2010), and non-prescriptive talk therapies (e.g., Bollas, 2013, 2016; Epstein, 1995, 1998) offer spaces where patients can inscribe their meanings and work through their experiences either individually, in formal group therapy, or in peer-support groups such as those pioneered by the Hearing Voices Network.[5] The notion of *bearing witness* is well established in psychoanalysis, for example, as a means of offering a receptive space where traumatized individuals or groups might begin the process of examining and speaking through their own life stories (e.g., O'Loughlin, 2007a, 2007b, 2013, 2018b). The speaking and naming of psychic distress is a key first step in pulling together the parts of a narrative that may have fragmented, and this can result in a *re-storying* of experience so that a new or re-told life narrative may be crafted that incorporates the experience of the psychic crash which temporarily foreclosed the making of new meaning. Discussing the rupture that is trauma, O'Loughlin used the metaphor of darning a sock to illustrate this re-storying process:

> I have vivid memories from my childhood of my mother, who was skilled at knitting, darning our socks and sweaters when they wore threadbare. Darning is a fabulous process of repair in which a patch is artfully woven in such a way that the rips and tears in the garment are skillfully patched by reconnecting the strands of wool in a seamless manner. If trauma cuts the threads of speech as Lacanian psychoanalysts suggest, then a society needs a host of darners who can skillfully braid strands of severed speech and social linkages together in ways that endow citizens with new capacities to come to terms with the ancestral lineages and inheritances of their pasts—as opposed to being overdetermined by their pasts. (O'Loughlin, 2018b, p. 11)

In *Ethical Loneliness*, Jill Stauffer (2015) draws on the writings of Jean Améry and on the philosophy of Emmanuel Levinas to identify the catastrophic effects of forms of social isolation and indifference on suffering people. Her work holds echoes, perhaps, of Agamben's notion of *bare* life (cf. Agamben, 1998; Fassin & Rechtman, 2009), a condition in which a whole group of people are reduced to a non-status so that processes of dehumanization and even annihilation can be enacted without qualms. Such an ascription can certainly be applied to the suffering of large sociopolitical groups such as Holocaust survivors (Agamben), refugees (O'Loughlin, 2016), and trauma survivors (Fassin & Rechtman). Stauffer defines ethical loneliness as follows:

> Ethical loneliness is the isolation one feels when one, as a violated person or as one member of a persecuted group, has been abandoned by humanity, or by those who have power over one's life possibilities. It is a condition undergone by persons who have been unjustly treated and dehumanized by human beings and political structures, who emerge from that injustice only to find that the surrounding world will not listen or cannot properly hear their testimony—their claims about what they suffered and about what is now owed them—on their own terms. So ethical loneliness is the experience of having been abandoned by humanity compounded by the experience of not being heard. (p. 1)

Stauffer notes that "stories without an audience do not survive" (p. 2), and she says that "unintended ironies surface whenever institutions designed for hearing fail to hear well, and I show how the effects of those ironies tend to weigh most heavily on those with the least power to endure bad outcomes" (p. 6). Her book is replete with examples of people with power and the best of intentions failing to hear or hearing only the confirmatory thoughts they expected. As Lucy Newlyn, quoted earlier, said, we must learn how to LISTEN! In what follows, we will discuss the methodological considerations entailed in seeking to listen well in a research context, all the while acknowledging the power asymmetries and ethical conundrums such a context necessarily entails. While we lay out our theoretical position in this introduction, in presenting the narratives, we have sought to privilege the phenomenological accounts of participants over psychologically or clinically-interpretive description and analysis. Our desire is to leave the space open, as far as possible, for readers to bring a new ear to the stories and to formulate their own opinions of the narratives that are presented. We believe that too little is known about deep psychic suffering to do otherwise. Just as good therapists let their patients be their teachers, we hope that our readers can let the participants in this project be their teachers. With their dignity and humility in the face of chronic struggles, they have taught us much.

CONCEPTUALIZING PSYCHIC DISTRESS: RECLAIMING THE SUBJECT OF PSYCHOLOGY

Perhaps there is no area of medicine where the debate about treatment and nomenclature is as fraught or as polarized as the area we choose to call severe psychic distress. Despite sustained criticism by people who suffer from extreme psychic experiences—experts by experience—and sustained scholarship and advocacy in critical psychiatry,[6] the medical/biological model holds sway in Western medicine. Sustained critique over more than half a century from writers in the anti-psychiatry movement such as Peter Breggin (1991), David Cooper (1967), Erving Goffman (1961), R. D. Laing (1969), D. L. Rosenhan (1973), and Thomas Szasz (1961, 2008), as well as more recent critiques by Richard Bentall (2003, 2009), Bonnie Burstow (2015), David Healy (2012, 2019), Joanne Moncrieff (2013), Darby Penney & Peter Stastny (2009), Louis Sass (2007, 2017), Robert Whitaker (2001, 2010) and others appears to have had little impact on the day-to-day practices of psychiatry. In *Crazy Like Us: The Globalization of the American Psyche*, Ethan Watters (2010) points out that the medicalized, reductionist, disease-based, biologized model of psychic distress is gradually colonizing global psychiatric care, abetted by the kind of cost-conscious corporate implementation favored by neoliberal governments. Most troubling of all, perhaps, genealogical research by Lisa Cosgrove and colleagues (Cosgrove & Krimsky, 2012; Cosgrove & Wheeler, 2013) into the money trail reveals the powerful influence of monies from the pharmaceutical industry in shaping the ideology of the influence-makers who have shaped the Diagnostic and Statistical Manual [DSM]. The DSM is produced and marketed by the American Psychiatric Association. In its latest iterations [DSM IV; DSM-5], it has shifted its allegiance completely in favor of a disease-based/biologized/medicalized model of psychic distress as disease—a condition for which pharmaceutical and other medical solutions become the inevitable—and frequently the sole—solution. Nefariously allied with the profit and cost imperatives of neoliberal corporate healthcare and Big Pharma, medication becomes the vital partner of a psychiatric "care" system that requires that sufferers be "stabilized" and revolve out of the hospital in the few precious days that insurance coverage allocates as the approved time-limited treatment window.

We refuse the disease-based, objectifying, and pejorative terms "schizophrenic" and "psychotic," and we worry that terms such as "mental illness," as well as the many specific "disorder" descriptors in the DSM and ICD classifications—e.g., bipolar disorder, borderline personality disorder, schizoaffective disorder—serve to reinforce the idea that mental distress constitutes a biological illness in a form analogous, perhaps, to an infection or a cancer. Irrespective of whether there is a genetic or epigenetic component, acknowledgment of the vector of stressors that cause some people to experience situations of extreme distress is surely called for. Beyond the capacity of psychotropic medications to stabilize persons in extreme states of dysregulation, we believe that it is critical to understand the psychosocial and familial contexts from whence such distress emanates, and to combine detailed history-taking with the provision of respite and psychosocial supports that can enhance recovery.

For many years, Michael O'Loughlin has been a persistent critic of the normalizing and pathologizing effects of psychology, acknowledging the failure of psychology, as Amodeo Giorgi (1970, 2009) suggests, to achieve its potential as a human science. Writing in 2002, and drawing on Chambers' (1996) essay on the colonizing uses of power, for example, he noted:

> In words that might be a *fetishschrift* for the everyday practices of psychology, [Chambers] talks of the power of the decontextualized and supposedly neutral discourses of Western science to objectify and control those seen as other: ". . . the power to name, identify, classify, domesticate and contain that simultaneously doubles as the power to obliterate, silence and negate. For the recognition of other histories, of other people, of other languages and sounds, of other ways of dwelling in the same space that have been confined to the shadow, obliterated by the bright light of the unswerving beam of 'progress,' also invokes the recognition of their place, however obscured and repressed, in the very constitution of our own histories and culture; in our national and individual identities, in our psychic and social selves." (O'Loughlin, 2001, pp. 179–80)

O'Loughlin later posed the fundamental dilemma of representing human experience from within a normalized, privileged, Western psychological worldview this way:[7]

> Psychologists traffic daily in distinctions between the psyche and the social; between essentialist and multiple notions of subjectivity; between the idiosyncratic and the universal; between autonomy and acculturation. How much are our ways of framing therapeutic and research interpretations governed by unexamined notions of privileged Sameness and aberrant Otherness? (2002, p. 182)

In her theatrical accounts of her own troubling experiences with institutional approaches to handling the extreme states she continues to experience, Professor Erin Soros (2015) suggests that the institutional blinders of psychology and psychiatry can engender what Stauffer calls an ethical loneliness—a sense of misrecognition that is nothing short of catastrophic for the psyche of a person who is in an extreme state (cf., Bollas, 2013; Charmaz, 1983) and desperately seeking what psychoanalysts call emotional holding and containment, or even the needed respite from the world that William Styron (1990) discussed in *Darkness Visible*.[8]

Elsewhere, O'Loughlin offers a critique of the accelerated rush toward medicalized treatment of children and seeks to expose the vested interests behind this unseemly and dangerous trend. Drawing on the writing of Françoise Davoine and Jean-Max Gaudillière (2004) in *History Beyond*

Trauma, he suggests that instead of seeking to eradicate symptoms viewed as pathological, we ought to pay close attention to the gaps in communication that persons suffering extreme distress experience, because these gaps and ruptures contain the concealed story that needs to be named, spoken, and claimed, in order to ease the sense of abandonment—of ethical loneliness—and thereby create opportunities for regenerative restorying of psychic experience:

> Davoine and Gaudillière (2004) point out the appalling reductionism involved in articulating an intrapsychic notion of clinical practice that takes no account of history, ancestry, and intergenerationally transmitted or buried trauma. Instead of seeing the difficulties of an individual as reflecting individual pathology, Davoine and Gaudillière argue that we must pay attention to the gaps and ruptures of individual experience because these are symptoms pointing us precisely to the moments of history that have been erased. They suggest that we should recognize severe symptoms such as psychosis and major depression as signifiers pointing back to lack or rupture from the historical crises of trauma. Persons with such symptoms, therefore, need our assistance to "bring into existence zones of non-existence wiped out by a powerful blow that actually took place." (O'Loughlin, 2012, p. 283)

In *Six Moments in Lacan*, Derek Hook (2018) explains why Jacques Lacan was derisively opposed to behavioral and cognitive psychology, and to many forms of psychoanalysis which, Hook suggests, have been "effectively psychologized" (p. 3). Psychologization, here, refers to a shift from acknowledging human subjectivity to seeing the subject as object, "including the idea that psychology is 'objectivistic' overly ego-focused, that it wrongly presumes natural scientific, biological, developmental and adaptive perspectives" (p. 10). Here for example, Hook uses a quote from Martin Murray's (2016) recent book to point out the objectifying functions of cognitive-behavioral therapy [CBT], an approach to psychotherapy that is rapidly establishing hegemony in neoliberal hospital environments because its positivist roots are embraced as supposedly demonstrably "evidence-based."

If there is any doubt that Lacan's critique is of current relevance, consider Murray's (2016) comments:

> Representations of human life as mechanical are even evident in . . . psychology now, in the twenty-first century. A popular contemporary example is cognitive behavioral therapy (CBT), which "forces" patients to relinquish self-destructive thoughts and "trains" them to adopt more positive ones . . . human psychology is taken to resemble animal behavior in reacting mechanistically to instinctive impulses. Behavioural psychology . . . still takes . . . this kind of positivistic and causal view of the human as a sort of animal that is also a sort of machine. (quoted in Hook, 2018, p. 178)

The argument here, of course, is whether psychotherapy and psychoanalysis should be "adjustment therapies," or whether, as Lacan (2006) would claim (see also Van Haute, 2002), we should take a stand against adaptation to conventional notions of normalcy. Nowhere are the stakes in this discussion higher than for persons who experience conventional society as intolerable and for whom coercion to adapt to normalcy, however imprisoning and claustrophobic society may be, can only be viewed as what Comaroff and Comaroff (2003) and Kleinman, Ramphele, and Reynolds (2000) would suggest is an act of violence. As Hook notes, any form of objectification inevitably involves a misapprehension of the subject (p. 182). Instead of seeking to understand, to impose coherence and a state of meaning, Lacan suggests an epistemology of *not-knowing* (p. 182). Quoting from Bruce Fink's (2014) *Against Understanding*, Hook summarized this negative epistemological stance thus:

> Such a stance is explicitly premised *against understanding* for, as Fink (2014) warns, the process of understanding can be seen to reduce the unfamiliar to the familiar, to transform the radically other into the same, and to render the analyst hard of hearing. Our ability . . . to detect the unconscious . . . is compromised by our emphasis on understanding and can be rectified only by taking as our fundamental premise that we do not understand . . . (quoted in Hook, p. 182)

In Adam Phillips' (2007) *Winnicott*, the author compares Kleinian and Winnicottian work with children in ways that echo the Lacanian concerns just described. While the focus in Phillips' discussion is on child therapy, the point he makes in contrasting Klein's heavily interpretive and external approach to Winnicott's more invitational approach—an approach that gives the child a space to reveal his or her understanding—applies equally, we think, to work with adults with psychic distress. To put it simply, is the child [or adult] patient to receive pre-formed understanding of its condition, as Klein would have it, or must the analyst wait for the child to make him or herself known to the analyst, as Winnicott would suggest? Phillips described the choice this way:

> But having worked out the basic constituents of the child's internal world, the risk for the Kleinian analyst was of seeming to know beforehand all there was to know about the child. Klein's apparently comprehensive knowledge of the child's unconscious could be used as a blueprint. From the very beginning, Winnicott would represent himself as less knowing than Klein as an analyst; and he would stress the importance, as an analyst, of being able to tolerate not-knowing. Klein had described the child's wish for knowledge—what she called the "epistemophilic instinct"—as integral to his [sic] development, and this led her to overvalue the insight gained from interpretation and analysis. Winnicott would never insist on Klein's equation of development and the

> acquisition of knowledge. And in his later work he would replace the capacity to know by the capacity to play. (pp. 46–47)

Winnicott assumed, Phillips notes, that "the child has a primary wish to be understood, indeed 'longs for someone to bring understanding'" (p. 51) and he further states, "the Winnicotttian child tends to be a collaborator rather than an antagonist" (p. 52). What this points to, of course, is an attitude of receptivity and deep listening, and a commitment to understanding the history and context of the presenting human experience, however puzzling or fragmented it may be. Do we owe suffering fellow human beings any less?

A NOTE ON THE ROLE OF NEGATIVE LIFE EXPERIENCES

A reader of a prepublication copy of this book worried that the tone of the work embodied a polemic against conventional psychiatry and further worried that drawing forth participants' life stories risked being exploitative. To make our position abundantly clear, this book is not "anti-psychiatry" in any broad-brush sense. What we are opposed to is (1) the attribution of *all* causality for psychic distress to biological and/or chemical factors; and (2) the treatment of psychic distress *exclusively* and for the long term by pharmacological means. The purpose of sharing the stories which, as the discussion in chapter 15 illustrates, some of our partners at Fountain House experienced as overwhelming in their depictions of suffering, is to illustrate precisely the psychosocial complexity of the events that contribute to psychic distress. Our hope is that we can raise awareness of the psychosocial backstory of psychic suffering so that comprehensive treatment approaches are developed that can include psychosocial supports, as well as peer support and individual and group psychotherapy. While pharmacological symptom reduction has its place—particularly for florid symptoms—we believe it is misguided to look to pharmacology as either the sole remedy or the long-term solution to all psychic distress.

By way of brief illustration, consider recent research by Vallath, Luhrmann, Bunders, Rakivant, and Gopikumar (2018). The authors present a report of a study that explored the relationship between what were termed Negative Life Experiences and voice hearing, for which they use the conventional psychiatric term, Auditory Voice Hallucinations. They suggest that research has recently shifted from a nosolgoical (i.e., DSM/ICD classification) approach to a more contextual, phenomenological, and functional understanding (p. 3). Invoking the stress-vulnerabilty model articulated by Zubin and Spring (1977), they suggest that an understanding of voice hearing must be grounded in "understanding the content of voices and lived experiences of the individual . . . since they influence almost all parts of an individual's life—personality, coping and vulnerabilities" (p. 3). Negative life experiences are most likely to be significant, they note, though they point out that many adverse life events (e.g., bereavement, abandonment, homelessness) do not rise to the clinical level of trauma, and hence are rarely studied in the context of severe psychiatric symptoms. In their study, many participants suffered from adverse life events which stemmed from "sociocultural and psychosocial contexts, such as dysfunctional family, marriage, social control, social schemas, loss, abuse, or failure" (p. 5). Most important, they note, "the individual's subjective appraisal of the (negative life experiences) often determined the content of the voices" (p. 5). Their conclusions, coming from a complementary research tradition, offer validation for the posture we adopt in this work that negative and stressful life events contribute greatly to severe psychic distress in some people, and are therefore deserving of our attention. They conclude:

> This research finds that hallucinations are often meaningful and relate to one's psychological and sociocultural context particularly the experience of [negative life experiences] and related events. . . . Voices were found to not only be meaningful but also to have functional properties, especially in coping with [negative life experiences] . . . (pp. 10–11)

While acknowledging the interaction of biological, social, and psychological factors in psychic distress, the authors argue ineluctably for the need to provide therapeutic support to examine negative life experiences that are frequently found to be contributory to psychosis:

> Psychotherapy must thus focus on treatment of trauma [negative life experiences] while treating psychosis. The design of this study does not allow for causal inferences to be drawn. But it is clear that there is an association between [negative life experiences], distress and hallucinations, as discussed above. (p. 13)

DOING RESEARCH THAT MATTERS WITH PERSONS WITH PSYCHIATRIC STRUGGLES

Origins of the Project

This work grew out of an ongoing collaboration between Marilyn Charles and Michael O'Loughlin that began some ten years ago at the Austin Riggs Center. That collaboration has yielded a number of publications that offer background to the present work (e.g., Charles & O'Loughlin, 2012; O'Loughlin & Charles, 2012; O'Loughlin et al., 2014). In an earlier publication, here is how we laid out the origins of the current work:

> Austen Riggs Center (ARC), nestled in the Berkshire Mountains of Massachusetts, has been providing intensive psychodynamic therapy to what are described as "treatment-resistant" patients for almost a century. It is a haven of last resort for patients who often have chronic and intractable psychiatric difficulties, and it is renowned for its humane and intensive treatment of psychic terror. Michael O'Loughlin began collaborating with Marilyn Charles at ARC in 2008, studying videotaped interviews collected by other researchers over a series of years with ARC patients. While we described some findings from that work in a recent essay (Charles and O'Loughlin, 2012), we are only gradually grasping how to fashion a narrative from the data. This is, after all, research at some distance. The interviews were performed by other clinicians, who were not acquainted with the people they interviewed. As viewers of the archived interviews, we were twice removed. Despite all of this, the arc of human suffering was inescapable. We listened to poignant interviews with patients who had their personal and professional lives inexorably disrupted by the intervention of persecutory and delusional thoughts, by ungovernable anxiety, and by intractable depression. We were witness to young people still struggling with restitution narratives, or seeking bemused refuge in psychiatric diagnoses, while watching life as they knew it slip through their hands like grains of sand. Some had decided that life as they knew it was over; they failed to pick up the narrative threads. We learned to trace the lineage from early traumatic events, and even from intergenerationally inherited trauma, to eventual catastrophic breakdown. Burdened with knowledge from the medical records of the outcome ten years later for each of these patients, we were left with heavy hearts. Could any good come of our turning this private suffering into public experience? We worried about betrayal and exposure. We worried about our own voyeurism and about provoking voyeuristic responses in future readers. We witnessed patients struggling to articulate pain and hope through a haze produced by massive doses of psychotropic medications, and sometimes through the confusion of the battle between delusional thought and rational thought. We lived with evident dread—the fear of breakdown. Were our attempts to bear witness well intentioned or were we being foolhardy or exploitative? (O'Loughlin et al., 2014, pp. 100–101)

For the current project we resolved to carry out our own interviews. Furthermore, we recognized that ARC is a highly privileged environment. The hospital caters to person of means and therefore the sample skews toward an affluent white demographic. We wondered what chronic psychic struggles were like for those less privileged—those who did not have access to therapy and those who were economically marginal or indigent. Could we tell their stories with fidelity, and what might they teach us about what they could find most useful to live their lives with greater ease?

GETTING THE STORY: ETHICAL AND METHODOLOGICAL CONSIDERATIONS

There is a profound disconnect between the existential experiences we, therapists, have when we engage in intensive therapy with patients, and the kind of experience René Muller (2008) describes in *Doing Psychiatry Wrong.* Muller notes the profound mismatch between the stories his patients offered, and the official diagnoses assigned to them at intake. A narrative approach is etiological and privileges the patient's narrative of his or her world while a DSM-based approach is necessarily categorical, decontextualized, and ahistorical. The calamitous disjuncture between the two is evident, for example in Joäo Biehl's (2013) study of Catarina, a destitute woman suffering severe psychiatric distress in Brazil. As far as institutional psychiatry was concerned, Catarina's obsessive dictionary-building was gibberish . . . until, of course, under Biehl's anthropological scrutiny, it proved to contain meaningful communication. A foundational knowledge source for us, therefore, in developing our inquiry was information that was phenomenologically near to the human experience of patients. This included published patient narratives and research into the existential experience of being a psychiatric patient (e.g., Biehl, 2013; Charmaz, 1983; Corin, 1992, 1998; Corin & Lauzon, 1992; Estroff, 1981, 2004; Haslam, 2000; Hunter Jenkins & Barrett, 2004; Pandolfo, 2008; Sass, 2007). That the relatively straightforward work of Jaako Seikkula and colleagues (Seikkula, 2001; Seikkula & Olson, 2003) in developing Open Dialogue, a psychosocial approach to treatment in Finland—an approach that privileges the embedded narrative of the patient in family and community contexts—is regarded as pioneering, is a powerful indicator of how far the biological and DSM-based discourses of psychiatry have shifted understanding away from the patient as a whole person, embedded in nested contexts of belief and ideology, family and community. Instead, patients are stripped down to the *bare life* (Agamben, 1998; Fassin & Rechtman, 2009) so familiar to anybody who has ever surrendered their personal possessions and donned a generic hospital gown. Nancy Scheper-Hughes (2003), addressing the dehumanization of her own frail elderly parents in a nursing home, suggests that such institutionalized dehumanization amounts to *invisible genocide.*

Our intent, therefore, was to seek to develop a qualitative research methodology that was sensitive to context, culture, being, and connection. We were striving to acknowledge and work around power asymmetries and privileging systems in the hope of expanding the discourses of psychic distress—often pejoratively labeled "schizophrenic"[9] or "psychotic"—beyond the simple dualisms of the biological and the social, the sane and the crazy, the doctor and the patient, the researcher and the researched, to reach for the deep humanity of the person suffering psychic distress.[10] Our methodology has been influenced particularly by three specific ideas.

First, with respect to overall orientation, Michael Jackson's essay "The prose of suffering," from his book *Existential Anthropology* (2005), has been influential in framing our overall purpose in seeking to "do justice to the way others experience the world, and whatever is at stake for them." Here is the challenge of developing "sustained communion," as Jackson sees it:

> What it means not to "give in" is very much at the heart of ethnography. It means coexisting with the subject of one's concern, sustaining an engagement over time in his or her place, on his or her terms, and trying not to escape into consoling intellectualisations, sympathetic identifications, or political actions that reduce the other to a means for advancing an academic career, or demonstrating what a compassionate person one is, or changing the world. It is a form of sustained communion. And though . . . its analogue is conversation, words are not essential to this dialectic. Moreover, its aim is not to take upon ourselves to redress the injustices of the world but to do justice to the way others experience the world, and whatever is at stake for them. As I see it, this necessitates placing oneself in the situation of the other—a sustained, intimate, and often silent involvement in his or her everyday lifeworld that inevitably transforms one's own worldview and may involve the other seeing his or her situation from a new perspective. In this sense, the ethnographic method seeks not some form of abstract knowledge but through the mix of osmosis and dialogue understands the other in oneself *in other circumstances*, and sees both self and other from the unsettling and unsettled spaces of "the subjective in-between."

Jackson continues, posing troubling questions about the ethnographic enterprise:

> Consider Arthur Kleinman's view that we do violence to others, not only in the way we act toward them but in the ways we speak and write about them. Kleinman argues that subjecting the experience of suffering to anthropological theorisation we violate that experience in much the same way as medicalisation delegitimates the existential reality of illness. These 'professional transformations' turn an 'experience-rich and—near human subject into a dehumanized object—a caricature of experience.' The suffering should not be seen as patients or victims, nor the violated 'romanticized or cynically deconstructed.' Our task is to describe 'what is at stake for particular participants in particular situations. But the trouble with making 'lived experience' and 'what is at stake' into measures of interpretive adequacy or authenticity is that these terms are as abstract and general as any other. *Whose* experience is to be prioritised—the sufferers or ours? And so do we privilege what is at stake for the liberal spectator or what is at stake for the sufferer—for the issues are seldom the same? With the best will in the world it is as difficult to distance oneself from one's own assumptions as it is to embrace the experience of the other. (pp. 152–53)

The importance of "sustaining an engagement over time in his or her place, on his or her terms," will be explored further in the afterword, in which Montana and Secil will meditate on the importance of their deep interpersonal engagement with participants in producing the kinds of conversations escribed below.

Arthur Frank (1995) wrote *The wounded storyteller* about his own extended experiences as a hospital patient after two catastrophic medical events. As we discussed elsewhere (O'Loughlin et al., 2014), Franks speaks of the narrative rupture caused by catastrophic illness, and he has looked at the ways in which people who have had such experiences resume, or fail to resume, the narrative trajectories of their former lives. As we noted, "Many cancer patients in remission . . . are participants in a secret society—people who appear to go on being, but who often live with unspeakable narrative shards and dread at the core of their being" (O'Loughlin et al., 2014, p. 99). Ultimately, after the initial shock of an illness crisis, Frank suggests, patients often subscribe to a *restitution narrative* where they cling to faith in a cure; if their hopes for a cure are not realized, they may unconsciously dwell in what Frank calls a *chaos narrative* and continue to live their lives thoroughly preoccupied by illness and suffering. However, some patients will work to incorporate the illness crisis into their identities and, through what Frank calls *a quest narrative*, develop a capacity for a regenerative re-storying of life experience and renewed pursuit of a purposeful life.

We have adapted Frank's work to conceptualize a severe psychic crisis similarly as a rupture in narrative . . . a collapse of the fundamental capacity for speech and for *going on being* (cf., Winnicott, 1960). Frank's work also provided us with a reminder that, in important respects, suffering is socially produced, and that any inquiry into psychic suffering, as well as considering the existential experience of distress, needed to focus too on the psychosocial origins of such distress, as well as the ways in which interactions with medicalized care (i.e., diagnostic systems; hospitalizations; pharmacology; electroconvulsive therapy; presence or absence of psychotherapy, etc.) contribute to people's understanding of their own suffering.

Cognizant of the reservations in the literature about the hazards inherent in telling someone else's story (cf., Behar & Gordon, 1995; Britzman, 1995; Fine, 1994; Patai, 1987, 1991), but also drawn by the compelling power of human narrative as exhibited in Jackson's and Frank's writings, we set out to develop a phenomenological methodology to engage in conversations with persons with chronic histories of psychic distress. We drew generally on Interpretative Phenomenological Analysis (Smith, 2011; Smith & Osborn, 2003; Smith, Flowers, & Larkin, 2009). Smith and Osborn summarize the method this way:

> The aim of interpretative phenomenological analysis (IPA) is to explore in detail how participants are making sense of their personal and social world, and the main currency for an IPA study is the meanings particular experiences, events, states hold for participants. The approach is phenomenological . . . in that it involves detailed examination of the participant's lifeworld; it attempts to explore personal experience and is concerned with an individual's personal perception or account of an object or event, as opposed to an attempt to produce an objective statement of the object or event itself. At the same time, IPA also emphasizes that the research exercise is a dynamic process with an active role for the researcher in that process. (2003, p. 53)

Our interview method and analysis was also influenced by the detailed protocol for clinical dynamic interviewing detailed by Christopher Fowler and Christopher Perry (2005). This protocol, which Marilyn Charles and Michael O'Loughlin have used to study interviews at the Austen Riggs Center (Charles & O'Loughlin, 2012; O'Loughlin & Charles, 2012; O'Loughlin et al., 2014), is distinctive in that, in addition to eliciting open-ended narrative and reflection, the interview seeks to elicit the unconscious subtext underlying the words that are uttered.

NEGOTIATING THE RESEARCH PROCESS IN THE FIELD

We received an introduction to Fountain House courtesy of Jay Crosby, a graduate of the PhD program in clinical psychology at Adelphi University. The research team at Fountain House consisted of staff and members of the Fountain House community. They were enormously protective of their community and, for the reasons discussed earlier, suitably suspicious of a bunch of psychologists who might wish to classify, judge, or categorize the members of their community—or, at a minimum, think of their lives in narrowly clinical and possibly pathological terms. An early suggestion by team member Elliott Madison was enormously valuable. He said, in effect, that if strangers came in and asked questions, prospective participants might not be forthcoming, and further, how could we possibly know what to ask if we were not immersed in the community? He had zeroed right in on the credibility issue. In response, we proposed that doctoral students Montana Queler and Secil Arac-Orhun would immerse themselves in the Fountain House community one day per week for at least six months before any recruiting would take place. We also expressed a desire to develop a *collaborative interpretive community* (Gilchrist et al., 2015; Millar et al., 2004) in which community participants, both members and staff, could join with us in interpreting the interviews and writing up the final research narrative. We were successful in convincing the University Institutional Review Board that we had sufficient safeguards in place to create an environment that was safe enough to engage in this collaborative process. We originally had visions of a grand collaborative process, in which all members of the team shared in discussion of each of the thirty-nine hours of video interviews that we collected from thirteen participants. The exigencies of life intervened, particularly when Michael O'Loughlin had to recover from an auto accident and later a serious illness, and so this more ambitious plan was shelved. In the end, after some initial collaborative viewing of video interviews, we took a more expedient route and the Fountain House team members proposed to hold a focus group to discuss the book. An edited transcript of that discussion is presented as chapter 15 (below). It is notable too that Fountain House became sufficiently invested in this project to offer generous stipends support to Montana and Secil, as well as offering compensation to all members who participated in interviews. Further details of the *working community* philosophy and practice of Fountain House are presented in chapter 16.

THE INTERVIEW PROTOCOL

We developed an interview protocol designed to be implemented in three approximately one-hour sessions. While the broad parameters of the discussion were laid down in the protocol, the meetings were considered more as life conversations rather than as formal interviews. Participants were invited into conversation with open-ended questions, and specific follow-up probes were only asked if the participant had difficulty sustaining a narrative stream. The first conversation focused on the participant's current psychic state, their struggles with psychic distress, and their understanding of their own experience; the second conversation focused on family history and psychosocial stressors; while the third conversation focused on interactions with institutional and medicalized systems including diagnosis and the use of DSM labels; experiences in hospitals; effects of pharmacological treatments; experiences with electroconvulsive therapy, etc. Here are the guiding statements [written for our use] and initial questions [posed to participants] that we prepared in order to orient ourselves toward each interview. The complete interview protocol is presented in the appendix:

> *In the* ***first conversation*** *we are particularly interested in what Arthur Frank calls "the wounded storyteller" narrative. We are interested in when the participant first experienced psychiatric difficulties; what effect that interruption had on their life plans; what the long-term effects of the psychiatric interruption was on the participant's long-term life plans; and the participant's ability to revise the life plan and develop a new purposeful life plan subsequent to the interruption.*

- If it is OK with you, I wonder if we could begin by talking about your life, beginning perhaps with why you are here at Fountain House?

In the ***second conversation*** *we are interested in understanding the matrix of familial, societal, and inherited factors and stressors that may have either produced the initial psychiatric crisis or contributed to the difficulty the participant had in adapting to and mastering that crisis. The second part takes up from where the first interview left off, with the emphasis this time on participant's understanding of psychosocial supports and stressors, relational successes and failures, and understanding of the origins of current and past social and psychic strains.*

- I'd like to remind you again that this interview is open-ended, you can say anything about yourself that you would like.
- Could you perhaps start by telling me a bit about where you grew up and what you remember of your mom and dad?

In the third conversation we hope to understand the support structures and services that have been facilitative for the participant, as well as the participant's response to institutions and services that they found unhelpful. Here we have in mind psychiatric services, hospital in- and out-patient programs, partial hospital programs, community and government agencies, as well as the services provided by the Fountain House community. The third part takes up from where the second interview left off, with the emphasis this time on participant's understanding of the nature of the psychiatric difficulty and their feelings about the courses of treatment they have received, and their interaction with agencies, hospitals, therapeutic communities, therapeutic residences, bureaucratic agencies, social service systems, etc. Of particular interest, in relation to the latter is their sense of the therapeutic facilitation or limitation of the various contexts they have experienced.

- I'd like to remind you again that this interview is open-ended, you can say anything about yourself that you would like.
- Could you perhaps start by telling me about when you were first hospitalized or treated for psychiatric issues?

In all, we collected thirty-nine hours of interviews from thirteen participants. The participants ranged in age from their early twenties to their seventies, and they were diverse with respect to gender and ethnicity. In the following reports, identities have been disguised and details, names, and locations have been changed to protect participant privacy, as recommended, for example, by Clifft (1986).

We have been humbled by the suffering our participants have experienced, as well as by their deep generosity in sharing their stories with us. It is our hope, that by working as a collegial interpretive team to put forth these stories, we can contribute to increasing the place for narrative understanding both in researching human lives and in treating the psychic distress to which all of us as humans are subject from time to time.

A BRIEF NOTE ON THE TEXT

Then doctoral students Secil Arac-Orhun and Montana Queler conducted all interviews after a lengthy immersion at Fountain House. As part of their dissertation work, each chose to write about the lives of four participants. Chapters 3, 8, 9, and 14 originally appeared in a different form in Secil's dissertation, and chapters 2, 5, 7, and 10 are adapted from Montana's dissertation. For this book, preliminary accounts of the remaining cases were written by Marilyn Charles (chapters, 4, 11), Michael O'laughlin (chapters 12, 13), and doctoral student Veronica Ozog and Michael O'laughlin (chapter 6). All writers were encouraged to hew to a phenomenological line as much as possible, and to avoid excessively clinical interpretation or potentially pathologizing terminology or ways of framing experience. A slightly different version of chapter 3 was originally written for publication elsewhere (O'Loughlin & Queler, 2019).

The reader will also note some variation in the structure of the narratives. The chapters that were adapted from previously completed dissertations have a more monological structure, in which the participant's views are mainly represented by quoted excerpts from the participant's words. The later chapters are presented more dialogically, with lengthy excerpts from the dialog included, to convey more of the profoundly dialogical and interpersonal nature of the interaction. This discrepancy was pointed out to us by our Fountain House colleagues (see chapter 15), who worried that the deeply personal and existentially deep relationship between Montana and Secil and their interviewees might be lost. As a result of this discussion, in the afterword, Montana and Secil will explore in some depth precisely what those existential encounters felt like and why they were so crucial to the quality of the interviews.

NOTES

1. From *Diary of a Bipolar Explorer* by Lucy Newlyn (2018, Signal Books). Used by kind permission of the author and publisher.
2. See, for example, Remembering Mad Pride, The Movement That Celebrated Mental Illness. Retrieved from https://www.vice.com/en_uk/article/7bxqxa/mad-pride-remembering-the-uks-mental-health-pride-movement on 8/16/18.
3. The reference is to the poem *Two Loves* by Lord Alfred Douglas, published in 1894 and now in the public domain.
4. For an extensive list of survivor narratives compiled by Dr. Gail Hornstein and current as of 2011, please see http://www.gailhornstein.com/files/Bibliography_of_First_Person_Narratives_of_Madness_5th_edition.pdf.
5. For peer support, see, for example, https://www.hearing-voices.org/, http://www.intervoiceonline.org/, and http://www.hearingvoicesusa.org/.
6. Michael O'Loughlin's (2017) podcast on Mad in America, *Exploring Narrative Approaches to Psychological Distress*, offers an overview of the issues discussed here: https://www.madinamerica.com/2017/09/michael-oloughlin-exploring-narrative-approaches-psycho-

logical-distress/. For a hospital talk seeking to explain a critical psychiatry perspective to medical residents and physicians, see O'Loughlin (2018c). For links to a frequently updated list of critical psychiatry and psychiatric rights websites, please visit http://michaelologhlin phd.com/human-rights-and-social-justice-projects/psychiatric-rights-issues/. Mad in America contains an extensive range of blogs and podcasts by leading contemporary critics of medicalized psychiatry: https://www.madinamerica.com/.

7. In *Dark Continents: Psychoanalysis and Colonialism*, Ranjana Khanna (2003) raises similar questions about the capacity of bourgeois Western psychoanalysis to ever capture the experience of its Others.

8. For similar perspectives, see the Ted talk of psychologist Dr. Eleanor Longden, addressing the ethical loneliness of her extreme psychic suffering until she met psychiatrist, Dr. Pat Bracken. Bracken summoned his humanity and the capacity to hear her and acknowledge her humanity in a true existential meeting: https://www.ted.com/talks/eleanor_longden_the_voices_in_my_head; also Catherine Penney's story of her recovery from a catatonic state through her work with Dr. Daniel Dorman is described in Dorman's (2003) book, *Dante's Cure*. Penney offers accounts of her experience here: https://www.youtube.com/watch?v=Cac8AieCgto and also in Daniel Mackler's film *Take These Broken Wings*, viewable here: https://www.you tube.com/watch?v=edaxwaiIrQU.

9. Brian Koehler has started an international petition to the American Psychiatric Association seeking to eliminate the stigmatizing term "schizophrenia." Details may be found here: https://www.change.org/p/american-psychiatric-association-apa-drop-the-stigmatizing-term-schizophrenia.

Here is Brian Koehlker's rationale for the petition:

The term "schizophrenia" has become synonymous with dangerousness even though it is a very small minority of persons with this diagnosis who violently hurt others and this may be explained better by the following factors: male gender, young adulthood, misuse of substances, homelessness, having been exposed to violence, sense of powerlessness, helplessness, stigma, etc. The term is also associated with non-recoverability. Dangerousness and non-recoverability seem to be hard-wired into the diagnosis. The term encompasses a heterogeneous group of people with different symptoms, etiologies, course and outcomes. It is a static, traumatizing and stigmatizing term for those persons given it. It often takes away hope and a sense of agency because people are told that they have a genetic brain disease. Hope, ongoing social and peer support, and a sense of agency and self-efficacy are needed to facilitate recovery. Nine world outcome studies and the World Health Organization studies on "schizophrenia" demonstrate substantial recoveries. People have a better chance of recovery when given good care that is acceptable to them. Perhaps, many of the neurobiological findings in "schizophrenia," which are often non-specific and can not be used for diagnosis, could be better explained to be the result of chronic stress, relational and social traumas, social isolation/exclusion, social defeat, economic adversities, low self-esteem, stigma, prenatal stress, migration (particularly from a non-white to a white environment), urban birth/living, low impact SNPs & CNVs (single nucleotide polymorphisms and copy number variants), epigenetic changes to gene expression, the effects of first- and second-generation antipsychotics (e.g., the Iowa Longitudinal Study), etc. African Americans are about 3-fold more likely than whites to be diagnosed with "schizophrenia." Social adversity can become biologically embedded and result in epigenetic changes to gene expression, which may be potentially transmitted across generations. Japan (integration disorder), Hong Kong and Taiwan (cognitive-perceptual dysregulation/dysfunction) and South Korea (attunement disorder) have dropped the term "schizophrenia" from their psychiatric nosology. Surveys in Japan have shown that service recipients and professionals alike are pleased with the change. Prominent psychiatrists such as Robin Murray in the UK and Jim van Os in The Netherlands have presented strong and convincing arguments as to why this term should be dropped. The editor of the prestigious journal *Schizophrenia Bulletin* has also recently wondered whether the term should be replaced. I believe the time is now to drop this stigmatizing, hope-disabling, scientifically controversial term which is saturated with various myths about non-recoverability and dangerousness.

10. For further detail on our work at Austen Riggs Center and how it shaped this project, please see Marilyn Charles's discussion in chapter 1 of this volume.

Chapter One

Thinking Psychosocially about Psychosis

Marilyn Charles

We are living in a time in which the meanings of even basic principles such as truth and justice are in question. In such a time, these meanings must be renegotiated in order to find a common language and also to ensure that we are working towards a common goal, a common good. In an era in which we seem to have lost touch with the moral fiber that is also at our roots, we need more than ever to hold fast to the moral compass at the core of any research project that attempts to better understand the experience and the suffering of others. We need to listen better to one another in order to accomplish that task without violating the very person we would hope to assist. Towards that end, we need research methods that will help us to find and to re-find the heart of any project in which there is actual engagement with the individuals under investigation.

In this era of pressured movements towards standards that are based on group evidence rather than individual meanings, it is useful to consider Lacan's (1977) warnings about an external Authority that we are in danger of becoming lost in, in relation to which we must learn to locate ourselves and our own desire, and also our own moral authority. This admonition is in line with Levinas' (1998) appeal to an ethics dictated precisely by the call from the other that invites a deeper self-reflection than we can find in any dogmatic rule. In between those two vantage points lies the possibility of an ethics that is based on personal responsibility in relation to common principles and also to the call from the other that makes a legitimate demand upon us to face that call and reflect on it respectfully as a thinking/feeling subject, to not de-authorize anyone as the primary knower of his or her experience and, in that way, to impose the *ethical loneliness* (Stauffer, 2015) described in the introductory chapter of this volume. In order to be ethical, we, as researchers, must be willing to find our common core, an ethical center that is based on the call from the other that organizes, reorganizes, and dictates our work.

At the heart of my work at the Austen Riggs Center has been a collective allegiance to a self-reflective, interpretive space that heeds and is mindful of the call from the other, committed to collectively and individually interpreting those calls, in order to move beyond the hazards of self-interest towards deeper understandings. That focus has been girded in the language of psychoanalysis and group-relations theories. Although those tools are useful—and perhaps indispensable—to the mission, as we have known it, those tools also hold space for a larger truth. That larger truth has to do with a deep commitment to an ethical responsibility that we both hold and hold dear, a commitment to listen to how the other person is right while also being willing to reflect further, to expand what might be known or thought, and to be willing to learn more than we thought we had known. That is the place where we can potentially find one another in a common cause, to attempt to learn within those contexts in which we work, and to share what we learn with one another as best we can, so that we can all benefit from the work that we do individually and collectively.

That mission is in line with a general attitude towards "knowledge as research" (Levinas, 1999, p. 14) that undergirds the current project. But Levinas goes further, positioning research within an ethical frame that must move beyond a phenomenological approach that is based on an authentic encounter with the other, to recognition of an encounter that has already been structured by the society in which violence has been done. The challenge, suggests Dykeman (1993), is to envision a new paradigm, one in which "In every moment I act as researcher, I can act either to reduce the Other to a servant of my own needs (narcissistic or political) or to empty myself and take on the Other's needs as my own" (p. 13). Levinas invites us to move away from ethics that are based on abstract principles, turning rather towards an "ethics of alterity—an ethics for others. . . . For Levinas, ethics is a responsibility to other people that is involuntary and singular" (Vermeylen & Clark, 2017, p. 504). From this perspective, an ethics of care demands that we not reduce the other to simply being like or unlike us. We must rather, inquire into the inevitable alienness—the strangeness of the other—rather than avoiding it.

Vermeylen and Clark (2017) invite us to take seriously our responsibilities as researchers: "The researcher should be affected by the interpersonal relationship and so become self-reflective. S/he ought to challenge (historical) power relations when exposed to asymmetry and discomfort. Ethical sensibilities cannot be anticipated; they emerge only through encounters in the field. . . . Ethics is more than just predefining the researcher's ethical behavior in the field; it is an experience of awaiting the call of responsibility that leads the researcher to be affected by others" (p. 508).

THE RESEARCH CONTEXT

The current study grew out of a previous interdisciplinary investigation undertaken by Michael O'Loughlin, myself, and several other colleagues, in which we attempted to gain insight into the experiences of those participants in the Austen Riggs/Erikson Institute Follow-Along Study who had been labeled psychotic. That initial project grew out of an investigation I had begun on creativity in which, in looking for participants from our data pool, I was struck by the discourse of a woman who, time after time, seemed to assert the same statement, which did not seem to rest but rather needed continual reassertion. Was this a sign of her psychopathology? Or did it represent a personal truth that could not sufficiently be lodged and therefore needed repeated reaffirmation? How might her assertions be seen as attempts to speak back to the investigators beyond the layers of meanings imposed by whatever presumptions underlay their own project?

These questions became the impetus for our original study of individuals labeled psychotic from the Follow-Along Study data. In that study, we used transcripts of one-hour dynamic clinical interviews to try to understand what those individuals might be trying to tell us beyond what the investigators were seeking. We hoped, in this way, to allow the individuals to speak in their own voices about their needs, feelings, and experience, as best they might, beyond the perceived or structural demands of the situation. Notably, individuals at the Austen Riggs Center have often been labeled *treatment resistant,* which we take to mean that *treatment as usual* has failed them. The irony that individuals are labeled—and often, by inference, blamed and shamed—in this way when the treatment offerings have failed is not lost on us.

In that initial study, we employed psychoanalytic and narratological methods in an attempt to look beyond our preconceptions and listen more carefully to what "treatment resistant" patients might be telling us about what "caregivers" have failed to hear. Our preliminary task was to get to know our sample and our data set using the Ward Method of creative consensus (Schielke, Fishman, Osatuke, & Stiles, 2009). To this end, we began first to listen to (and to watch, where videotapes were available) interviews, noting differences across individual patients, interviewers, and the interviews themselves (preliminary structured clinical interviews were also available for each person). Salient in our minds in this initial stage was a question regarding what we might hear from the participants regarding factors that facilitated or impeded their constructive use of psychotherapy to explore and make meaning from their lives and experience.

At the core of our work is an allegiance to research as an ethical process in which the stakes are always very high, on the one hand affording the possibility of obtaining information that may be of value but, on the other hand, running the risk of doing harm in that process. We find Levinas' perspective particularly useful because, in the words of ethnographers Benson and O'Neill (2007), "His philosophy is concerned with questions of responsibility and justice . . . questions of objectivity and the legitimate, ethical, or even violent dimensions associated with the knowledge of other people" (p. 30). Such concerns can also be seen through the lens of what Fricker (2007) calls *epistemic injustice,* the problem of the privileging or delegitimizing people as potential *knowers.* I will speak more to some of those issues later in this chapter, after describing our research process.

THE ORIGINAL PROJECT

In our original project, we worked at understanding the narratives of forty-four individuals who had participated in the Austen Riggs/Erikson Institute Follow-Along Study. We learned a great deal from watching videotapes and reading transcripts of the interviews collected across time in that study, which informed our ideas about the current project.

Beyond the explicit questions, there were demands of the research situation, and the clinical environment in which it was embedded, that impacted the speech of participants. Perhaps most notably, the interviewer's style had a major impact on his or her ability to invite speech from the participant. We noticed a trend, for example, for the male participants in our study to respond better to interviewers who maintained both physical and emotional distance, whereas the female participants responded better to greater warmth and relatedness. The best interviewers, from our perspective, were those who were able to accommodate their style to the perceived needs of the subject, rather than remaining caught in an impasse driven by their own lack of flexibility.

We learned that medical systems and structures had a major impact on many of the participants, including the offerings of Austen Riggs, itself. The initial interview often occurred directly after the initial case conference, during which the subject had received a diagnosis. One young man, for example, who had been given a diagnosis of thought disorder, engaged quite cogently in the interview until the point when he began to discuss the diagnosis. At that point, his thinking became overtly disordered and his narrative broke down. The diagnosis seemed to provide, not a useful context for recognizing and working with his symptoms but rather a stumbling block that further impeded his ability to make use of his mind. Another individual defined herself exclusively in diagnostic terms until the interviewer inquired past the medical jargon into her subjective experience. That inquiry seemed to afford her an avenue through which to circumvent the stumbling block she encountered in trying to relate to her diagnosis rather than her experience. If the "experts" contextualize experience through diagnostic categories, then that framework governs the currency of value, prioritizing medicalized jargon over human meaning or experience.

We could also see other ways in which the larger context had an impact on the participants' perceptions of themselves. As patients in a psychiatric hospital, there were implicit and explicit meanings in relation to their place in society and also within the smaller social structure of the hospital and in the interview process itself. Meaning structures and power dynamics were each at play, dictating who has the power to create meanings and to impose them, and who is at the mercy of those imposed meanings. We could see how even the idea that meanings *might* be imposed grossly and profoundly affected the discourse of the participants. For example, the young woman mentioned previously initially appeared quite dull, which we might have attributed to a lack of intelligence, drugs, or other impairment, but she also showed, through her language structure, that there was something more to her. The interviewer seemed to recognize that greater capacity. He worked hard to meet her in a place other than where she was positioning herself by opposing the medicalized jargon with his own thoughtful, reflective engagement with her offerings.

Our efforts have been driven by our recognition of the fundamental difficulty that arises in being labelled as a psychiatric patient when clinicians are "invested with the power and authority to define and legitimate certain social norms" (Tranulis, Corin, & Kirmayer, 2008, p. 229). Demands for accountability can lead to evidence that has the *appearance* of validity without necessarily being relevant to the subject under scrutiny. Further, attempts to manage behavior may not only be dehumanizing but also interfere with self-management, thereby reinforcing the type of stigma that can impede recovery over the long term (Charles, 2009; Lysaker, Roe, & Yanos, 2007; Ritsher & Phelan, 2004).

The dilemma of dehumanization through "treatment" can be particularly problematic in relation to individuals with psychotic symptoms. I am defining psychotic symptoms roughly in terms of symptoms that are so individually encoded with meaning that they are difficult to understand from the framework of consensual reality. Our assumption in our work is that meanings become coded in this way because they are in some sense unspeakable in relation to social relationships and structures that do not recognize the suffering and attendant meanings. In spite of research findings to the contrary, there is a tendency to equate psychosis with a lack of insight (Amador et al. 1993; David, 1990). Clearly, these standards are lodged within a model in which the assignation of "insight" depends on the extent to which the individual's self-assessment would agree with that of a healthcare provider (Kirmayer, Corin, & Jarvis, 2004).

In trying to understand the types of dilemmas that might be unique to the personal struggles of the patient designated psychotic, there were some major areas of learning. First, we could see histories of relational difficulties marked by striking gender differences. Whereas the women recounted yearnings for intimacy and engagement, the men shared a common theme of social awkwardness, alienation, and impotence that seemed to lead towards a desire for a sexual relationship with a woman.

We also saw histories of limited achievements or sense of mastery, and histories of trauma or neglect that are likely implicated in the extent and chronicity of the symptoms. The attachment literature shows quite profoundly ways in which the type of disorganized attachment linked to disrupted mourning across the generations can result in severely disrupted development in families where the parents seem to be "good enough" (Liotti, 2004; Main & Hesse, 1990). We had been interested in further study of psychosis because it marks trauma in a particular kind of way. With trauma, it is often the *gap* that marks meaning in a story that is told and untold at the same time. As such, we tried to listen past the structural barriers of the research process itself and also those barriers that our participants placed against making meaning together, to try to understand those very barriers as attempts at both self-understanding and self-protection. As noted previously, we could see that diagnosis became both a tool for understanding and for mis-understanding self and experience, much like the research process.

Clearly emerging from this study was the very tenuousness of meaning, itself. We could see how easily engagement can be subverted if the interviewer is not sufficiently sensitive and responsive to the person they are with. Communications at times may be highly coded, perhaps better conceptualized as questions regarding the ability of the other to actually attend to particularities of speech and meaning. Interpersonal space can also be very important; one person may demand a great deal of distance, and may only be able to talk in abstract terms, whereas another may demand a great deal of intimacy. Eye contact can be intrusive or necessary and a given individual may be unable to engage in conversation without first setting up the rules of engagement, so that the ensuing conversation may have a very different quality depending upon the interviewer's ability to respond to overt or subtle cues.

In this interplay, we could see the type of negotiation that Winnicott (1971) describes in terms of *the use of an object.* If we think of diagnoses as transitional objects, then we could see ways in which meanings were being negotiated. If we think of trauma as a disruption in the developmental flow, then we could consider our participants as individuals caught in a developmental impasse, searching for means to move beyond the impasse without accruing further harm, and yet not necessarily having much reason to trust a stranger.

We know that identity develops through the interchange of meanings between one person and another. From that perspective, we can think of the interview process as a potential space for learning *but* one in which learning itself has not been without its hazards. And yet, the form of the Dynamic Interview was such that the interviewer was not only obtaining information but also trying to offer something back, to offer a trial interpretation and see if that offering might be useful to the person being interviewed. In our opinion, the best interviews were those that moved past the language of doctor/ patient or diagnosis and disease into a narrative that illuminated the contexts in which an impasse had occurred that resulted in seeking treatment. In such instances, there appeared at times to be a meeting of minds such that relief and learning seemed possible.

LESSONS LEARNED

What emerged most notably was the relational quality of meaning, itself. We saw interviews where the "fit" had been bad, and the interviewer's push for information shut down the conversation. There were also, however, interviewers who could lean in or out, depending on the perceived needs of the interviewee, meeting the person in a place of most comfort rather than insisting on preserving their own space. Through that vantage point, we could see how profoundly vulnerable an individual in trouble can be, in the hands of authoritative others who in some ways have the power of psychic life and death in any given moment. Power and privilege can be used for good but can also be extremely destructive when wielded mindlessly. The researcher has tremendous power and privilege, which demands our greatest humility in approaching someone who might feel demeaned precisely because of the ways in which the experience is structured.

Because of our observations, we became interested in the research process itself, which both allows an individual to speak and also constrains and directs that speech. The interview study at Fountain House grew out of our frustration in not being able to ask our own questions of the participants. As a result, as described in the introduction, we developed two further interviews in addition to the Dynamic Interview, one in which participants were asked about life and family histories, in order to obtain a better sense of the contexts in which their troubles had evolved. We hoped, in this way, also to be able to see the *trauma trails* (Atkinson, 2002) that might illuminate the contexts through which distress and dis-ease had arisen. In the other new interview, we asked about the person's treatment experiences, hoping, in this way, to collect data regarding which offerings had and had not been helpful to these individuals, and in which ways help—or harm—had been done. The complete interview protocol can be found in the appendix.

Central to our investigations has been a recognition of ways in which trauma is transmitted across the generations not only at the individual level but also the levels of family and society (Charles, 2000). This perspective contrasts fundamentally with the disease model so prevalent in relation to human suffering today (O'Loughlin & Charles, 2012). We can trace in the stories of the individuals who share their lives and experiences in these pages the type of relational disruption that underlies psychosis and other forms of chronic distress (Liotti, 1999). Attuned parenting builds resilience as the child's distress is moderated through soothing tone, gesture, or touch, providing an experience-near sense of recognition and understanding. Harsh or inconsistent parenting, in contrast, interferes with the internalization of effective soothing functions and the development of effective coping mechanisms, which also undermines the ability to form relationships with others (Main & Hesse, 1990; Myin-Germeys & van Os, 2007).

Experiences of social exclusion and marginalization lead to social humiliation and shame, a virulent and self-perpetuating emotion (Birchwood, Meaden, Trower, Gilbert, & Plaistow, 2000; Charles, 2013). Because of its inhibiting effects, shame not only impedes social interactions, but also impedes new learning and mastery experiences, leading to the types of cognitive and affective difficulties associated with severe and chronic distress (Tangney, Wagner, & Gramzow, 1992). Experiences of mastery, in contrast, invite further exploration, helping to build not only positive self-regard but also metacognitive capacities, the ability to reflect on one's own thoughts and feelings in relation to the thoughts and feelings of others, and to make use of those thoughts towards greater mastery in relation to life's challenges (Lysaker, Erickson et al., 2011).

Identity develops within the context of meanings passed between parent and child that become the background melodies through which we develop our own life story (Charles, 2014a, b, c). What is known and valued can be passed along directly, whereas whatever has been hidden or repressed returns to haunt us. Shame becomes the vehicle through which whatever has not been faced in previous generations returns to haunt us in ways that are difficult to get hold of precisely because we do not have the language or opportunities through which to make sense of the enigmatic meanings that are communicated nonverbally across the generations (Abraham & Torok, 1994; Apprey, 1993; Laplanche, 1997). These are the types of stories that are told in coded form through symptoms of trauma, such as those associated with psychosis (Davoine & Gaudillière, 2004).

Structural oppression results in feelings of *abjection* at the *social level* that are experienced as a shame-inducing inferiority by the individual (Kristeva, 1982). Because the source of the distress is cultural, it is difficult for the individual to work through the problem. Shame turns our glance downwards, and we stand accused and alone, unable to look back at our oppressor. It is difficult to face such intense suffering in another, particularly in a culture in which "self-esteem" is linked with success rather than good fortune and the idea of "equal opportunity" is turned on the disadvantaged as an accusation. Splitting at the level of culture invites us to not-see ways in which we are implicated in ongoing abjecting processes, aided by our willingness to turn on others who are lost and vulnerable as a way of distancing ourselves from their distress. Psychosis is frightening precisely because we can all be driven mad by life experience. Marginalizing those who are suffering helps to avoid recognition of ways in which we might be implicated.

DISCUSSION

My intent in this chapter has been to introduce the context from which the Fountain House project evolved. Crucial to that project has been a social justice perspective that makes a demand on the researchers to attempt to be as respectful as possible to the individuals whose stories are being told. At the heart of any idea of social justice is the ethical imperative imposed by the call of the other. Our mission, then, is to attempt insofar as possible to be true to that call. In doing so, we need to be able to recognize that each person's perspective is both unique and driven by context. With that idea in mind, we can, perhaps, actively attempt to discern factors giving rise to that individual's perspective without doing violence to the person him or herself. In relation to that charge, we have addressed our attention to each individual in turn, so that we might open up their discourse in an attempt to discern possible meanings without clouding their experience with our own. To further that effort, in the chapters that follow we will use quotations directly from each individual, so that the reader might better track along with us in our explorations, and perhaps notice more or other than we have been able to see.

If we take seriously the Levinasian idea of research as an encounter (Benson & O'Neill, 2007), then you can see the Fountain House project as a series of encounters. First we have the interviewers' encounters with the environment in which the participants are living, then the interviews as more direct engagements with the persons themselves, and then the project of encountering, more deeply, possible meanings that might be mined from those layered encounters. In this way, we try to be true to an ethics that privileges the primacy of the other, and the process rather than the product, grounded in the premise, not of equality between researcher and subject but rather of a responsibility to the other demanded by an unequal and hierarchical encounter (Benson & O'Neill, 2007). It is only in recognizing our own power and privilege that we can counter the often-invisible arch of epistemic injustice that can skew or even eviscerate meanings, rendering personal truths invisible or seemingly irrelevant (Fricker, 2007).

In this type of study, suggest Benson and O'Neill, there is the potential for "change not simply for the self and its interests, but rather for the sake of new kinds of affiliations across interpersonal and intercultural boundaries" (2007, p. 31). Our contention would be that the experience of psychiatric diagnosis and treatment takes place within a context of marginalization that tends to be further marginalizing for precisely those people one might intend to "help." As such, in crossing that cultural boundary, the researcher risks an encounter that makes demands we cannot fully anticipate precisely because we are in unknown territory. In that sense, the research has value because it becomes possible to know more than one had previously known. It performs the mission of seeking knowledge.

Because one is learning through the other, a particular ethical challenge arises that legitimately makes demands on the researcher to justify the research, not through one's own aims and intentions entirely, but in relation to the needs of those we encounter. If we are willing to take on this challenge, then the purpose and product of the research are always beyond whatever we might have intended, because part of the purpose can only be articulated or brought to light by the participants themselves. In the act of engagement, we invoke ethical dilemmas beyond those that can be anticipated in a prospective protocol but rather in terms of what Guillemin and Gillam (2004) call an *ethics in practice,* in which the researcher is charged with interacting "in a humane, nonexploitative way while at the same time being mindful of one's role as a researcher" (p. 264). *Reflexivity,* mindful engagement, is proposed as a means for acknowledging and engaging with ethical considerations as they arise in the encounter with a thinking, feeling being who has been invited into an experience with you and by you.

This ethical dilemma is at the heart of any psychosocial research, where various "goods" may be juxtaposed against one another. In reference to this problem, Fabian (2012) suggests that we "redefine cultural anthropology as a science of human survival" (p. 449). From that perspective, the current study can be seen as precisely such an investigation, in which there is a particular type of survival at stake; the possibility of developing oneself as a unique subject. In a world in which difference too easily becomes marginalized and disparaged in ways that can fundamentally affect one's life, mind, and being, it is important to recognize that development can be subverted through systems of care that deny, in essential ways, not only one's personhood but also one's right to have and to know one's own mind as a precondition for becoming oneself (see Fricker, 2007). From Fabian's perspective, the purpose of such research is to obtain knowledge "that changes the knower as well as the known (p. 449). We can all be misled by "good intentions" that lead us astray because we are not open to the very learning needed to organize and refine our understanding.

Through research that is open to new learning, there is development at both the individual and the social levels. That complexity is highlighted by Castañeda (2006) in his distinction between *morals,* which reference the social group, and *ethics*, relating to the individual. He suggests that morals and ethics need to be understood in the context of "a hierarchical relation in which morals refer to a larger field of imperatives, norms, rights, duties, and criteria, whereas ethics refers to the application or embodiment of these principles in action or the evaluation of action" (p. 123). Anthropological ethics are relevant for our purposes here because of the attention on criteria of *the good* in relation to a specific group, "an appeal to external criteria of good based in the value of cultural otherness, specifically the difference of human groups" (p. 127). Anthropologists are well positioned to recognize the legitimate variations of meanings across cultural differences and thereby to also recognize the potential for "epistemological and moral violence of knowledge writing, and representation" (p. 128) in ways that are crucial for psychologists and psychoanalysts as well, who also must have in mind a public good that may at times compete with other moral imperatives at play (Wertz, 2011).

Following Sontag (1978), Scheper-Hughes and Lock (1986) note that "the societal and cultural responses to disease create a second illness in addition to the original affliction, what we are calling the 'double'; the layers of stigma, rejection, fear, and exclusion that attach to particularly dreaded diseases. This happens the moment we say to ourselves and each other, 'this person *is* a schizophrenic' . . . (with all that this implies for specific historical and cultural reasons)" (p. 137). The problem, then, these authors contend, is "an *excess* of meanings, most of them humbling, demeaning, and grossly stigmatizing" (italics in original; p. 137). Reification of "disease" processes has led to a certain type of dehumanization generally, through which "ill-ness" and medicine can become forms of social control (Taussig, 1980). Schizophrenia, in particular, has been used to point away from the problems in living that are linked to the symptoms marked by that term (Charles & O'Loughlin, 2012; Read et al., 2005; Varese et al., 2012). Attempts to move away from this term, however, and to focus more directly on the problems of those diagnosed in this way, threaten to lose sight of the actual experience of those so diagnosed (Morgan, 2010).

To meet the challenge of respectfully engaging with individuals who have in many ways a different experience than our own, and also of trying to offset the power imbalance that might inhibit or constrain others' ability to speak, we have tried to be transparent in our process, both with the institution in which we were working and also with the individuals who were asked to participate, so that participants were invited into a process that we hoped would have a public good. Because of our awareness of the complexity of the diversity of ethical imperatives in this project, we have tried to stay very close to the discourse of our participants, to track their stories respectfully, and to discern, as best we can, what they are telling us about their own experiences of navigating some of the hazards in the society in which we live, that might be instructive for those who would like to ameliorate some of the factors that are iatrogenic in our various systems and methods of "care."

Welch (2000) describes an *ethic of risk* in which researchers confront the possibility that nothing will change as a result of their work. "The ethic of risk is propelled by the equally vital recognition that to stop resisting, even when success is unimaginable, is to die." Such a death, she proposes, is multidimensional, including, perhaps most profoundly, "the death of the imagination, the death of the ability to care" (p. 46). To care in the face of the other's pain, and the limits of what one might be able to do to ameliorate such pain, is what my training as a psychoanalyst has afforded me. I have found that it invites respectfulness to the suffering of the other that can be, in and of itself, a healing force. Such care, suggest Benson and O'Neill (2007), "creates room for an ethical sensibility rather than a moral model . . . an ethics of risk that respects the impossibility of the human ethical condition and takes this impossibility as a starting point" (p. 49).

Power and privilege inevitably have an impact, which makes it important to use well those tools we have at our disposal, most particularly "our ability to listen carefully and with empathy and compassion" (Scheper-Hughes, 1995, p. 418). In spite of the many problems, or perhaps in *facing* and trying to be mindful of the multiple layers of ethical risk, ethnographic methods can "be used as a tool for critical reflection and human liberation" (p. 418). We hope that in the act of engaging respectfully in the research and interview process by first working alongside the participants and then listening deeply, that we have affirmed our hope for a process of mutual exploration of the struggle to make a life under difficult circumstances in which we are all implicated.

Levinas (1987) writes that "meaning is situated in the ethical. . . . Morality does not belong to culture: it enables one to judge it" (p. 100). In line with our own project, for Levinas, the provenance of morality is to discover the lived experience, the embodied reality of the other. Inherent in a research project that is attempting to be ethical in this kind of way, suggests Scheper-Hughes (1995), is the possibility that part of our reports, our investigations, "can be a site of resistance," a place where we use our power and our privilege to take a stand on behalf of those whose voices have not been heard (p. 420). From this perspective, it is likely important to view ourselves not as "neutral" or "objective" observers but rather as witnesses who "are accountable for what they see and how they fail to act in critical situations" (p. 419).

It is in this spirit that we offer our reports from the interviews with the participants from Fountain House.

Chapter Two

Faith

A Woman Interrupted

Montana Queler and Michael O'Loughlin

Faith, a sixty-one-year-old Caucasian woman, said that she "knew she had a problem" when, at twenty-three, she found herself waist deep in the Pacific Ocean, miles from her home, without any conscious recollection of how she got there.[1] This, she reported, was when she realized there was something "odd" about her:

> I mean, there was one morning, in 1970 it must have been, yeah, I was in grad school . . . I got up one morning, this was when I knew I had a problem. There was definitely something wrong with me. I got up and I walked ten miles without even knowing I walked ten miles until I woke up in the Pacific Ocean and all I had on me was a quarter, and I called my husband who was still in bed at that time. I must have gone sometime in the early morning, and I walked not stopping until I walked and woke up in the Pacific Ocean . . . I was just manically driven and I couldn't stop. I just had to keep on walking right, and then I woke up waist deep in the water, and it was about oh, I guess, six o'clock in the morning and I only had a quarter, and I called my husband and he came and got me on the motorcycle.

Faith's flight reflects the profound impact of trauma on her psyche. Gifted in her creative capacity and exquisite sensitivity, as we will illustrate below, Faith's trajectory represents the courageous efforts of someone who has been able to rely on her extraordinary talents to survive, share, and transcend her pain. However, Faith's ascent to great heights has also meant bearing the pain of many psychic crises, and, in these moments, her extreme fragility has been laid bare.

TRAUMATIC ORIGINS OF PSYCHIC COLLAPSE

Reflecting on her childhood, Faith noted an instability that came to be characteristic of her life:

> I was born in a small town on the West Coast . . . my dad got a job as a travelling salesman and we spent my first five years in the car. We went all over the country, living in hotels and motels and trailer camps and trailer parks and by the side of the road. Um, that's what I remember as a child. And we had a Mercury called Telula, and then we had a Dodge called Telula the Second, 'cause it . . . my dad was very drunk and he plowed into a bull and totaled the car, so we had to wait in that town for the wire money to come in. I was used to sittin' in the front seat on the floor where all the state maps were, and I'd drool, and I'd wake up with a fish print on my face or a map print on my face from me drooling, and my dad would sleep across the front seat, and my older brother and my mom slept in the back . . . Dad was arrested a lot for driving while impaired, and we got pulled over in like [State] and lived in jail, which I thought was wonderful 'cause I had a cot, I had a real bed. And so I shared the jail cell with my dad. . . . And we spent three days because we couldn't afford the ticket, you know, for the speed trap, and I did everything from pick cotton and peel it, you know, to earn money . . .

Faith's early life was defined not only by transience and alcoholism but also poverty and untreated health issues:

> I used to get terrible, terrible ear infections, um, and started drinking actually before the age of one. My mom used to, it's like colic, it was just I had terrible drainage from my ears, I had an infection but we couldn't afford a doctor . . . and so she used to dip my diaper into bourbon and honey and then get me so I could sleep. So I started actually drinking before the age of one. My father was an alcoholic, my mother was an alcoholic. I was probably about five then, but I started to lose my hearing when my mom and dad separated. By the time I started first grade I was deaf. What had happened was that my scar tissue had grown over my ears from the infection. And my mom realized why I was doing so bad and why she was always grabbin' after me, 'cause I couldn't hear her, I didn't know, you know . . . So they put me on a tissue shrinkage pill in [City], and I went to a special school for hard of hearing and learned to lip-read

and all that stuff. Well it took about a year and a half for the pill to work so that I was just hard of hearing.

Further, Faith's earliest memories bear the scars of her father's sexual abuse. During the interview, she related memories of her father penetrating her with objects, as well as pouring alcohol inside of her. She also remembered being raped by him while the carousing of his fellow-drinkers drowned out her screams. The abuse continued until Faith was in the first grade. She shared that at times the abuse was so physically painful that she would mentally "go away":

> I thought I had done something wrong, you know why he would get the way he'd get when he got very drunk. And that's when I would just go away. I would melt into the . . . I had a little sock doll called Mr. Navy, and I would turn Mr. Navy away, and I would just go away. I would go into the magazine or the paper I was drawing, or I would go away, and just not think about it. You know, I just remember the burning, the burning I remember.

Here, Faith offers a poignant illustration of the way dissociation protected her from the pain of bearing witness to her own incestuous victimization by her father, protecting her not only from the pain of the experience itself, but also from having to fully engage with the awareness of her father's depravity. Winnicott's (1974) idea that psychotic breakdown stems from early, unintegrated trauma, a precursor to more contemporary theories of the traumatic origins of psychotic experience, as we discuss below, helps to illuminate Faith's journey into psychic collapse. Although Faith articulated the experience of her abuse, it emerged in snippets of memory and flashbacks, as well as through pangs of guilt and self-reproach. Reflecting on how the abuse impacted her relationship with her father, in keeping with so many child victims of incest (cf., Garland, 1998; Gartner, 1999; Herman, 1997), Faith took the blame into herself in order to preserve an idealized father image, "I loved him so much. I still loved him, you know, I thought everything that had happened was my fault."

Faith described her vulnerability and the relational instability and danger in her early life—a life in which her father became her predator—as follows:

> I remember my first AA meeting. I was about four years old, and it was in the middle of the country in some bar and there were like wagons and cars, and there was smoke everywhere. You couldn't see above the tabletop, you know where all the cakes and the pies and the Kool-Aid and all the women were, and the room was full of smoke. And you'd hear like "Hi, my name's Mike, I'm an alcoholic" (imitates grunting/cheering noises in response), and all the kids and us would be playin' in the stables and, you know, doin' penny throw into the um like little sandbox and

> stuff like that. And uh, I have a lot of stories about my childhood, about being raised. And when my parents couldn't take care of us, we would go stay with her mom and dad, my grandma and grandpa, and we'd stay there a couple weeks, you know, while they would go off to [State] or go down to [State]. I do remember one time my dad started having um sexual relationships with me when I was about two, mostly it was just with a bottle and objects. And I remember this one time in [City] I was about four, and I used to get special Shirley Temple drinks, and I used to dance in the bars, so they'd throw money, and the money would pay for his drink and I'd get a free plate of you know um, um like crawfish chowder or somethin', and I remember distinctly this one bar, you couldn't see above the lady's hips and stuff, but they were all dancin' on the bar and there was a brown man in the corner playin' a funny horn. And I remember they scooched the piano chair to the tables, and I was sitting on top of this music, and there was this image of this woman, which I never forgot, with her mouth open and singin', and I later saw that same image and it was Lena Horne, so it was a sheet of music from one of Lena Horne's albums.

Sadly, Faith's relationship with her mother was similarly fraught, leaving Faith with no place to turn to, and setting her up for a lifetime of vulnerability and insecurity. Her mother abused her through manipulation and neglect, depriving her of a stable, loving, good mother—a *good object* in psychoanalytic parlance—the thing she most desperately needed:

> She used to call me Miss Jones. She never called me by my real name. She said, they played a game all during the time I was in the car about, "We're taking you home, Miss Jones. You're not our little girl, you're not our daughter. Mr. Jones is waitin' for ya." And I'd say, "No, I'm Faith, I'm Faith." And they'd say, "No you're not. You're not our little girl. We're just keepin' you till we find Mr. Jones." And then one time, um, I must've been three or so, and it was very flat, must've been Kansas or Missouri or something. It was a dusty road, and a hot, hot day, that kind where you stick on the seats and it burns. And um, my mom had my dad pull over to the side of the road, and there was a shack leaning on the side of a hill, through dried corn stalks, so it must've been August, it must've been late August or somethin'. But it was very hot and uh, she opened the back door where I was, she picked me up, and she put me into the dirt on the side of the road. She said, "There's your home, Miss Jones, Mr. Jones is waitin' for ya. He's got supper on. Now you go on up, you go see Mr. Jones." And so, she got back in the car, and they were all laughin' and gigglin'. And my brother had an air rifle and shot it out the window at me, and they drove away. And I remember running after the car, but I had that

> kind of cry where you can't cry, you know, and I fell in the dirt, and the dirt was swirlin' all around me. And I watched the car, and it took forever to drive outta sight. And all I remember was that I couldn't hear very well. I crawled into the gulley. I had Mr. Navy, my sock doll, with me. And I remember the twinks of twilight. I must've been there, I don't know, for hours. And uh, no cars went by, it was just a two-lane country road. And I didn't go up to the shack, but I got on the other side of the broken cowboy fence, and I just sorta hid out in the stalks and cried and cried, and just kept sayin,' "I'm not Miss Jones, I'm not Miss Jones." And then um, I remember I saw headlights coming back and it was twilight, and the stars were out, and you could hear the crickets in the field a little bit, not too clearly but there was obviously something out there. And I walked into the gulley, and the car approached, and all I remember is feeling that I was being lifted up and put into the car. I remember that I didn't talk for a long time, and they never played that game again . . . And um, I just uh, I don't remember having a relationship with my mother after that. I mean, she would brush my hair really hard and . . . You know, but everything was "Yes, ma'am," "No, ma'am."

The absence of that *good object*—a stable loving parent—and the persecutory destructiveness that characterized Faith's early life had a shattering effect on her psyche. Faith was deprived of any positive mirroring that could have reflected back her internal goodness. Nothing buffered her from the conviction that her abuse was deserved. This combined with the need to depend on her parents in order to feel some sense of security produced a psychological landscape in which she was thrust into a position of guilt (cf., Fairbairn, 1954). There is considerable evidence that incest and the kind of destabilized early relationship patterns Faith experienced are strong predictors for later psychosis and other severe psychological disorders (Read, Goodman, Morrison, Ross, & Aderhold, 2004; Read & Gumley, 2008; Read & Ross, 2003; Read, Van Os, Morrison, & Ross, 2005).

Faith's parents separated when she was in the first grade. Faith and her brother lived with their mother, who began dating and eventually remarried when Faith was in the sixth grade. Faith's stepfather was professionally successful. His relative financial stability allowed for luxuries Faith had never known, and she explained that this was the first time she got to live in a house. While she appreciated these new physical comforts, her stepfather travelled much of the time, and in his absence her mother became a full-fledged alcoholic. Faith's relationship with her mother was continually strained. She shared that, in hindsight, she believed her mother was always jealous of her talents and skills. Her mother regarded her as a maid or servant, dictating rules and expectations without ever truly engaging her. As a result, Faith never developed warm or positive feelings toward her mother.

Faith remembered seeing her father infrequently after he and her mother separated. Although she wanted a relationship with him, her mother forbade her from inviting his threatening presence into their home:

> I remember Dad would come over and just beat the shit out of her when they were drunk. And he picked her up by her heels and was banging her head on the floor, and she hit him with a cast-iron skillet and broke his glasses and nose, and blood was everywhere. The police came and arrested him, and took him away . . . I was horrified because I had asked him to come over, and he promised that he would be gone before mom got back. And I woke up on the couch with them screaming at each other 'cause she had been out with one of her dates, and they were already into it. And it was my fault.

On another occasion, he came to their house intoxicated and enraged:

> Then my real father came back in one day and almost killed my brother and I. He was totally stark naked. He and my mom had some kind of physical thing, and she was out in the yard, totally drunk with a hose, and he had a knife, and he was coming after my brother and I. And if it wasn't for my brother pulling me from the window, you know I wouldn't be here. 'Cause he got very violent when he was drunk.

Owing to these experiences Faith lost contact with her father for stretches of time. When she saw him again during high school, he was sober and had remarried. However, his wife was aware of his previous incestuous relation with his daughter and terminated contact between them, reinforcing Faith's conviction of her culpability in the incest she had experienced.

In addition to her father's early sexual abuse, Faith fell victim to sexual violence on a number of occasions later in her life, and each time she felt guilty for her part in the events and did not report them. Here is one example from her narrative:

> I was accosted in [City] by this really big, burly man when I was sixteen when I was working. . . . I was going to march in a parade that day. And you . . . I don't know if you've been in tragedies like this . . . it happened when I was in an earthquake. All of a sudden, everything got really quiet. You don't hear any birds. You don't hear anything. And all of a sudden all of the traffic cars went away. All the sound went away and then all of a sudden this big man with the pockmarked face jumped me and pushed me into the bushes by the science center and started ripping at my blouse, and I had bought from the food service some clogs, some wooden clogs and the tops of my feet were so sore because I'd never worn them . . . worn them that all I could think about while he was accosting me was, I'm

going to lose my clogs! So I took one of my clogs and I started pounding him on the back, and as I started pounding him on the back, um, all of a sudden car noises came in, and I could hear people talking and stuff and he got up and ran away. I never reported it. I never reported it. I went to the fair, and I did a parade and two shows that day so I never, never really thought it happened to me, you know?

FAITH'S CAPACITY FOR ADAPTATION

Faith was introduced to performance art when she was fourteen years old. Performance offered a vital path forward for a vulnerable young girl who was painfully shy due to her hearing loss, compounded by a tendency to stutter. Throughout her life, performance would prove to be an important outlet for Faith, who had no other means of processing or integrating her traumatic life experiences:

> I found out when I was performing, I could be everything that I couldn't be offstage. I wasn't me. I was somebody else. I was able to talk. I was able to use my physical skills. I had some dance training. Um, I . . . I wasn't me and I think that was a godsend for, especially being bipolar, I . . . I didn't have to live in me. I had an access, a way to use the energy, use the depression . . .

Faith's description of the link between her inner emotional life and her acting work suggests that performing allowed her to experience dissociated or split off self-states that were otherwise too uncomfortable or unsafe to feel. In this way, Faith's art fostered a reparative process that allowed her to experience parts of herself that she otherwise could not consciously connect to.

Consistent with the path many children with inner resilience choose, Faith managed to find someone who could serve as a good object—a substitute parental figure—who helped her experience her own agency and creativity. In Faith's case, this took the form of a young man who became her first husband at an early age, and who clearly allowed her to begin the difficult process of imagining herself *otherwise* (O'Loughlin & Johnson, 2010):

> And in August of that summer a guy named Robert had graduated—he graduated the year before I did—I found out that if you were married for fifty cents you could get fifty-two dollars' worth of food stamps. So I said to him, "Let's get married so I can get some food stamps." So, and he loved me—he was, you know, infatuated with me and whatever, I mean all we ever did was kiss, you know and uh, so we went and bought a dime-store ring, cost a dollar, six cents off those little finger poles, you know they have your sizes. And we got married—somebody loaned us

> twenty-five dollars for the marriage license and justice of the peace. . . . That's how I went through my senior year of high school. But because of Robert we . . . he applied for college. We got scholarships to [University], and that's where we went for our undergrad degrees. And then we got scholarships . . . I mean, I never ever thought of college. I just thought, I didn't think, you know. And if it wasn't for him thinking that far . . .

Robert's presence in Faith's life proved invaluable. He became the good object that she needed in order to develop a sense of internal goodness and worth. He opened Faith's imagination to possibilities for her future, inspiring her to aspire to professional heights. They applied to college together and both received scholarships to college and subsequently to a graduate program in performing arts. Reflecting on their relationship, Faith noted ironically that she was the more ambitious of the pair. After completing her MFA, Faith taught at a university and subsequently worked as a touring performance artist. Her husband remained at home, where he took advantage of local professional opportunities. Sadly, while Faith benefited from Robert's goodness, she was terrified of her own sexuality and her potential for motherhood, and this eventually led to psychic collapse.

PSYCHIC COLLAPSE

Faith was thirty when she first attempted to take her life. Unable to agree on whether to have children, Faith and her husband decided to divorce after fourteen years of marriage:

> He really wanted children, and I didn't want children at all. I didn't want 'em to go through what I had gone through, I had my tubes clamped . . . this was during college. In college I had my tubes clamped . . . he really wanted children, and I said I can't have children now, you know . . . I just had no . . . no drive, no want, no need, and in my profession it would have been in the way of my independence, of doing different shows and touring and stuff. And just . . . and even today, I'm terrified of children. And I'm a little bit jealous they have things I never had . . . a house, a bike, dolls, a school that they went to you know for a length of time, friends . . .

The prospect of having children conjured ghosts from Faith's early life that she had up until that point effectively staved off through the stability of her marriage and professional success. However, without an inkling as to how she might construct a different kind of life for a child than the one she had experienced, Faith could only imagine herself as the mother she had—envious of all the good things that she never had as a child. In her fantasy of motherhood, Faith simultaneously embodied her embittered, alcoholic mother as well as her childhood self—a deprived, angry child. Within this fantasy, Faith's husband became the father she grew up with, who she both loved and fervently feared. During the interview, Faith spoke candidly about her inability to engage in physical intimacy. She stated that she "hates sex" and that it "feels like rape," though she could not reconcile this with her conception of what it meant to be a good wife, a role she defined in very stereotypic patriarchal terms: "[S]ex had a lot to do with me drinking because I felt so bad about not being a good wife and . . . hating it so much and . . . and a wife should be, you know . . . good about things . . ." Her language echoes the internalized conviction of her badness, which was repeatedly tied to her sexuality, undoubtedly linked not only to her experiences of incest as a child but also to the sexual abuse she suffered as a young girl and woman.

Faith learned as a child that her body's intended use was for the enjoyment of and exploitation by others. Her induction into patriarchy was traumatic and set her up to repeatedly submit to the demands of others at the expense of her own needs and desires. Nevertheless, loss of the containing structure that her platonic marriage had once provided, compounded by deterioration of her hearing and its deleterious effects on her career as a performer, culminated in her first suicide attempt:

> I was getting very lost in myself and very paranoid. And then I decided *I'll just kill myself*, so I went back to my apartment. It was late in the evening. I picked up a jug of Gallo burgundy wine and I picked up some speed and some Quaaludes and some other pills from the street seller, and amphetamines. And I went back to my apartment and I cleaned it all up and I wrote on the bottoms of everything where everything was to go, um I only had a little tub sink, and I showered and put on a clean nighty and fresh underwear because my mom said always have on fresh underwear, you never know what people will find . . . And um, and I didn't know what to do with myself so, um, I had a little army cot in my room—because it was so tiny—as my bed, and I lay down on the little wooden mat the, the place mat, the flooring, the Gallo wine and the amphetamines and black beauties and the speed lined up, and then I just proceeded to situate my backside in between two pipes to hold me up and I just started going through all the pills and all the liquor and the next thing I knew um, there was like shards of shiny, and I felt bumps. I'd evidently fallen off the gurney in the ambulance. The door was busted down by cops. My friend called the cops and they put me in an ambulance and sent me to hospital, where they gave me charcoal and I puked and was very, very sick—but they saved my life.

Faith said that at the time she thought that suicide was "the right thing to do," though in hindsight she recognized how depressed she had been. Given the tremendous emotional deprivation and cruelty to which Faith had been subjected as a child, the reappearance of these demons at the prospect of experiencing herself as a sexual being, not to mention the prospect of becoming a mother, was enough to engender psychic collapse. According to Fromm-Reichmann (1954), the kind of deprivation Faith experienced in her early childhood would have set the stage for a regressive preoccupation with a sense of "badness" and fear of uncontainable aggression. Unable to contain these feelings, Faith turned her aggression toward herself for the unlovable person she believed herself to be.

Describing her depression, Faith stated, "I just remember I went inside and I couldn't find a way out. I was way at the bottom of my feet and that's when I went inside and I went away." Faith remained in the hospital for approximately three months, and she captured the abjectness of her psychic state this way:

> It was a suicide attempt, and I was so depressed that I couldn't look at anybody, and I only knew people by their shoes, and I would be under tables and things and I couldn't talk. I didn't talk for three months but I started . . . drawing pictures of the rooms and the people and I called the staff door keepers because they would come in, and they would bring door people through with white shoes and stuff and that became a voice for me . . . I, all of a sudden, was drawing from my own inner self and putting it onto the page.

The similarity in the language Faith used to describe her depression and her experience of incest is striking. The experience of "going away" from the present moment and into some private psychic space is apparent, and it is not hard to imagine that this is because her depressive self-state took root in the boundary violations she suffered. It is also not surprising, then, that through sustained contact with her depression, her early sexual abuse, which had been repressed for several years, resurfaced. The reemergence of these memories, evoked by her husband's desire to have children, engulfed her in the pain of her dissociated and repressed past. Trapped between feelings of fear, rage, and her own fundamental badness, Faith saw suicide as not only a release but as an ethical act. Before her overdose, Faith ensured that Robert was on the path to having children by successfully matching him with one of her close friends. Describing her mindset as she planned her suicide, Faith noted:

> I thought I was just doing the right thing. It felt very normal to me. It felt . . . I knew I was putting everything right . . . and everything was taken care of. Robert had a new girlfriend and a wife. I had the divorce papers so I knew I didn't owe him anything else now because he's going to have kids.

During her first hospitalization, Faith experienced the institutionalization of her suffering as a mental disorder. She was diagnosed with bipolar disorder and began taking Lithium and Thorazine, as well as receiving electroconvulsive therapy [ECT]. The severity of her psychic collapse was evident in her description of her hospitalization:

> And I was, I entered in the locked ward, after they just let me in and I stayed in a room with two other ladies who kept getting ECT, electric convulsive therapy, which I didn't know what it was, I just knew they're being electrocuted. And I couldn't, for months look at anybody or talk. I'd crawl under tables, I wrote in the journal and I remember one time they left a glass in the sink, and I broke the glass because I heard God in my head and I had to let God out. And I cut off all my hair and I started to cut my scalp, so they put me in the pink room in a straitjacket, and I was there for I guess a while because I remember them bringing in trays of food and unstrapping me and all I had was a mattress on the floor, and they started shock therapy with me in the hospital three times a week. But I had this most euphoric feeling that God was talking to me and I had to let him out, I had to let him out of myself.

While Faith stated that she felt safe in the hospital, she recalled leaving after about three months without improvement. It is notable that during her hospitalization, while she received copious amounts of medications, as well as ECT, she could not recall ever receiving psychotherapy or psychosocial support during her stay. Nevertheless, she was sufficiently stabilized that she was able to resume her career as a performer.

Although Faith went on with her life as an artist, she continued to suffer from periodic psychic breakdowns. On one occasion, for example, she attempted to take her life by overdosing on Klonopin, a psychotropic medication known for its sedating effect. She remarked that her suicidal impulses had most often been triggered by feelings of failure or a lack of self-worth. She was particularly vulnerable to interpersonal loss or professional setbacks as, lacking self-confidence and self-soothing capabilities, she was totally dependent on external validation to maintain her emotional equilibrium. Faith related having been hospitalized about two to three times per year for the past thirty years. Her most recent hospitalization occurred just weeks before the first interview:

> And, um, and when I went back to see how the last year, I went to make amends on their graves, I couldn't find my father's but I made amends to my other two stepfathers and my mother and to some people which made me feel better. You know, that I was sorry, whatever I'd done to hurt you and that whole thing. And that's why I went back, and then I was hospi-

talized in August for three weeks, I think. It was too much for me, you know doing all that. But that was my last hospitalization was last August.

Faith felt compelled to seek reparation from her parents, and that very impulse then triggered traumatic memories that resulted in psychic collapse. Overwhelmed by the trip home, Faith began cutting herself, something she had engaged in at times in the past. Regarding her periodic retreat into the hospital setting, Faith stated, "I sometimes just want to be taken care of, you know, in a safe place . . . I just feel it's a safe place to go where I won't hurt myself, when I get overwhelmed . . ."

WITHIN THE KALEIDOSCOPE

Faith's experience of the cycle that at times carried her to the highest heights and at other times crashed her to the deepest depths reflects the kaleidoscopic shifts of her internal world. For example, while suicide seemed to have a consistent place in Faith's psyche, her feelings about death morphed in accordance with a more pervasive shift in affect. While in both mania and depression Faith experienced a longing for death, this yearning assumed different meanings depending upon her emotional state—either as a welcomed respite or as deserved punishment:

> When I get high, I want to hurt myself. When I get very manic, I get like death is a beautiful thing, you know? It's not bad thing. It's a beautiful thing. It makes me joyous. It makes me feel enraptured. It's like . . . when I'm depressed I want to die also but . . . it's . . . I mean I have my will all made out. I know where I'm going to be cremated. I've made all the plans and all the arrangements so nobody has to worry about anything. I took an overdose when I lived on 20th Street and walked over to the police precinct and sat on the bench and sighed, waiting to die with my address on me and my note with where the will was, but they found out and they took me away by ambulance because I passed out there . . . but I took a lot of Klonopin and just had my stomach pumped.

Faith's depression at times caused her to tumble into a catatonic state, unable to speak for protracted periods. However, in contrast with her overt appearance during these times, Faith described her internal experience as a process of self-reflection. This is consistent with Sass and Parnas's (2003) assertion, and a similar assertion by Ellen Corin (1992) that what are commonly identified as the "negative symptoms" of psychosis are often not accurate reflections or an analog for what is happening internally. During her first hospitalization Faith did not speak for three months—the entirety of her stay: "I just remember I went inside and I couldn't find a way out. I was way at the bottom of my feet and that's when I went inside and I went away." Similar to what William Styron (1990) reported in *Darkness Visible*, the isolation and disconnection from the outside world created a space in Faith's head for a kind of introspection that connected her with early experiences normally kept out of awareness.

While in contact with the agony of her repeated victimization, Faith was plunged into a depression that severed her ties from a world whose injustice had made her its target while accentuating its inflicted pain. The high of the manic state existed to counter the agony of such painful experience. It shifted the kaleidoscope's focus from the ugliness of poverty, neglect, and abuse to the splendor of the world, inspiring love and fascination. Unfortunately, the cost of these extreme oscillations was their self-perpetuation. Without the possibility for integration, Faith continued to slide between dissociative poles, acting out an early psychic rhythm that helped her survive but also led her repeatedly to the precipice of annihilation.

SPLITTING AND STITCHING

Faith acknowledged the importance of artistic expression in managing her inner experience. Through her art, Faith was able to channel facets of herself that were too difficult or painful to integrate. "I can do anything on stage. I could be nude on stage . . . it's like I'm protected. I'm like totally protected and I can be all things." This observation evokes questions regarding which parts of herself Faith needed protection from. Her examples of displaying her nude body and performing her sexuality, while being unable to actually engage in sexual intercourse, suggested that she managed her psychic needs through a split in her subjectivity. Within the circumscribed space of performance art, Faith felt free to connect with her sexuality. However, outside of this protected space, expressing her sexuality was too dangerous. Reflecting on the culpability induced by her experience of incest, she was preoccupied with trying to understand her role in the production of her father's incestuous actions: "Must've been something I did to encourage him, I don't know. But he was always such a double person when he was drinking. I didn't like the person he was as a drunk. I couldn't control him." This conviction of culpability would relegate sexuality to the realm of taboo and as too dangerous to allow into the "unprotected" territory of sexual enjoyment.

However, while only a partial solution, her capacity to experience her sexuality while performing served a soothing function and perhaps preserved some possibility, however remote, of working through some of her emotional constriction: "And I find that I take the feelings that I have, and I put them into my work, and my work brings about how I'm feeling. So it's sort of like a mirror to what's going on inside me, so it's been very gratifying . . . it soothes me." Performing, therefore, served as a partial substitute for the mirroring that Faith had failed to receive in her childhood, offering evidence of her capacity for resilience.

These stratagems, however, could not fully compensate for the relational deficits Faith experienced in her childhood. Throughout her life she had an ongoing dependency on external mirroring for registering her inner experience, and her continuing parasuicidal behavior, alcoholism, self-injurious behavior, and binge eating suggest that her battle to experience the integrity of her own subjectivity and to stave off collapse was ceaseless. For example, Faith reported that she began cutting herself before the age of fourteen after she stumbled upon the feeling of relief that self-harm provided:

> I burned myself really bad on the ropes in gym class. And . . . it looked like it hurt really bad, you know, and I was feeling . . . was seeing my stepmom, my real father, and I didn't want to see her because she was really a drunk and didn't want me to see it. I burned my, my thing and it felt good. As I slid down the ropes, I burned my arm and it felt good and there were like little tear marks in my arm. . . . And it felt good. I could feel the pain. I couldn't feel it inside but . . . feeling it outside makes me feel it inside. I guess that sounds weird but when I cut . . . I'm in control. And I could see that I must be in pain. So I recognized that. . . . And when I can't feel any pain, that's when I cut. But um, 'cause I wanna see the . . . I feel the . . . I don't feel the pain, but I know I'm in pain. And if I see myself bleed I know that I must be in pain . . .

From a Kleinian perspective (Klein, 1946), early failure of the maternal function had left Faith with unmetabolized aggression, leaving her vulnerable to periods of self-persecution and fragmentation. Kohut (1984) viewed experience of this kind of fragmentation as an inevitable consequence of early abuse and neglect, leaving people such as Faith with a vast deficit in the ability to self-soothe, to tolerate anxiety, and to experience a continuous, cohesive sense of self. Cutting, therefore, can be viewed as representing Faith's attempt to define the boundaries of her physical being as a counter to the feeling of fragmentation. Faith's statement that she would revert to cutting a couple of times each year is indicative of the fragile state of her ego and the constant struggle she has had just to *go on being*, to use Winnicott's (1974) phrase. It was times like this that that led her to return to the hospital for inpatient treatment, a place where, just as Styron (1990) had, she could safely fall into collapse:

> I just go inside, I go to that place that special dark place and just hang out, try not to cut myself, try to get active, but it's very hard. I sometimes just want to be taken care of. You know in a safe place . . . They let me go

> low. They [hospitals] let me go to the bottom. And I know I won't hurt myself there.

UNSUSTAINABLE LOVE

A few years after her divorce, Faith met the man who would later become her second husband. Although married for several years, their work often separated them geographically. When together, their relationship was haunted by the demons of their respective pasts. For Faith, this manifested in self-harm, alcohol abuse, and multiple suicide attempts. During the interview, Faith spoke about the difficulty she continued to have with sexual intimacy and with conforming to societal expectations of her as woman and wife:

> I wasn't a good sexual partner. And it's funny, well it's not funny, but all the roles I played on stage were mostly sexual. I could be sexual on stage, I could be naked on stage, but I couldn't be in real life. 'Cause I had such a, I hated my body, I hated what it was, I hated what it became, and I couldn't imagine anybody wanting it . . . I just hated it. And I've been very fortunate, I married two wonderful men who have seen me through my insanity, and I mean I've talked to my [second] husband about it, "Go have an affair, have a relationship, you know, please. You know, I can't imagine you living like this with me for twenty more years. You know, I just can't." I can't do it, Montana. It feels like rape.

Faith shared that she would attempt to engage in intercourse but that it often triggered flashbacks of earlier episodes of sexual abuse. These would emerge as fragmented memories crystallized in the way they were originally experienced, with dissociated emotion. "[I]f I get a flash of something . . . It's mostly memories. I have no feelings about those things. I just have memories." While seemingly contradictory, the constriction of affect that Faith described is also a hallmark of the psychological effect of trauma. Herman (1997) refers to the vacillation between memory intrusion and affect constriction as the *dialectic of trauma*, which she views as a consequence of the inability to integrate past traumatic experience. After twenty-seven years of marriage, alcohol ultimately drove the most tangible wedge between Faith and her second husband. In an attempt to manage the psychic scars of past abuse, Faith broke her sobriety. She reported that her husband became verbally abusive when inebriated, and that in her own intoxication her rage would surface:

> I had rage and my husband was just uncontrollable. He was fallin' down drunk, and, and I could've killed him. . . . I could've killed him with no, no feeling whatsoever. You know, I could've just gone ahead and just

> stabbed him in the back. And I knew I had to get out of there. And then when he accosted me and tried to choke me, I just said "I gotta go."

Faith's resentment toward her husband stood against the backdrop of an early life with two alcoholic parents toward whom she was unable to feel or express anger. Having internalized her own culpability for the acrimony they directed at her, Faith had no outlet for the sheer hate she, in turn, aimed back at herself. Later in life, her alcoholic partner became a trigger and convenient target for these feelings that nobody had ever helped her to work through. In an act of self-preservation, Faith decided to separate from her husband. This is what led Faith to live at one of Fountain House's affiliated residences, which became a stabilizing and containing structure for her. During the interview, Faith related that she continued to worry about what would become of her marriage. She stated that her husband "will not give her a divorce," though she also appeared ambivalent about whether she would want this. This unresolved ambivalence reflects the culmination of a life without a good enough object—a dependable person who can mirror back her own goodness. As a child, Faith protected herself through consciously seeing herself as bad while preserving the goodness of the other, and therefore never having to truly acknowledge the cruelty of those who were meant to protect and cherish her. While this divide in Faith's psychic experience allowed her to produce remarkable artwork, it also prevented her from sustaining intimate relationships. This seemed to be the tragedy of Faith's life, as no amount of professional success could compensate for the lack of love, trust, and human connection she experienced in childhood. Relationships inherently threatened Faith's ability to contain what she called her "crazy parts." She had to manage her perpetual urge to flee, culminating in a manic rush, which then inevitably crashed her back into the depths of herself where her "crazy parts" reside. This appeared to have been the cycle of her adult life.

TRAVAILS IN THE MENTAL "HEALTH" SYSTEM

Faith's experience with the mental "health" system was extensive. She reported having seen the same psychiatrist for the past twenty years and that she continued to take a cocktail of psychotropic medications. In addition, she related that she had continued to undergo electroconvulsive therapy [ECT] periodically, since her first hospitalization twenty years prior, in spite of "hating" it. She stated that her psychiatrist was a proponent of ECT but that she felt it had led to memory degradation. Faith reported that she was previously on an antipsychotic medication that caused her to gain eighty pounds, as well as on another medication which caused significant organ damage.

Overall, despite the drawbacks, she believed that the medication had helped "lift" her "suicidal impulses" in addition to helping her sleep.

At the time of the interviews, Faith reported that she had just begun to engage with psychotherapy for the first time. The absence of psychotherapy in Faith's treatment over prior decades is alarming, though hardly surprising given the changing landscape of the North American mental health field during this time (cf., Estroff, 1981; Bentall, 2009; Moncrieff, 2013; Whitaker, 2001, 2010). However, juxtaposed with the medical interventions she received, psychotherapy could offer Faith the opportunity to integrate past traumas into her narrative of suffering, something that would seem essential to her healing process. When asked about whether she saw a connection between her difficult past and present suffering, Faith stated, "I don't see a connection, I just see them as all stories, snippets but I don't know what the connection is. . . . But the past, my present acceptance has made me who I am. You know just the overall palette." This response reflects a gap in Faith's narrative, and particularly a lack of the kind of integration that would save her from living in the shadow of psychic collapse.

In *The Wounded Storyteller,* Frank (1995) notes that the medical system privileges objective and technical thinking over the production of meaning from the experience of illness. Rather than addressing Faith's experience in relation to her past and future, Faith's treatment provided intervention almost as if within a vacuum. This vacuum did not consider the social and traumatic origins of her suffering, nor did it attend to questions of the kind of person she might like to be in the future and how these might be shaped by her unique strengths, talents, and vulnerabilities. Rather, her treatment seemed a perfect setup for what Frank refers to as a "chaos narrative," one in which fragments of a personality are patched together without much interest in the kind of integration or re-storying that would lead to robust psychic health. Faith's use of the word "snippets" to describe how her life story is organized reveals just such fragmentation. Against all odds, Faith consistently managed to look forward to new projects and professional endeavors. However, her capacity to progress was not related to a quest or purpose that was tied to her suffering, but rather seemed split from her narrative of trauma, psychic suffering, and hospitalization. These two narratives, the one of suffering and the other of her professional accomplishments, seemed to run along separate corridors in Faith's mind, intersecting minimally and most frequently in terms of a recurrent cycle: work, hospitalization, work, hospitalization. This is certainly one potential outcome of an atomistic approach to mental health care that fails to acknowledge narrative or context. From this perspective, psychological distress is a product of a chemical imbalance that requires first and foremost pharmacological intervention. To some proponents of the disease model for psychic distress, the chaotic or disjointed form of Faith's narrative might reflect the symptomatology of her supposed psychotic condition. While the precise etiology of Faith's condition cannot be determined retrospectively, the kind of treatment she received—a treatment that did not value Faith's life context or deeply traumatic history—while, perhaps, containing and managing her condition, did not provide the kind of narrative arc that could have led to a potentially helpful re-storying and integration. Rather, Faith was given a diagnosis of Bipolar I, a diagnosis that, while not clearly understood by her, provided something concrete to cling to:

> I didn't understand the diagnosis, I just understood that I wanted to die . . . Um I never, even though I knew I was bipolar, I never associated it with my suicide attempts or anything, I just, it was just some wording that would give me a certain kind of prescription, but I didn't understand what it was.

When asked about how her understanding of the diagnosis changed over time, Faith's response was consistent with the psychiatric treatment she had received:

> That it is a mental illness, and that I can see my manic, when I get manic and when I get depressed as part of the symptoms of my disease. I see it as a disease . . . a mental disease, which implies stigma . . .

The language that Faith used to describe her psychic pain illustrates the power that the disease model holds in shaping personal experience. Within this conceptual frame, symptoms are "natural objects" that are "discovered" through trained clinical observation. With circular logic, these observed symptoms serve to corroborate a neurochemical model of the mind (Rose, 2003). By this logic, the gestalt of the person's life history and present context are not relevant to understanding psychic suffering. Faith's narrative captures one inevitable consequence of this paradigm. She internalized a belief that the etiology of her suffering must be rooted in a "disease." Disease is the sole cause of her pain, and the disease is solely hers to bear. Faith's statement that disease "implies" stigma also touches upon something that is rarely if ever acknowledged—that the disease model is itself responsible for creating the social stigma that it disclaims. Having individualized and pathologized her suffering, the disease model turns Faith's pain into a product of faulty neurophysiology. This notion not only pardons her abusers for their part in her suffering, but also adds layers to the sense of internal badness that the abuse had planted within her. She is not only the bad little girl who deserved to be battered and neglected, she is also biologically defective with no tangible hope of recovery. From this perspective, intermittent stabilization is the most that Faith can hope for, assuming that the right amalgam of medication and electroshock therapy can be titrated.

However, Faith's story illustrates a potential that transcends this limited prognosis. Her multiple achievements are a testament to her resilience, in part attributable to her remarkable artistic talents and narrative capacity, and, in part, perhaps, to the capacity of her hospitalizations to stabilize her decompensatory slides. What the medical model missed in its diagnosis and treatment of Faith are the beautiful gifts she offers, even while in the midst of her suffering. Faith's sensitivity to the vast spectrum of feeling has not only rendered her fragile and vulnerable to breakdown but has also allowed her to transmute her experience into profound works of performance and visual art. Faith's multiple hospitalizations, continued medication, and repeated exposure to ECT failed to value her robust internal resources, and to assist her in understanding the ways in which her suffering relates to a history of chronic and acute trauma. Unlike so many others who find themselves in the thrall of psychic breakdown, Faith discovered forms of self-healing that helped her to survive and, in many ways, to thrive.

In *Mothering Without a Map*, Kathryn Black (2004) describes the dilemma for girls raised by mothers who lacked the containing capacity, mirroring, and receptivity, to keep their daughters in mind and thereby to allow their daughters to gain a sense of their own capacity to be, to feel, to self-soothe, to trust, and to get their relational needs met without abjection or abuse. Faith's journey was compromised by the lack of such an inner map, compounded by catastrophic sexual abuse from her father and later from others. These failures were further magnified by living more than six decades of life without ever being offered a therapeutic relationship or a restorative home, until she was fortunate to arrive at Fountain House, where she has experienced a containing, supportive environment and where she was finally offered access to therapeutic services. For Faith, first as girl, then as sexual woman, then as wife, the tragedy is compounded in that inflexible, implicit patriarchal norms for what counts as girl, woman, and wife, are inscribed in such a way as to leave her feeling empty and a failure despite her considerable success and the admirable pockets of resilience she exhibits. Her story raises troubling questions not only about the lack of interest in history and narrative in contemporary institutional psychiatry, but also about the straitjacket that norms of "femininity" impose on all girls—norms that are particularly difficult to manage and negotiate for somebody who experienced the kind of trust and sexual boundary violations Faith suffered. Surely, as a society, should we not strive to do better?

CODA

In *Trauma and Recovery*, Judith Herman (1997), drawing on Sylvia Fraser's (1987) memoir of incest, reminds us that in earlier times Fraser "might well have been condemned as a witch. In Freud's time she would have been diagnosed as a hysteric. Today she would be diagnosed with multiple personality disorder" (Herman, p. 97). Trauma theorists (e.g., Garland, 1998; Gartner, 2001; Herman, 1997) describe remarkable progress in the psychodynamic treatment of survivors of sexual trauma. Recent work has depathologized suffering, documented the narrative etiology of traumatic suffering, and helped articulate therapeutic approaches that prioritize safety and containment, and hold promise for allowing sufferers to symbolize their suffering and strive to integrate their traumatic experience and live life fully. A challenge that remains, however, is to bear in mind the possibility of sexual trauma when women present with symptoms of madness. Just as Freud regrettably abandoned his seduction theory in favor of the pejorative label of *hysteric*, we run the risk of marginalizing sexual trauma survivors as crazy, thought-disordered, bipolar, psychotic, etc., simply because we chose not to listen carefully for the backstory that produced such a catastrophic flight from reality. Our goal in this narrative work is to draw attention to backstory, context, trauma, and loss, so that we avoid a rush to treatment, and instead seek fuller understanding of what lies beneath the terrifying experiences that drive people to a position of madness.

NOTE

1. This chapter appears in a slightly different form in M. Brown and M. Charles (Ed), (2019), *Women & the Psychosocial Construction of Madness*, published by Lexington Books.

Chapter Three

Mary

Surviving "Head Traumas"

Secil Arac-Orhun and Michael O'Loughlin

Mary, an African-American female in her late forties, holds a college degree in Business Administration and had previously worked as an employee in business, although she expressed a desire to be an actress. Prior to the conversations, Secil had volunteered in the clubhouse for eight months, and Mary was familiar with her. Whenever she saw Secil, she had a sincere smile that lit up her face, and she greeted her with an enthusiastic "Hi." Yet, this sense of familiarity was not enough to relieve her anxiety about telling Secil about her depression and her experience of hearing voices.

Mary began her story by describing her most recent suicide attempt:

> Last year I tried to commit suicide three times. Um, just one day I felt depressed and later when I kind of found out I had severe depression and also was hearing voices telling me to kill myself. Um, like I said before, I tried three times trying to kill myself, I . . . I swallowed a few coins . . . I drank boric acid and that's what made me, um, and I also tried to slit my wrists. That also made me . . . upset because I wasn't achieving my goal, and the goal was to . . . to die.
>
> The first time I tried to kill myself, I was put in a hospital, I think it was [Hospital] that, you know, I went through, uh, through the whole procedures there . . . just have me think a minute, it's been a while [smiles, then laughs]. Um, I went through the whole procedure, the doctors checked me out and what have you, and then I was discharged. At the time I thought I was okay, but when I got home, everything started to come on to me again, the severe depression, the laying down and not getting out of bed,

> not wanting to see people, and all of that. Again I was rushed to the hospital, and this time I was, uh, in . . . [Hospital], and I did the same thing again. I took the medicines that they gave me, but this time I . . . did a lot of isolating.

The suicide attempt and the profound depression led to her first encounters with psychiatry and treatment, and since it was a year ago, it felt fresh in her mind.

CHILDHOOD TRAUMA

Mary's life was characterized by severe depression and a childhood with multiple traumatic experiences and unprocessed feelings. She grew up in a household with an alcoholic mother and a drug-addicted father.

> M: Did I have a father image?
>
> I: Mmhmm.
>
> M: Uh . . . no. (Laughing) Not really. 'Cause he k- he kept leaving. . . . he only bought me one toy, it was a bicycle. And, I didn't see it for a while, and I was asking my mother what happened to the bicycle? She said your father took it and sold it. So um, he could have money for his drugs. Yeah.

She witnessed recurrent conflict and domestic violence between her parents. Mary was the oldest of four siblings; she grew up with three younger brothers. Two of her brothers carried a diagnosis of schizophrenia, and one was developmentally disabled. Mary's memories of childhood were filled with parental arguments. She witnessed her mother being physically assaulted by her father. Her mother made repeated attempts to flee with Mary and her siblings, but Mary's father always found them. When Mary was eight years old, her father died of a heart attack while he was using heroin. Mary stated that alcohol abuse also ran in her family. She remembered her mother getting drunk, sometimes to the point of falling down:

> M: Yeah, her drinking, yeah . . . It was usually with a group of people or with someone else. 'Cause that's how she used to drink with my father. Um, yeah she used to get really drunk sometimes. Yeah.
>
> I: What would she do?
>
> M: She would fall down. Yeah. Um, passing out. Yeah.

I: How did you feel?

M: I thought she was [laughing] dead.

I: You thought . . . that's a scary feeling.

M: Yeah, yeah. Yeah. So. She . . . she survived it. Yeah.

Mary said that she and her brothers grew up without a father figure, partly because of his untimely death and partly because, before that, her father often disappeared for periods of time. When he was around, Mary wished he would leave again, because she felt that this was the only way her mother would be safe. In contrast, Mary remembered her brothers being angry with their mother for not leaving their father. When asked about how her brothers coped with the violence at home, Mary related:

> They didn't . . . for some reason they didn't pay much attention to it. Um, they just started just to accept the fact that they're fighting and this is the way it's supposed to be, this . . . they're growing up with that idea in their head. You know. Now that they've grown, um, they realize now that it wasn't right. Right, my father was sick. And what have you. And they had resented my mother for a long time because . . . they resented my mother for a long time because they felt that she could have done something. Fight him back, hit him back, or something like that. I didn't think that way.

Mary also spoke of how, as a young adult, she became involved with romantic partners who were emotionally abusive or had drug or alcohol problems. She acknowledged her attraction to men who were similar to her father. She simultaneously feared male figures in her life and found herself attracted to them despite their negative attributes:

> Um, I had bad relationships . . . all my—most, or all my boyfriends—were interested in getting high all the time. I guess I do gravitate towards them because something I was picking up from my childhood. About my mother and father used to drink together. So in some ways I was like looking for that, looking for a little father image and hating it at the same time.

Mary recalled wanting closeness, but also fearing the repercussions intimacy could bring. Her exposure to domestic violence during childhood set an unhealthy model for both Mary and her brothers. She recounted:

> M: But all this time, this is always, was some sort of stress. My brothers, um, became violent with each other, they'd play games, like you know, sword fighting and guns and stuff like that. All of that coming from my mother and father and what image they left. So all this time I still, I was unhappy.
>
> I: You were unhappy?
>
> M: Yeah. My mother used to leave us at home, ah and that's when my brothers used to go crazy, used to do crazy s— . . . like sword fighting, um they broke doors [laughing] down you know. So it's, the violence . . . would continue. I, I tried to tell them to stop.

UNRESOLVED EMOTIONS

When left unresolved, anxieties and splitting may result in severe psychic difficulties including psychosis (Klein, 1946). In Mary's case, caregivers in her life were not constant. Her father, for example, frequently disappeared for indefinite periods of time. The memories that Mary had of her father were conflicted. On the one hand, she recalled her father being the only parent who played with her, and at other times, he was neglectful and deceitful. Mary began by describing her relationship with her father as positive, yet the story took a different turn as she recounted the circumstances:

> My relationship with him was, eh, pretty cool. He, um, he never touched any of us . . . which was surprising, and all of the disciplinarian work was . . . was either by my grandmother or my mother. Um, when I was little, he, he used to you know play with me and stuff. He only bought me one toy, it was a bicycle. And I didn't see it for a while, and I was asking my mother, "What happened to the bicycle?" My father took it and sold it so, he could have money for his drugs. Yeah . . . I thought it wasn't fair that he would take my bicycle . . . It wasn't there that long [laughs], you know, he just, like, bought it for me, and then sold it right, you know, immediately afterward. Yeah. So, and then at—after that I was just quiet about the whole thing, how you know . . . not saying anything about the bicycle. I just stopped asking about it and what have you. Yeah. I don't know, it was, it was like, I was really pissed off . . . I stopped talking to him. Yeah. Not too long after that he, he died.

In a similar fashion, Mary's view of her mother shifted between negative and positive perspectives throughout the three interviews. When asked about her present relationship with her mother, Mary stated:

We're best friends now . . . [laughs] Yeah. She still wants me to come live with her, and that I won't do. I think, I think it made me sick in the, you know, the first time. The dysfunction . . . would be coming out of her. And then, I think about that, and then I would get depressed, and this is when I first got sick. I fell into a depression. I guess it had a lot to do with not . . . coming out and sharing things with—with people. But it caught up to me. And I became depressed, and I tried to commit suicide. And went to the hospital and all that, and that's how I ended up here [laughs]. You know. So, I can't really, like, live with her again . . . we would talk and what have you. What not. I didn't realize how much, um, negative effect it had on me. I didn't know what was wrong. My mother's . . . it would never really get caught on, until she had to come to the hospital. Never really caught on that I was sick, which was very strange [laughs] to me. Because that was the only thing I was doing was lying down and not getting out of bed.

Wilfred Bion's (1967) notion of a "willfully misunderstanding object" comes to life through Mary's relationship with her mother. According to Bion, sometimes a mother, because of her own struggles, cannot soothe her child and takes away any potential substitute that the child may find (Bion, 1967). For example, Mary talked about her grandmother as the figure in her life who provided her with good mothering, love, and a safe environment. She spoke fondly of her grandmother and the way she used to cook for Mary and her brothers, do their laundry, and demonstrate her love for them. Mary reported that her mother became envious of her children's love for their grandmother. According to Mary, her grandmother was better than her mother at everything. "She was almost perfect." Mary recounted:

M: So, I sort of like, took my grandmother as being my mother, you know, a little bit. And then that changed once we moved away. My mother would get jealous of the fact that I would want to stay with my grandmother than with her [laughing]. So she didn't see it that way.

I: How did you know that she was jealous?

M: Um, she'd get angry. She would say, "Don't take too much things from your grandmother because she might spoil you." . . . stuff like that. I didn't feel like I was spoiled [laughing]. I didn't feel like I was spoiled, but my mother did. Yeah.

I: How did she express her anger?

M: It was, sometimes, she would hit us. Other times, just yelling. And then she called us up one day, and said that—you know, she shouldn't be

> hitting her children. 'Cause that's what my father did to her . . . Yeah. Yeah. So, I don't know, she's—she just, didn't like the fact that, you know, I was coming closer to my grandmother than with her.

The memories Mary shared of her mother were usually painful. For example, Mary remembered her mother telling her, "I wish I had a boy first." Hearing this was devastating for Mary. Not surprisingly, Mary explained that she became what she called "sick" because of her mother. Initially, Mary described her current relationship with her mother as positive, stating, "we are best friends now." Later on she talked about how her relationship with her mother had a negative effect on her: "the dysfunction . . . would be coming out of her . . . I fell into depression."

According to Bion (1962/1988), if a mother is not available and therefore cannot accept her infant's unwanted feelings, those intolerable feelings become a "nameless dread," meaning that the unwanted feelings are intolerable initially for the mother, and then for the infant, and as a result, the infant cannot name and make sense of the feelings. In Mary's case, the negative effect of her relationship with her mother and the experiences of her childhood took the form of nameless dread. What Mary referred to as "head traumas" appeared to be the undigested, unprocessed feelings that became nameless dreads because they were never symbolized (Bion, 1962/1988). Mary explained these as the conflicting voices in her head, some telling her to kill herself and some telling her to save herself.

> I don't . . . go through head traumas like I used to . . . I call it head traumas, the conflicts in my head. I used to have a lot of that. Just go ahead and do it you know, or not. The biggest conflict is, like I said, the voices telling me to kill myself. That was, like, the last conflict of that, it was huge, you know. I think, the whole experience, I think that going through it puts you into in reality . . . very quickly. I used to never deal with reality, but going through the schizophrenia and all that, once you come out of it, it's like a weight has been lifted off of you. Um . . . like I said before, in some ways it's a good thing.

Mary indicated she could not recall a lot of memories, and she declared that it must have been because she had been sick:

> M: Yeah. But I still can't re . . . I still can't remember a whole lot. It bugs me now. Now it bugs, it bothers me.
>
> I: You can't remember?
>
> M: That I can't remember, yeah. I th . . . 'cause I'm saying that I mus . . . I must have been sick from childhood. You know.

I: By sick, what do you mean?

M: Um, you know in the head. Traumatized to the point where I can't remember.

UNPROCESSED TRAUMA

On several occasions during the interview, when asked about the events that led to her hospitalization, Mary seemed unable to offer much reflection:

I: Can you tell me when was the first time that you started feeling it?

M: Uh, when was the first time?

I: . . . very depressed or isolated?

M: Uh . . . it was last year.

I: It was the first time?

M: Yeah (nods). It was the first time. Last year this whole thing has been a year-long thing.

I: Like can you like imagine what happened that maybe precipitated that?

M: I think I ju . . .

I: feelings?

M: . . . 'Cause I I guess because I I keep think in my head a lot, at that time . . . and, I think I was uh upse-uh upset because I didn't have a job at the time.

Mary was initially hospitalized in her thirties, which was after her first suicide attempt. She remained there for a brief period, got discharged but got readmitted as she continued to feel very depressed and she had two subsequent suicide attempts over that year. In the initial interview Mary appeared to be defended against the painful origins of her struggles and talked about her psychic difficulties as if they were new phenomena that had surfaced during the previous year: "Just one day I felt depressed, and later when I kind of found out I had severe depression and also was hearing voices telling me to kill myself." When asked when she started feeling depressed, Mary answered, "It was last year . . . Yeah [nods]. It was the first time. Last year, this whole thing has been a year-long thing." However, in the second interview, as Mary managed to get more in touch with her painful childhood experiences, she began to identify some of the early origins of her depression and voice hearing.

Mary described the first time she heard voices when she was in her early thirties. "It was very scary. I always had a stomachache because it was tied up in knots, 'cause I was nervous . . . Yeah, I couldn't get it, them, out of the, out of the head." Mary elaborated:

> Hearing the voices, and finding out that there was no one there. That kind of thing that shocked me . . . Yeah. Really scary 'cause it seemed so real. Yeah. And, um, one night I had left the, my mother's house [clears throat], like real early in the morning, and was walking the street and the voices would come, and I really thought they were up there in the sky somewhere just making—making me, pushing me t-to jump off the roof or jump in the lake or something like that. So tha-that was a really big thing. Mm-hmm . . . they would tell me go . . . go find a lake or something and jump in . . . they said they were here to take care of me, and then it started . . . they started instructing me on ways of killing myself. Yeah, you know, and it was it was, it was like, "take some rat poison and something" or "slit the wrists" type of thing, yeah. So that was . . . that was a really traumatic experience.

Mary reported feeling disconnected from her emotions. She described not being able to feel anything. She learned from her mother that crying signaled weakness, so she never cried. When asked, "Were you able to cry?" Mary replied, "No. And I still have a problem with that to this day. No, the tears wouldn't come." She could identify her childhood struggles as very painful, yet her lack of tears revealed a disconnected emotional state. Further, when Mary expressed anger toward her father, love for her grandmother, and when she described her sense of hopelessness, she expressed them in a generally detached manner, while she had an uncomfortable laugh. For example, speaking of her father's death: "He died a couple of years later. And I was happy about that. Because he took my bicycle (laughing). I was happy about that, he was awful. Yeah."

Mary identified not being able to express her feelings as one of her current struggles. She said, "I think that's part of my problem today. Carrying all those . . . carrying feelings and emotions that I kept to myself. It still affects me." As a child, Mary kept her feelings inside, but over time, because she had no opportunity for expression, she lost contact with her emotional experience. On several occasions during the interviews, Mary talked about keeping quiet, not saying anything, and further, not feeling anything. She internalized the importance of "keeping quiet" from her mother. Further, when Mary described being unable to cry, she recalled that, as a child, she was afraid that if she cried, her father would physically assault her mother.

Psychosis can be viewed as a state of insecurity. The individual deals with this insecurity and the resulting constant threat by withdrawing to her inner self. As Laing (1960) noted, at that point, the inner self may become detached from the external world. Mary found herself in a bind. Her tears were so powerful that, if they were seen, they might have caused her father to hurt her mother. The powerless parent, helpless to protect her children from an abuser, may actually incite more anger in the children than the abuser does (Herman, 1997; Garland, 1998). For example, Mary described her brothers being upset with their mother for not leaving their abusive father. Mary was severely hurt by her mother and felt the lack of a protective figure in her life. In childhood, she wished she could have had an older brother as a protective figure. However, this wish was multifaceted. Was her wish based on her need to have a protective father-like figure in her life? Or was it to fulfill her mother's contemptuous statement to Mary that she sometimes wished she had a son instead of Mary? Her mother's words affected her deeply:

> I don't know if I'm saying this, saying that because my mother said she always wanted a boy first, instead of a girl. And she used to say that and that used to make me angry . . . It's like . . . I don't want you and I'd rather have a boy instead of a girl. That kind of thing, that's what I used to think.

Later on, as she talked about the fights between her parents, she described a sense of helplessness and passivity associated with keeping quiet. When asked about the feelings, Mary said:

> Oh, the, the way he used to treat my mother. We kept quiet about that. We didn't explain what he did and what have you . . . and, and that—you know that way, everybo . . . we would keep quiet about it. It would be all kept inside, and—and when you think about it, it hurts a bit. It hurts a lot. Yeah. Yeah, but we never really screamed or yelled or anything. When it was going on . . . I think that's part of my problem today. Is that carrying all those . . . carrying feelings and emotions that I kept to myself. Um, it's you know it's, it still affects me. It does.

When asked how keeping everything inside affected her now, she related, "I keep quiet also. Things that should bother me does not bother me . . . let's say if somebody gets, ah, hit or something, um, I wouldn't wince or anything. Just look and just keep quiet about it." The traumatic environment in which Mary felt she could not express her feelings created disconnected memories and established a pattern of dissociation and numbing. Mary's silent stance and inability to remember is a typical response to trauma. For example, she did not remember her grandmother's funeral:

> I was doing one of those, um, blank stares, you know, kind of thing. But then now that you mention it—I don't remember. I just remember going into the church. And . . . seeing lots of people, and then I must have walked away from it because I don't remember going to her funeral. So, I was really upset about that.

Mary related that when she tried to remember her childhood, she could only remember certain aspects; she could not remember the entire narrative.

Growing up in such a stressful situation induced a sense of powerlessness. Mary's feeling of helplessness as a child continued into her teenage and adult years. For example, she assumed a passive role in her relationship with her mother. She felt as though she could not pursue the career she wanted in the arts, and instead, felt compelled to follow her mother's advice. It makes sense, then, that as an adult, when Mary was in the depths of depression, hearing persecutory voices, she did not know how to ask for support. Rather, she silently hoped that somebody would help her. Mary recalled:

> M: I couldn't do it [commit suicide]. No I couldn't do it. Something just made me not do it. I tried. I even tried walking in traffic, and then all of a sudden I would hear this voice, and then I'd pull back. You know, and I was like running up and down the streets saying that I don't want to kill myself. Yeah.
>
> I: So you, a part of you was, like, "no"?
>
> M: That's right. And that little piece of me kept me alive. Yeah. I think . . . I wanted, I need help, I wanted, I wanted help. Yeah.
>
> I: When was the first time you asked for help?
>
> M: I didn't.
>
> I: No?
>
> M: No [shakes head]. I just, um, was hoping that people would help me.
>
> I: Would find out?
>
> M: Ye-yeah. Yeah.
>
> I: So how did they find out?

M: Um, 'cause the things that I would do, I was doing . . . I was banging my head against a grating laying on the floor, and that's when somebody, you know, people came and helped, and they, you know, they j-just, they uh, said that I think she's trying to kill herself or something [nods], yeah.

DEPRESSION AND PSYCHOSIS

As an adult, when Mary realized that her life had not turned out the way she wanted, she fell into deep depression and psychosis. Mary reported that not having a successful life, continuing to live with her mother and not having a place of her own, and not having the kind of job that she sought, were precipitating factors that led to her first psychotic break.

Grotstein suggests that individuals who experience psychosis are "orphans of the real," because they do not have experience with attuned relationships or with symbolization. These are required to create a protective shield against the "horrors that inhere in the world of the 'real'" (Grotstein, 1995, p. 288). Mary stated that during her depression, her mother would tell her, "You don't know what you are doing with your life." Mary said, "The voices sound like my mother, the voices were things she might have said." It would seem that some of those voices echoed years of trauma that had not been worked through. Mary also internalized her mother's harsh, critical tone. She explained that she could be very hard on herself, just like her mother. She reported:

M: She would say something, "You don't know what you're doing with your life." She didn't understand when I was sick.

I: Toughest time for hearing criticism.

M: Yeah.

I: Did she criticize you before that too?

M: Uh, yeah. Yeah.

I: The same kind of things about your goals for the future and why you weren't moving in a particular direction?

M: Yeah. She didn't for a while. Yeah. I don't know, maybe the voices sound like my mother. The voices were just, things she might have said. Yeah.

Mary related that currently she hears only one voice, which she believed was her own critical voice. It appeared, however, that this was an internalization of her mother's critical voice. Mary talked about feeling resentful toward her mother, sacrificing her desires to become what her mother expected:

> I: So can you tell me a little bit about your job? What made you pick business administration?
>
> M: Oh, it was my mother [laughing]. My mother had visions for all of us of what we should do. And, um, yeah, my mother controlled a lot about our lives. She wanted . . . the only thing she wanted me to do was to become a secretary and work in an office. And she kept saying that, you know, and I used to try to tell her this: "there's a lot more, uh, things to be done, you just . . . " she said, "No, you just go and everything will be fine, you should . . . you'll get your degree and . . . " [laughs] what have you. So then she sent me to . . . to another all-girl college, [City], and so. And then she expected me to have a job, doing business, doing business in an office. And that came, and after a while, I said this is not what I wanted. This is what my mother wanted. And . . . and I just thought about it and I just kept on going with it, all the time hating all the jobs that I had, basically. 'Cause I wanted to do what I wanted to do. I wanted to do performing arts, you know.

Mary really wanted to become an actress and singer and she talked about her experience acting at a local theater. The way she described this contrasted starkly with the sense of lifelessness she felt during her depression:

> At this this old theater called [———], and we put on . . . me and my brother, produced the play and so he wrote me in as one of the lead characters [laughs] . . . He said I did well and stuff. It was fun . . . I just remember the feeling that I got when I stepped on the stage . . . I just felt like all of a the sudden, like my heart opened up you know. And . . . and I started talking and I said, I can't believe it, I'm actually doing it. It was fun. Yeah. Well, it's fun when you produce the play yourself [laughs].

Mary internalized her mother's comment that she could not do other jobs and that she was destined to work in an office as a business administrator. She spoke of her growing resentment toward her mother:

> I: When she had you go to college for Business Administration, how was your schoolwork?
>
> M: Oh, it was pretty good. It was pretty good, but at that time I was really feeling resentment against my mother. And I sort of, like, retaliated by not doing as well as I could have done. You know. My whole life when I was younger, um, it always seemed like I was just doing things just to be

> doing things or doing things just for my mother. And the real me was hidden inside. And so, our relationship at that point—me and my mother's relationship at that point sort of got strained, became strained. She started saying that, "You're not listening to me [laughing]. You never wanted to do what I always ask you to say, and you can't go outside" [laughing]. So one day I went outside and defied her [laughing]. Yeah. Yeah. So, and then it goes on and on [laughing] you know. Until I realized one day, "Wait a minute, there's a pattern." It was a pattern to what I was doing. Underneath I was just not liking any of my jobs because my mother told me to do it. And I went on for a long while doing it, which was . . . should have been . . . I shouldn't have done that. Yeah. She's domineering.

As Mary spoke about the factors that led her to experience depression, she identified not having a job in which she could pursue her own desires and aspirations as one of those factors:

> M: Yeah, yeah, yeah, and then my life didn't turn out the way I thought it would, so that too.
>
> I: What did you want to turn out to be?
>
> M: Um . . . just . . . maybe work a little bit at a job I love doing, which I could never find . . . and then having my own place, is, and just, you know, doing more things that I like to do. Yeah, and that sort of made me depressed also, 'cause I couldn't seem to get a way into the into the . . . the workforce, to accommodate that need for me, so, so those were, those were depressing things. I think it all just builds up one day, you know.

MAKING SENSE OF HER LIFE NARRATIVE

There were many gaps in Mary's narrative. She appeared disconnected from her emotions. She was unable to manage her inner critic, which included the internalized voice of her critical mother. The schizophrenia diagnosis she was given during her hospitalization gave her an explanatory structure to create some meaning to explain what she had endured. Because Mary felt she did not know how to stop this critical inner voice, she said, "I would like to know which part of the brain it is coming from." Medication helped what she called her "head traumas"; it allowed her to be more focused, helped slow her racing thoughts, and provided some emotional stability. Still, the medication did not help her work through many years' worth of unprocessed traumas.

Although Mary accepted her diagnosis, in some ways, the diagnosis of chronic schizophrenia was not helpful for her and actually made things more difficult. She said, "I thought I was going crazy . . . I saw myself being in a straitjacket . . . The voices would get crazy just thinking that I'm just crazy and I am never gonna get out of the hospital." She continued, "Mental illness is a major handicap, you just feel like a half person or not a person at all." Yet the only model Mary had for constructing meaning of her struggles was embracing her diagnosis, perhaps because that was the only explanation that was offered to her. The demoralization and loss of hope often experienced by those diagnosed with schizophrenia underlines the important role of clinicians in raising hope (Sullivan, 1929). Yet, she was not offered long-term psychotherapy to process her struggles in hospital nor after discharge. On several occasions during the conversations, Mary discussed having a "mental illness." Unfortunately, when a person's struggles are explained only through medicalized diagnosis, it is sometimes difficult to distinguish the diagnosis of "schizophrenia" from the person who is struggling with it. Mary talked about her fear of going crazy, and she felt the stigma of mental illness—both within her family and on a broader social scale. She recalled the derogatory way her family spoke about mental illness:

> Well . . . I'm using crazy in a sense the word, um, like growing up we would say people were crazy. My mother would say something like, a psycho ward. She used to refer to some people. Growing up with that, is like when I say I'm crazy is coming from the way we, the way we used to talk about people who weren't well. So it's . . . it's coming from family, generations of it.

Mary stated that a lot of good had come out of what she called "being sick." For example, she suggested that receiving a diagnosis allowed her to be less hard on herself. However, the diagnosis and the stigma attached to it made her self-conscious. Throughout our conversations, her inner conflict between compassion toward herself and unease about the stigma attached to the idea of mental illness was evident. For example, at many points during the conversations, Mary described the way medication helped her; yet, at other points, she voiced her ambivalence toward medications and said she would sometimes rather not take them: "Some days, some days I don't feel like taking medicines, but I have to get over it very, very quickly." She did not feel that she had the option of not taking her medication, even though at times she thought about stopping.

Similarly, the diagnosis of "schizophrenia" engendered mixed feelings. On the one hand, it allowed her to make meaning of her struggles:

> Yeah, yeah, 'cause it helps me get to the realization that . . . that I'm, you know, that I have a mental illness. I was blocking that out a lot, yeah . . . I

think it will affect my life through my whole lifetime. 'Cause it was really a traumatic experience that I was going through, yeah.

In addition, the implications of the diagnosis were a wake-up call to Mary, reminding her of the need for self-care. She explained:

> Before I got sick, I just used to ignore my feelings . . . and . . . and just . . . just move on to the next thing. Not ever taking any time to think about myself, investigate myself, and what have you. Just everything was . . . just everything was just okay, and [quick laugh and smile]. I'd go to sleep and the next day do . . . it would be better. But sometimes that didn't happen, you know . . . um, yeah . . . I was just thinking. So, after the illness, the major part passed away. The depression went away, and the voices went away. And then that sort of cleared my brain up to start investigating myself. Now, I just look at things a little differently than I used to . . . Um, and then I appreciate life more now. I didn't used to do that [shakes head]. You know, so it can, it came out when I got ill, but, so it's a lot . . . a lot of good came out of it, you know, it's the first time I said that a lot of good came.

At the same time, the diagnosis was frightening for Mary. The aspect of the diagnosis that scared her the most was her belief that it meant she was "crazy":

> Yeah, like I was put into a mental ward. I mean, other than the one I've gone to. I saw myself being in a straitjacket . . . The voices would get crazy just thinking that I'm just crazy and that and I'm never gonna get out the hospital, and I will stay like that a month or two months. Um, just being in fear and nervousness and anxiety.

Even though hearing voices was extremely traumatic for Mary, the diagnosis offered her a narrative framework for what she was experiencing. On the other hand, heavily influenced by the biological/medical model of psychiatry, which she experienced, she attributed her depression to genetics, precluding exploration of how her early experiences caused her psychic difficulties:

> So, it was like, the beginning of a birthday or something that sort of, like, triggered this stuff for happening, and my family does have a history of mental illness. Yeah, yeah, I . . . I never thought that that was wrong with me, but in this particular case, was sort of like a genetic thing, hereditary. So, and my . . . both my brothers had a . . . are schizophrenic, and, I have another brother, he is developmentally disabled. So, and I think I was the last one to get it in the family [smiles]. Yeah.

Although psychiatric treatment provided some explanation and meaning, it came with a cost. Mary's hospitalization helped her survive recurring suicidal ideation, but she said that seeing other patients suffering scared her:

> Just seeing people that you don't know, seeing other mentally ill patients . . . and, you know . . . if you're like that, if I was like that also. So, I think the patients in some of those places, it was . . . it was kind of scary to deal with, yeah.

The possibility that she might hear voices for the rest of her life—the chronic nature of her condition—was disconcerting for her. She also subscribed to society's view of "schizophrenia" as a permanent disability. In order to protect herself from the stigma, Mary did not share her diagnosis with others. However, she could not hide from the stigma, even within her family. Although her mother suffered from hearing voices herself, negative views of mental illness prevailed in her family. Mary also shared that she was mostly treated with medication, which was helpful to quiet the voices, yet, it was not enough to help with depression and the relational difficulties she encountered with her mother and romantic partners.

Mary survived multiple traumatic life events in environments that did not allow her to express her feelings. However, as she got some psychiatric treatment, as she began to work, as she sorted through her desires, and as she felt more confident about herself, Mary wanted to let her story be known to others. In fact, Mary also spoke about her desire to become a peer advocate:

> I like to always share with other people my story, and hear about theirs too, and maybe um, it would be a big help. It would be a big help for me 'cause I, you know, I like hearing other people that may—may have the same problems that I did. It would just give me more, it would give me more of a better understanding of [her struggles].

CONCLUSION

Mary's desire to voice her story and to become a model to others that are struggling the way she has speaks to her need to process and narrate a cohesive life story. Through all these struggles, she was able to complete her education, work, and have romantic relationships, all of which speak to her resilience and strong inner resources. Not surprisingly, one year after the completion of the interviews with Mary, she found a job as a manager in a company, where she was in the position of managing several employees working under her supervision. She became involved in a romantic relationship, and she was in a much different state of being. Mary said she had never talked about all the aspects of her life narrative with someone else before the interviews. Therefore, the interviews were experienced as both heavy and enlightening for her. Mary worked at developing insight, trying to take in the interview, and asking for my feedback and reflections regarding the causes of her difficulties; which again speaks to her desire to make sense of her struggles and her capacity and desire for insight into her life narrative. One wonders about how life would have evolved for Mary and how different it could have been, if she had been able to process her experiences through therapy at a much younger age. If she were to have been offered long-term psychotherapy, she could possibly have processed her trauma, gained an understanding of her complex family dynamics, and made sense of both her experiences and the struggles that were surfacing that led to her hospitalization. This could have saved her needless suffering and allowed her earlier access to a life-altering path.

Chapter Four

Jeff

Lost in Translation

Marilyn Charles, Michael O'Loughlin, and Secil Arac-Orhun

At the time of the interviews, Jeff was seventy-four years old. The interviews afforded an opportunity to reflect back on his experiences with his symptoms and also the mental health systems those symptoms invited into his life. From the beginning of the first interview, Jeff distinguished himself from the diagnostic categories imposed by those systems and also from the people who use the mental health systems. "I don't have psychiatric difficulties," he declared. As we listen to Jeff, a central problem emerges regarding the issue of who is looking and through what lens. He reported systematic, problematic responses from ostensible caregivers to the fact that he hears voices. "The usual response I get is 'do they ever ask you to harm yourself?' or 'do they ever ask you to harm others?' and my answer is always 'no' to both of those." In this way, Jeff highlights his relationship to doctors whose questions are addressed towards their own concerns rather than to him as a person. And yet, he also reported receiving needed supplies from those doctors. We can conjecture that the problem he cannot quite articulate, but becomes further embroiled in, is the gap we encounter repeatedly in his narrative between his desires and discovering a pathway by which those desires might be achieved.

Jeff reported first hearing voices at age thirty-nine but he was never hospitalized until 1990, when "a friend of mine got tired of hearing me say that I was listening to voices and so he brought me down to ______ Hospital one night." Jeff did not seem to blame his friend but also did not endorse his friend's actions. "I was a little resentful but I kept it to myself," he said.

Although he was "a little angry," Jeff recalled, "he was a very good friend and so I just went and stayed for about two months." Jeff's report of the hospital stay itself was benign, "pleasant," he called it. "The people there were very nice and the other people that I was living with."

At the hospital, he received a diagnosis that did not provide a pathway towards relief or assistance but rather named him as outside of the social order. The doctor "said I had a not very severe case of paranoid schizophrenia." Jeff reported that the diagnosis was not helpful to him because "It didn't mean anything to me. I didn't even know why. I vaguely knew what paranoid meant but I didn't know what schizophrenia meant." The medical diagnosis in some ways refused to recognize him as a human being experiencing a certain set of problematic symptoms, which complicated his sense of alienation from others. When asked how he thought people reacted to him, whether they were aware that he had what he termed a "disability," he responded, "I'm aware that if I can't make a living because of my disability, I'm someone different . . . Some people resent it or they don't want to be bothered with me . . . I think that there are people that probably don't want to know me." He spoke of having gone to a Catholic social club "where the idea was that everyone worked. Everyone was eligible for marriage." "But from my disability, my income was very limited. I didn't work like everyone else and I'm not as good as everyone else." Jeff felt excluded because so much of the conversation focused on work. He felt inferior to others and assumed that his relatives were disappointed in him because he was on disability and was "on the dole."

He did have mixed feelings, however, as the diagnosis also excused him from having to do whatever work might be needed in order to rejoin the ranks of those earning a living, a goal that had eluded him both at school and in job placements. Referring to the diagnosis, he said, "That helped me. I mean, before that I didn't know what I was doing in the hospital. And later on, at another point in time, he said 'You can have disability payment if you want it,' so I took it. Eventually when I got out I applied for disability."

I: So, in a sense, like, the diagnosis helped you, because it gave meaning to why you were staying in the hospital?

J: Yes, yes.

I: And it was a kind of economic help?

J: Well, it was more than an economic help, actually. Well, my uncle told me to, who I live with, I lived with my uncle. My uncle told me to apply for disability. He said "take the money," so I took the money.

In this way, Jeff received an accommodation for his struggles but was left with no way of contextualizing his difficulties. Rather, from his perspective, his symptoms appeared insidiously, with no precipitating event that he could recall. The first time he heard voices was in 1979. "I could hardly even hear the voice, it was more like a whisper, and I couldn't make out what they were saying most of the time, but it was just a few words at a time, not like now when they speak to me directly saying whatever they want as long as they want." When asked about the quality of the voices, he replied:

J: Sometimes . . . (leans in) Sometimes they're scary when they use bad language or, or tell off-color stories, something like that, off-color stories. (leans back)

I: Off color?

J: Yes, that means, uh . . . vu, vulgar.

I: Vulgar?

J: Vu- vulgar stories, yeah, yeah, vu, vulgar, vulgar sayings anyway.

I: Do you, do you know, like what- what's happening at those times that . . .?

J: No, I don't, I'm not aware of what's happening at those times.

I: Like, if something specific is going on in your life? You are maybe more stressed out or something like that?

J: No.

I: It just comes out of the blue?

J: Every now and then, yes.

I: Is there like, is there a specific time when the voices talk to you?

J: No.

I: It's just . . .?

J: All the time.

Jeff reported being confused about the voices:

J: I always thought that the voices would be resolved very soon, as soon as someone would tell me what was going on. At first, I didn't even realize that I was hearing voices. I didn't know what was happening. I went to my doctor . . . and I was confident when I went to him that he would tell me what was going on, that there was some sort of a game being played, or that, I thought maybe even he was responsible for them, you know, maybe he, just like a radio, just like having a radio in my head, but he didn't. All he could think of was . . . prescribing pills for me and giving me a needle in my rear end, so nothing was resolved.

J: I'm always expecting them to be resolved but that's going back probably thirty years now and nothing is resolved, so.

When asked if the voices disturbed him, Jeff replied, "Sometimes they disturb me. They prevent me from getting a good night's sleep. I wake up several times during the night usually." Initially, he said that the voices were like overhearing a conversation addressed to someone else. "Later on the voices were aimed completely at me." He described the voices as usually unpleasant or hurtful, and not related to how he is feeling at the time. Sometimes, when the voices were hurtful, he would address them. "Sometimes I say 'be gone, be gone Satan,' or sometimes if I'm hearing something or I'm about to hear something that's unpleasant, I say the name Jesus over and over again." When asked if that helped, he replied, "It helps a little and I give them the message that I don't want to hear what you got to say, you know, or what you're saying is trying to hurt me."

Without a way of contextualizing or managing his symptoms, Jeff reported a downward spiral. He was hospitalized twice in the following two years. "I stayed there about three months each time." Jeff lived with his uncle until the uncle, who was a widower, met another woman and moved in with her. "I became homeless. . . . My uncle gave up his apartment and I couldn't afford the rent myself, so there I was out on the street and one night I just decided, one night I went to the hospital. I didn't go with the intention of admitting myself, but that's what happened when I was there. The person I got in touch with, the person, the doctor who interviewed me said 'do you wish to be admitted?' and I said yeah, that's a good idea, you know, 'cause I was homeless anyway, I had no place to go, so I was admitted a second time."

For Jeff, the hospital had been a place of respite and of companionship, and also of care for his basic needs. "They arranged for me to visit ______ residence when I got out. They didn't release anybody unless they had a housing situation for them, and that's where I live still to this day." Companionship was important to Jeff, as was work. "Life is pretty good," he said. "I can't complain about where I live or coming to Fountain House is something

I enjoy doing also." When asked what he enjoyed about Fountain House, he replied, "I enjoy having something to do and I enjoy the people." Fountain House gave him a place where he could contribute. Speaking of the people in the horticulture department, he said, "They're all wonderful people and so I was glad to work here every day, doing different tasks." He added, "Plus, there's the possibility of getting a job. That's Monday, I think, I'm going for an interview."

Jeff described being invested in working but finding it difficult to sustain employment. "I think the voices had something to do with quitting my jobs." He thought back to those times. "I was not hearing voices all the time. At the beginning, I said, it was very, very slight, just very—I could barely hear the words, and just every now and then I could hear them and it didn't seem to have anything to do with me, actually. That's all I can say." When Secil inquired further, he replied, "Well, it was almost as if it was something I was overhearing, you know, just something I was overhearing." Jeff's reporting of his life seemed factual, without much emotional investment. "I didn't have anything in mind as far as a career," he said. "After I got a job working with the city, I expected to work there for the rest of my life."

Jeff reported first hearing voices at age thirty-two but not being bothered by them, "I like them," he said. He did acknowledge, however, "Sometimes they're scary when they use bad language or tell off-color stories." "I'm not aware of what's happening at those times." By the time that Jeff was first hospitalized, he was forty-six. He could make no links between his life and his symptoms, saying, "My memories are warm and happy." In striking contrast, he reported extreme childhood difficulties, including loss, disruption, and family conflict. Perhaps most notably, his mother died of cancer when he was six. "I was too young to remember. To remember much, you know. I was told she had died and that's it."

> J: Oh, well I grew up in the Bronx on ______ street and my . . . memories are warm and, uh, happy. I grew up with uh . . . three sisters and uh, I have actually two stepsisters and one sister and uh . . . my-my m-mom died when I was six. My father remarried and we were raised . . . we were happy. Uh . . . We were happily so until the time when I was about fifteen when, when I went to live just down the street with my uh uncle and aunt because my stepmother had moved out and uh . . . It was, It was, (inaudible) that was kind of a . . . Well, my stepmother moved out and she took her two daughters and my-my blood sister and I were went to my-my aunt and uncle's house and uh . . . that's all I can remember (inaudible). I finished high school uh, and then I went to ______ for college and graduated from there in 1970.

Jeff's maternal grandfather died the year after his mother's death, and then he lost touch "because all contact was cut off with them, of course, once my father remarried." Jeff had fond memories of his mother's parents, who were originally from another country. "They were love. They were a big part of love, okay? I can't say I remember seeing them many times."

Jeff's father's second marriage took place two years after his mother died, but then his stepmother left and the family was broken up once again. "When my father lost his job, my stepmother had to leave, had to leave and go out and go to work and support her two daughters and that's the way it was." Upon inquiry as to what precipitated his stepmother moving out, we heard more of the story.

I: Okay. And you said your stepmother moved out?

J: Yes. (folds arms)

I: Like, do you remember what precipitated that?

J: That's when my father lost his job. (inaudible)

I: Sorry?

J: He began drinking. That's always a bad combination—drinking and employment. So . . .

I: When did he start drinking?

J: When did he start drinking? He was always a drinking man (smiles) but he, in 1962, I don't remember what started it but he really went on a, he was drinking and stopped but this time he went on for till, for about seven or eight weeks. So he lost his job.

I: He lost his job? Yeah? And then your stepmother left?

J: Yes.

I: So, it should like, how was it at the time?

J: Well, (inaudible) when she left, my sister and I were told to go over to my aunt and uncle's house, which was just down the street, actually. So we did and we lived there happily, over there.

I: It should have been a big change, I guess, moving from your father's house to your uncle's house?

J: (leans forward) Not for me it was a big change. I was always a friend of . . . My aunt and uncle had one son and one daughter and the one son was two years older than I was but he was a good friend. He was always a good friend of mine.

We can see in this interchange the extent to which extended family has been protective for Jeff, both in terms of this aunt and uncle who took him in as a boy, and also the other uncle who took him in later as an adult. Jeff holds on to the good memories of holidays, family vacations, and "just running around in the streets playing ball." When asked if he recalled any sad memories, he denied having any. When pressed to consider whether there had been anything "a little more difficult," he responded, "Sometimes my father would drink. So, sometimes he would drink just for a few days and then there would be a big argument between him and my stepmom." When asked how the drinking affected him, he smiled and replied, "there was nothing I could do about it, you know." In contrast, when asked how the drinking affected his stepmother, he responded:

J: Well . . . I guess drinking always gets down to money.

I: Sorry?

J: Guess drinking always gets down to money. That's what costs money. And then . . . she. . . . It was always a bad thing going by, we were off, we would find him he'd been drinking and he'd be spending money, a lot of money. (Pause) So uh . . . How'd it affect my stepmother? (leans forward) Well, I guess it (taps table with both hands). . . . I guess it broke her heart. I guess I could hear that, hear that. I remember hearing that said a number of times. So . . . (smiling) so I don't have anything more to say about that.

I: How did, how did she say that? She, that it broke her heart?

J: Well . . . she'd say uh, my heart, my heart was broken, it's broken. She might have said it maybe during one of the arguments. A lamp would get knocked over and break and uh, I knew-I knew that. I remember one year we weren't allowed new furniture and uh . . . I can remember during the argument, the cup on the new lamps got broken. (inaudible) break them so, so she, she said, "My heart is broken. I try to have a house nice, a nice house and you kids," and uh, and uh . . . and that's not possible.

Jeff's contact with his father during this period of time was minimal. "I would see my father every now and then but my aunt and uncle weren't friendly towards him and they said he had to get a job." And yet, his father continued to live in the same apartment down the street "for about five years before the landlord finally threw him out, and that's how I saw him occasionally, not often." Jeff reported meeting his father either at the apartment or at "one of the local taverns." He described these meetings as uncomfortable because "I think the attitude was that he had to get a job and that was not easy." For Jeff, however, this was his father, who seems to represent both love and closeness. "I was always very close to my father." When asked what he and his father would talk about he replied, "Well, we'd love one another, that's all. That's pretty much it, you know what I mean? . . . We didn't argue or have anything to argue about, I don't know. I don't know what was on his mind, but . . ."

We discover later in the interview that "back when my mother died, I was living with my aunt and uncle, the same aunt and uncle at the time, because my mother was in the hospital for about a year before she died and uh and after she died, I was still living with my aunt and uncle. I started school there."

I: At what point did you move back in with your father?

J: Well, I, I moved back in with him, not my sister, my sister was at another aunt and uncle's yet, the ones that I haven't mentioned yet. But uh, I moved back in with him because my aunt found herself pregnant and I guess, I never knew, I never could, could answer that question, you know, why did you go back to your father, and I'd say, I'd have to say I don't know. That was something the grown-ups decided. But later on I found out that it was, that she, she found herself pregnant and uh, felt that taking care of me was too much.

I: Mm-hm.

J: So I went to, I moved back with my father and that was a very happy time, most of it, you know?

I: Mm-hm.

J: Well, I just, you know, he was, he was lonely, you know?

I: You could see it in the way that he was? Did he cry? Were there things he said to you?

J: I did see my, I did see my father cry once. I don't know what happened. He got something in the mail. I don't know what happened that made him cry like that but I remember that very much. And so I lived with him for about a year or two after moving out of my aunt and uncle's house.

Jeff spoke of having wanted to please his father, a bartender who was adamant that his son should attend college. He stresses the importance to his father of grades, recalling crying in front of his father once in grammar school "when I had gotten all C's. A lot of C's on my report card. I had never gotten C's before. I had always gotten A's and B's and he was appalled." In retrospect, Jeff was surprised by the grades, although he continued to struggle with grades increasingly over time.

In spite of his bond with his father, Jeff described life at the home of his aunt and uncle as "quite pleasant, really very pleasant there. . . . It was more calmer. Calmer, yes. I remember they would get *Time* magazine and *Life* magazine in the mail each week and that was a big thing, and I enjoyed reading, reading those things. We didn't get that over where I lived." That pleasure in reading also affected his choices during his college years. "My first year I studied business administration but then I switched over to liberal art and studied English." That change occurred in the context of having moved out of the home of his aunt and uncle into one of the houses linked with Opus Dei, a Catholic association. One of the members had told Jeff that liberal arts would give him "a broader education." He struggled in college. "I found it hard to keep up with the readings. . . . I could just barely talk my way through the final exam."

One high point that Jeff recalled was a part-time position on a school newspaper as a copy boy, but he never felt up to standard. Although he knew he was not really very good at it, he enjoyed being part of it. "I wasn't the bright light of the paper. What I did, for one year, I did write pretty much every issues they had, so I did work hard but . . . nothing ever came of that journalism." He thought back fondly on the people he worked with there. "They were all very nice. They were all very, very good people and three of them are working through the [newspaper] today. I enjoy everything on their . . . looking . . . looking at for their, for their biography, for their bylines, and I could see them." When asked if he kept in touch, he responded, "I hadn't, I didn't get, I never got a good job. I took the civil service jobs. They weren't bad paying but I never did get a very good job and that would make me worthy in their eyes, you know, in the eyes of the school newspaper people . . . I mean, I was just another, well, I don't know. Another, another ne'er-do-well."

This deep sense of never having quite come up to standards seemed to haunt Jeff. Although he could recall having had desires and aspirations, he had trouble achieving success in any of his endeavors and seemed to have no expectation of being able to receive assistance in working through the various impasses he encountered in education or work efforts. With no one to help him to think through possible solutions to the challenges he faced, he just needed to move on into an uncertain world. After college, he said, "I needed money in a hurry. I didn't have any money and so I went out and got a job with a publishing company and . . . it was alright . . . the first year of the job at least. I had some wonderful people I was working with and then the second year, it didn't go so well. They shut it down, in fact. They shut it down and I was unemployed . . . for about three months. Then they gave me a callback to come back and start working at a different (inaudible) but doing the same work for different people."

J: I worked there for another year, then I decided to go get a master's certificate in business administration and I got into the course pretty easily and by, once again the work was awfully hard and I didn't do well enough. I got C's and D's and F's and so I had to drop out. I couldn't take the second year.

I: Of master's degree?

J: Right, right. I didn't do well enough the first year, so, and then I lived in a different—a number of different situations. I lived there again in a house of Opus Dei for a year while I was doing my master's degree and after that I moved out. The house of Opus Dei was shut down in [University]. It was a residence in [University]. It was shut down and then I sublet an apartment with a friend of mine from some people who were going (inaudible) for a year and then after that I. . . . Well, that's pretty much it. Why don't you ask me something?

I: Sorry?

J: Why don't you ask me a question or something? I don't know when to stop.

Jeff was most discursive when thinking back over his adult years:

I: You mentioned moving from one place to another?

J: Yes.

I: Like do you remember what it was about? How it affected you?

J: . . .Well, one day this time, I was in touch with my father. He wasn't doing so well. . . . By that time, he was getting his social security pension, so he was living at, actually in the street for a while and . . .

In spite of his father's limits, Jeff recalled him very fondly. Even when his father wound up on the streets, Jeff would see him from time to time. "I would give him one dollar or another. I would find him."

J: One year I decided to, I had this idea in my head that I was going to, that I'd move out to the west and get a better job, and uh, and live out there. So I went to Houston, Texas, and I lived there for a year but there was nothing, nothing pretty much doing, doing for me. I didn't drive. I didn't drive. I didn't have a driver's license and you need that in Texas, in, everywhere. Everywhere there's a car. So I moved back and I . . . lived with my sister for, my biological sister, for four years. She separated from her husband. She hadn't seen him in a while and, well, that was alright and I wasn't working much. I took some civil service tests and I passed the tests and was called. Then I got a job working out in [area], working as an assistant assessor, tax assessor, and then I, like I said, there's nothing, I said last week that the first meeting that I got fired from that job. Well, I knew I was going to get fired but I quit and I couldn't understand, I couldn't give an explanation of why I couldn't get to work on time, why I couldn't get to work on time. And uh, maybe I should have moved to [area]. That's what I should have done, I guess.

I: [area]?

J: Yes, That's where the job was. There was a long, long drive from my sister's house [second area]. Well, not a drive, a long subway ride and after that I lived with my uncle. It's another one, not the same one, another uncle. I lived with him for nine years. And during that time, I applied for another civil service test and I got it. I was appointed. As I said last week . . . I had seen in the newspaper, it read that the Board of Education was offering teacher's jobs to people who aren't teachers if they would just take a course in the summer, in the summer. Take one course and then promise to take three or twelve credits, one three-credit course I had to take and then promise to take three other, three other courses within ten months and I'd be qualified to be a teacher but actually you could qualify to be a teacher after taking this one course, a summer course, and I did take that and I did, did apply at the local community board for, to be a teacher and I was chosen and I was a teacher for about two weeks but then I got called for this other civil service job, which was, which was a case worker, that's someone who does clerical, clerical work in the welfare offices and the shelter system, men's shelter system. So I was in the men's shelter system there and worked. It was a pretty tough, pretty tough job but I liked it and then I just upped and quit, just upped and quit. I don't know why I did that but I did because there's no other job for me on the horizon, you know.

I: You said because there was no other job for you in the horizon?

J: Yes. There was no, so that's why . . .

I: (interrupting) Is that why you quit?

J: No, I don't understand why I quit but I needed a job, you know, but after that I, my uncle closed down his house because he was getting very old. He was about eighty and he had taken up with a, with an old lady from the, wherever he had lunch. He stayed at the senior citizens' center around the corner from where he lived. He had met an old lady there . . . she lived right nearby . . . he moved in with her . . . I didn't have a job and I was out of a house. So I think I was homeless for about two weeks and then I, then I admitted myself to [hospital] . . . That was the second time I was in [hospital].

In spite of his repeated struggles to sustain employment over time, we see Jeff still longing for work, for a means towards being counted as one of those who matter rather than being relegated to the side. Meaningful employment seems to be the mark for him of a competent, respectable adulthood, something he has longed for but always seems to have been out of reach. Although he seems to have little understanding of how his symptoms affect his ability to work, he noted that before being hospitalized, "I was always looking for a job." After being hospitalized and being put on disability, things changed.

J: Uh . . . After that, I, I, after that, after that I was, uh, on disability, I didn't have to look for a job anymore.

I: So, how did your life got affected from when you first heard the voices up to the time of your first hospitalization?

J: Didn't, didn't affect it too much. I had a couple of jobs . . . So it didn't affect it too much.

I: You had jobs?

J: Yes, I had jobs. I worked for the city. I worked as an assistant assessor, tax assessor, for the city and I worked as a case worker, also, for the city and for about two weeks I taught school, so I was a substitute teacher for the public school system.

I: And did you like those jobs?

J: Yes, I liked them.

I: And . . . but you didn't continue?

J: No, I didn't. I quit uh, I don't know, I think uh, my voices had something to do with, uh . . . I think the voices had something to do with uh, quitting my jobs.

I: In what way?

J: Well . . . I think they interfered with my uh, with my uh, my ability to do the job. On the one job that I had, working with the city as a tax assessor, all of a sudden I couldn't get to work on time in the morning, no matter how early I left, no matter what I did, I, I couldn't get to work on time and eventually, uh, I had, I had to go before a disciplinary committee. And uh, about two days before I had to go, to go the disciplinary committee, I, I quit, rather than get fired, I thought I'd get fired, so I quit, and uh . . . So I think they interfered, interfered there, uh, uh . . . And uh, I also went uh, I had the job as caseworker working at [another hospital] and uh . . . And uh, there I one day just upped and quit, I called up and told them I was quitting. Uh, I don't think I should've done that, 'cause, 'cause I always needed a job, I always needed a job, and uh, but I did, I, so . . .

I: Do you recall why you quit that job in [second hospital]?

J: No, I, I don't have any good, very good reason, except that the hours were very rough, I was working from four to midnight and uh . . . Working on weekends also, so it, it was a pretty rough job.

I: Yeah, sounds like it was stressful.

J: Yes.

Much like his course in college, we find Jeff with no clear thread that he followed, resulting in various positions as "assistant assessor, tax assessor, for the city and I worked as a case worker, also for the city, and for about two weeks I taught school, so I was a substitute teacher for the public school system." Poignantly, we see in his comment about those with whom he worked on the newspaper that the common thread for Jeff seems to be a lack of worthiness, that he saw others' lack of interest in him as a legitimate casting aside.

We can see in Jeff's recounting of apparently kind and concerned medical personnel, ways in which current medical practice and ethical standards allow practitioners to think in such purely diagnostic terms. They avoid a more engaged encounter with the person who is striving to build a life under difficult circumstances. Such avoidance helps to distance us from the painful poignancy of facing the type of recurrent losses that often accompany chronic struggles such as Jeff's. When we consider Jeff's plight from a social justice perspective, we can consider what values are and are not present in the social structure so as to leave him positioned in this way, and whether these are, indeed, the values we intend to endorse. It is always important to be able to look beyond our intentions to inquire into the effects of our interactions on the other person.

We can also recognize ways in which shame and stigma accompany the diagnosis. When asked what he thinks about the label of mental illness or disability, he replied "Well my friends that I grew up with, if they saw how I was living now, they would say he's not mentally ill . . . I don't feel mentally ill myself . . . I seem pretty healthy. The people at Fountain House all seem pretty healthy." And yet, he acknowledged, "I must admit sometimes I feel ashamed." In spite of his aversion to the label, Jeff said that he felt most ashamed when he is "with a group of people who are not mentally ill. I get along with them. It's still a tough thing to say that I don't work, that I'm on mental disability." Jeff's intellectual capacities are apparent, which adds to the poignancy of his dilemma. His biggest regret seems to be not having been able to work for a living at something that was satisfying. "I wanted to get a job and work for money."

Although his diagnosis allows Jeff to sustain his life, providing for basic survival needs, those provisions do not address his need to feel like a competent, autonomous, related adult, nor do they afford him the type of insight that might help to answer the questions he has learned to gloss over. This is the type of epistemic injustice (Fricker, 2007) that can hide behind ostensible "care" when we fail to sufficiently recognize that failures in living can to some extent be ameliorated by providing information and supportive interventions. From this perspective, we can see that Fountain House recognizes Jeff's need, as an adult, to be able to sustain collegial relationships and to achieve some success in working even though he still cannot seem to break through the barrier of obtaining or sustaining gainful employment. Although Jeff can tell us that he has been happiest when he has been part of a caring community, his childhood seemed to teach him to accept what is offered and not to make demands. We hear that thread of making the best of what is offered running throughout his narrative.

In her book *Ethical Loneliness*, Jill Stauffer (2015) talks about the difficulty that is faced when a person needs help but cannot expect it. In the search for truth, as Levinas (1998) suggests, it matters what is shown and who is looking. Stauffer says that "something exists; its existence is intelligible, a truth, a given. And yet we still have questions about it. Such questions assume an interlocutor, someone who listens and responds and, in doing so, helps to confirm both the reality of the world and standards of shared living . . . Questions and their assumed interlocutors thus open up a whole world beyond curiosity and research, leading us fairly directly to conditions necessary for human beings inhabiting a shared world" (p. 16). If we allow ourselves to stand in the position of interlocutor in relation to Jeff's narrative, we are invited to imagine how we might register and confirm his truths in ways that open up further possibilities. Such imaginings may help Jeff's story to have ramifications for others whose lives we touch.

We hear in Jeff's narrative his pleasure at being part of a household in which participants engaged in learning more about the world in which they lived. Those early experiences in the home of his aunt and uncle taught him something about the pleasure in having an intellectual community, something he seemed to be seeking in the school newspaper position and also through his friend at Opus Dei. For Stauffer, this capacity to engage in intellectual pursuits is a communal endeavor, "what feels like intellectual solitude to a free person is already a form of community; research takes form as a question, and a question addresses itself to others. That is an existential as much as an ethical truth" (p. 17). Notably, Jeff found the interviewer's questions difficult to engage with, and yet, precisely at the point where he became most free in his speech, he stopped himself to ask for the question that would help him know what he *should* be saying from the other person's perspective. At that point in the narrative, his voice becomes truncated and his response seems to trail off into an abyss of silence. In that silence, we can perhaps feel most poignantly the weight of his wasted potential.

"Ethical loneliness begins when a human being, because of abuse or neglect, has been refused the human relation necessary for self-formation and thus is unable to take on the present moment freely," Stauffer tells us (p. 26). In Jeff's story, we find precisely such loneliness, as we see him both thriving in relationship—speaking more freely over the course of the three interviews—but also certain that knowledge is the possession of the other rather than himself. As we consider Jeff's plight, we can consider the distinction between wrongs versus harms, and recognize that, although prospective caregivers were not necessarily doing anything "wrong," they were, indeed, causing harm in the sense of not taking seriously enough and addressing more actively his developmental needs.

Jeff talked about his initial hospitalization in very bland terms, saying "it was a very pleasant place" though "I can't say it was helpful for me." This statement should be taken very seriously. How do we think about a mental health system that is pleasant but not helpful? Would such a system not further the problems rather than helping the individual learn how to more adaptively address them? What does repair mean when the harm is epistemic, in relation to the meanings ascribed to one's mind, actions and life, by people embedded in a social structure that has too much power in relation to that person? This type of problem cannot be resolved by adjudication but rather by illumination. To meet the challenge, Jeff's narrative suggests, we must be able to meet the individual, trying to make the person's perspective more visible, so that it might have an impact as a legitimate frame of reference, to be seriously considered in any deliberation.

Stauffer's work suggests that censoring oneself is a privilege afforded to those who have a valued place within the social structure. For those who do not, it may be more correct to say that one is censored by the various systems that circumscribe meanings and therefore the possibility of a speech that might be more fully one's own. In the story of Jeff and in the other narratives recounted in this volume, it will be useful to the reader to look for ways in which the speech of the individual subject has been censored or circumscribed, and what meaning we might therefore make of what is being offered, both in terms of what it directly signifies and also in terms of what it indirectly points to that is absent.

Both psychoanalysis (Lacan, 1978) and philosophy (Levinas, 1998) point towards a truth that is revealed rather than spoken. From that perspective, there is a truth that can become manifest even though it cannot be directly spoken. This would seem, in part, to be part of the puzzle of people's relationships to God or to Truth, with a capital T. How are we defined by and how do we determine meanings in relation to what is absent from our awareness and yet implicated in some way through what is presented? We do tribute to the gift offered by those who shared with us their life experiences in listening deeply to their stories; those who have struggled to find their way and who therefore have something important to say to us both about how such struggles evolve and also how they are helped or hindered by social forces and mental health systems.

Chapter Five

Dylan

Escape Artist

Montana Queler and Michael O'Loughlin

Dylan, a twenty-four-year-old African-American male, grew up in a large city in the Northeastern United States. He was the middle of three children, with one older and one younger sister. During the time of the interviews, he lived with his mother and younger sister. His parents divorced when he was about ten, and he continued to live with his mother, visiting his father on weekends. Dylan had some high school education but had not obtained a diploma.

During the interviews, Dylan conveyed a kind of childlike innocence. He spoke with conviction as he disclosed, for example, that dragons were haunting his life. His eager and earnest disposition during the interviews allowed for exploration of the elaborate and illusory features of his subjective reality.

Dylan was the only male and the youngest participant that Montana interviewed. In many respects, he proved to be a more challenging participant to write about because he exhibited salient features of flight from consensual reality. The content of his narrative had a vague and elusive quality to it, and the fantastical construct within which he primarily resided made it more difficult to obtain information that might help elucidate this need for psychic flight. As a result, in our attempt to understand Dylan's life narrative, we struggled to make meaning where integral information was lacking.

DYLAN'S ESCAPE FROM MATERIAL REALITY

Dylan reported that he began hearing voices sometime during childhood or early adolescence. He associated voice hearing with his eventual psychic breakdown:

> I: And what was going on with you before you started coming to the clubhouse?
>
> D: I've been hearing a lot of stuff in my head, at the, at, what happened, when I was out of control.
>
> I: What kind of stuff was going on in your head? What were you hearing?
>
> D: I've been hearing a lot of voices going on, like ghosts, demons, dragons, DVPs.
>
> I: What are DVPs?
>
> D: Dragon virus parasites.
>
> I: Hmm, what does that mean exactly?
>
> D: Well it goes in, it, it goes in your head when, it goes in your body, when, when something's wrong with you, when you're sickness and out of control.
>
> I: When did that first start for you?
>
> D: It was back from 2009.
>
> I: And what was happening around that time?
>
> D: Around that time?
>
> I: Yeah, that's when you started to hear the voices?
>
> D: Mhm.
>
> I: What was happening around that time?
>
> D: It was, it was about 2009, August, when I, when I was hearing a lot of stuff in my head, telling me what to do, destroy this, destroy that.

Dylan began having notable difficulties even as a young child. When asked about what he thought might have caused his voice hearing, Dylan related:

D: It was back from the beginning when I was a kid, they must've saw me, from the sky.

I: What saw you?

D: It was a dragon lord, a dragon lord voice. He was in the Saurian Empire.

I: The what empire?

D: The Saurian Empire, dinosaur empire, it was him from the beginning when I, when I was a kid, when I was a bad kid once.

I: Why do you think you hear voices?

D: I don't know. They just won't leave me alone.

I: Still they won't leave you alone?

D: No.

I: You still hear them?

D: Yes.

I: What do they tell you to do?

D: Just tell me to kill myself and just get rid of it.

I: They still tell you to kill yourself?

D: Yes, and I didn't want to do it, I refused. And they wanted me to kill my mom, too.

I: Mhm . . . That seems painful.

D: It was. It was led by a dragon lord named Lord Jagonis and his um, his general, Blassord, he did this to me. General Blassord did this to me.

I: Why?

D: He wanted me to kill my mother.

I: Why does he want that?

D: He just wants, he just wants me to be a bad guy, but I don't want to, so I refused.

Later during the interview, Dylan reported that he no longer heard the "bad" voices, but continued to hear more benevolent ones:

I: How do you feel about the voices having gone away?

D: I never seen them again, even I met the good voices that'll help me take my medicine every day, and never talk to nobody, just say hello.

I: The good voices?

D: Yes.

I: Those went away also?

D: They didn't go away, they helped me.

I: They help you, so there were some good voices?

D: They want me to take my medication every day and they want me to go to, go to Fountain House without any trouble, without problems, and they want me to, uh, move around here one day without fail.

I: So some of the good voices are left, were the good voices there before?

D: Yes, they were, yeah they were.

I: So there were good voices and bad voices, so now the bad voices have gone away and the good voices are still there?

D: Yes.

I: Do the voices sound like anybody that you know?

D: My old friend, Cyber 24.

I: What's his or her name?

D: That's his name, Cyber 24.

I: What's the 24 for, what does that mean?

D: It's a version, he's like a, uh, a robot.

I: Oh . . .

D: Yes . . . He use, he used to be part of the Hunter Force 3, I used to draw a picture of him, and then, uh, yeah he's a good friend. He also runs in my head, he also tells me to just go to bed, take my medication, wash the dishes, make dinner. He's a good friend, he's been helping me. I hear him in telepathy, though.

I: What do you mean?

D: Without, without speaking I can hear him in telepathy, he's very invisible but I can hear him.

I: You can hear him just inside your head?

D: Yes, I can't use my mouth. I can use my head by speaking to him.

I: How do you feel about still having the good voices?

D: Cyber 24?

I: Mhm . . .

D: He's still my friend, he helps me around the house, even when, even this week he wants me to clean up my . . . my messy room and, and be, become clean.

I: So the good voices, sort of, help you throughout the day and they're also protective of you?

D: Yes, they are, the bad voice who got me into this was uh, was a CO, my former CO. My former CO in my head was a bad voice, I got rid of him, he set me up, and he also was, and he also does everything to me.

I: Like what?

D: Like destroying things in my room, when I was uh, you know, doing my work, checking my, my, my, my messages. His name is uh, General Ice Feather. After he was uh, out of my head, I banished him for good, so Cyber 24 and I work together, so I could uh, you know, change my life, he just, he just told me no, not to talk to General Ice Feather no more, he wanted me to talk to his son, Colonel Davis Ice Feather, he wanted me to go to jail for him, he told me not to change my (inaudible) light between his, his father and Cyber 24.

These kinds of exchanges were common over the course of the interviews. Dylan's interpersonal life appeared to be populated primarily by video game and superhero characters, so much so that they seemingly substituted for a social life in the material world. Looking back over our conversations, Dylan spoke only briefly about people from the relational world of school and his neighborhood that he considered friends. Meanwhile, the majority of his stories involved characters from comic books and video games, such as those in the above excerpts.

Asked about his goals for the future, Dylan's response was similarly rooted in fantasy:

D: I have plans. I'm joining the King's musketeers.

I: What does that mean?

D: I did it on Facebook, that, after I start I, I just want to be a musketeer, a leader—

I: A musketeer's a leader?

D: [Pointing to his shirt] Yes, and lately, I just uh, wear a royal blue shirt.

I: Oh, is that what your shirt signifies?

D: Yes, it's the cross. It's a cross that the King's musketeers . . . it's in France and New York City.

I: And what does it mean to be a musketeer? What kind of leader do you become?

D: A hero, an officer.

I: And what kind of work does that mean then?

D: So, I protect people, like the police do, when there's trouble, I just call my police friends, say there's trouble, neighborhood watch in [City].

I: What inspired you to do this work?

D: When I was a kid I used to watch cartoons, when I was a kid . . . I wanted to become neighborhood watch with the musketeers.

> I: Did you know other people who were protectors like musketeers growing up?
>
> D: Like D'Artagnan, Athos, Porthos, and Aramis . . . Yes.
>
> I: Were there people in your everyday life who you felt were protective like those characters?
>
> D: Yeah, it's like the Ninja Turtles, Superman, Batman, the Avengers, Captain America, Thor, Ironman, all the, all those characters that I loved when I was a kid, and even MegaMan X.

Later in the conversation, Dylan commented on his desire to join the military: "I just want to be proud of myself, when I, when I'm getting um, you know, killed or something, I just want to you know, serve my country." This assertion captured Dylan's positioning between two worlds. Much like his use of real-world comic book and video game heroes to construct his fantasy life, Dylan's statement about joining the military carried a semblance of material reality, even while his ideas about giving his life to service felt largely embedded in fantasy.

The presence of Dylan's voices, and his division of them between "good" and "bad," can be interpreted as splitting and projection which serve as a means of managing anxiety and intolerable affects. From this perspective, the containing function of an attuned caregiver is what allows the child to develop the capacity for integrating good and bad feelings; without it, negative affects can become too powerful, leading to a projection out in an effort to preserve that which is good. Dylan's struggle to integrate the menagerie of emotions within speaks to possible limitations in his early environment to help him contain negative feelings. Unfortunately a heavy reliance on projection can end up reinforcing the need for an illusory reality, as an ensuing sense of emptiness places limits on a whole range of life experiences—both in the realms of love and work. Dylan's narrative illustrates his struggle to forge a sense of identity where large swaths of self had been expelled beyond reach.

NAVIGATING THE EXTERNAL WORLD

Dylan's interviews revealed significant struggles, both for Dylan and for the institutions charged with his care. Throughout our conversations, Dylan often alluded to having tremendous difficulty modulating his emotions. Lack of attunement and containment in early childhood left Dylan ill-equipped to regulate his own negative feelings. Further, his challenges identifying the boundaries between self and other and between fantasy and reality would have rendered him disoriented, confused, and at times terrified, particularly within the context of his school's social landscape. In turn, there were periods of extreme psychic distress that his school was not prepared to manage. Many times, Dylan's emotional outbursts triggered institutional reactions that inadvertently exacerbated his psychic distress. Dylan recounted multiple incidents from school that illustrated what seemed to become a pattern of mismatched needs and response:

> D: One of the teachers at my school called the police on me and tell them what I was doing is . . . I told them no police, I didn't do nothing, nothing. I had did nothing. The lady called the police, Ms. O called the police on me 'cause she think I was getting wild and one of the police officers came and then tell them what I was doing.
>
> I: And what did she report to the police?
>
> D: She, she, uh, Ms. O thinks that uh, she thinks that I um, was, was wild and crazy . . . And she called the police on me.
>
> I: So she thought you were getting out of control?
>
> D: Yes.
>
> I: Why did the teacher call crisis on you?
>
> D: They, they think I was in trouble, talking to everybody, what I did, they think I was hitting people.
>
> I: They thought that you were hitting people?
>
> D: Yeah and then they called me, I had to get out of there as soon as, quick as possible.
>
> I: Do you remember hitting people?
>
> D: No, I pushed them off the chair and they fell.
>
> I: Why did you push them?
>
> D: Because they were making fun of me.
>
> I: Mmm, so you felt like they were bullying you?
>
> D: Yes.

I: What were they making fun of?

D: They were trying to say my, my name is Special K, Special K they called me and I told them I don't like that name because that's not my name, it's Dylan.

I: Why were they calling you Special K?

D: Don't know, every time they would call me that, I just get upset.

I: So they did it just as a way of kind of taunting you?

D: Yes.

I: Did that happen a lot in school?

D: Yeah, it does.

Dylan later shared another incident that took place at school:

I: When you say you were a bad kid, what does that mean? What kinds of things were you doing?

D: I was cursing, I was, I was yelling, I was, getting out, getting wild.

I: Were you in pain at that point?

D: Yes I was.

I: How come? What were you feeling?

D: I felt I was about to run away, but I refused. I started tearing up my notebook, when I was a kid, I went all crazy and wild, screaming and yelling, I ripped out my notebook, I got all the paper I ripped out, when I was a kid, they took pictures of me, they showed them to my mother, I was very upset about that.

I: The teachers took pictures of you?

D: Yes.

I: It sounds like you were scared at the time?

D: I was.

I: What were you afraid of?

D: I was afraid of dragons and dinosaurs . . . I was afraid of those teachers, they would put me into a hospital, they were trying to call the police on me, they thought I was out of control, and I told them not to do that, 'cause I'm too old for that, going to jail like this (looks down). I will never, I will never forgive them for that, for what they did to me.

I: The teachers didn't understand that you were scared.

D: Yes . . . I felt all alone, too, Montana (looks up), I did have a few friends but they trying to make fun of me (looks down).

As these exchanges suggest, Dylan's inability to conform to the reality-based expectations of his school generated conflict with his teachers as well as with his peers. From his account, it seemed his academic environment was ill-equipped to respond to his difficulties and that the school lacked appropriate resources—in a Winnicottian sense, containing and holding spaces—that would have provided psychological support. At the same time, Dylan's powerlessness to better regulate his emotional tidal waves must have stoked frustration and also fear in those witnessing his outbursts. Unfortunately, this resulted in responses that further exacerbated Dylan's own terror.

There is evidence that Dylan's atypicality emerged early on. He recounted being in the third or fourth grade and already feeling ostracized by the other children:

I: What were people teasing you about then, do you know?

D: They called me idiot, they call me jerk, all the time.

I: Do you know why they said that to you?

D: That wasn't funny.

I: No, I'm sure that it was extremely hurtful.

D: It was.

I: And nobody should have ever said that to you.

D: Yeah, I know.

I: How did you understand why they were saying that to you?

D: Don't know.

I: Did you think that it was true? Did you start to believe what they were saying was true?

D: No, they just trying to make fun of me, that's all.

From Montana's experiences with Dylan, it was not difficult to imagine him standing out among his peers. His sensitivity, intensity of affect, and immersion in an illusory reality would have made him an easy target for teasing and ridicule. Fromm-Reichmann (1959) noted that in the need for emotional intimacy, the lonely child might find fulfillment in fantasy. She observed that this could ultimately reinforce isolation, as the ability to distinguish between reality and fantasy would not fully develop. As Fromm-Reichmann suggested, this can turn into a self-perpetuating cycle in which the need to escape from others' judgments engenders further withdrawal into isolation, further driving the need for fantasy and entrenching disconnection and isolation. Dylan's tethering to consensual reality was seriously compromised from early on; in consequence, the fabric of his social life never fully developed.

Dylan's struggle to adapt to his environment ultimately culminated in his hospitalization. He alluded to multiple occasions in which his inability to contain his distress resulted in inpatient stays:

D: I went, I went to the hospital a lot of times when I was out of control.

I: What was happening? What do you mean when you say you were out of control?

D: I was totally freaked out. They uh, they, they tried to cuff me, in handcuffs, tie me on to the gurney when I was out of control, they gave me some, some medication to calm me down when I was out of control, my anger and my rage, yes.

While in the hospital, Dylan had encounters that left him feeling similarly misunderstood:

I: What happened while you were in the hospital? What was that experience like?

D: I had to spend fourteen days over there.

I: And what did you do while you were there?

D: I was . . . I was sleeping all day and just talk to my doctor.

I: What was your doctor like?

D: Dr. S, that's her name.

I: And how did she treat you?

D: When I was bad and I was walking around the floor and sleeping there, I couldn't control it.

I: What couldn't you control?

D: My anger.

I: You were angry while you were in the hospital?

D: Yes.

I: What were you angry about?

D: I just want to go back. I just want to get out of here.

I: You wanted to get out of the hospital?

D: Yes.

I: How did it feel to be there?

D: It was very bad.

I: Could you tell me a little more about that?

D: Yes, I could tell you. I been there for fourteen days and I couldn't get out of there. When, when the door opened, I escaped and I was trying to get to the elevator. I went to a closet and I locked myself in until somebody comes and you know . . .

I: And found you?

D: Yeah.

I: How come you were trying to escape?

D: I just want to get out of here . . . One of the patients tried to, tried to touch me, when I was leaving.

I: Tried to touch you inappropriately?

D: Yes.

I: Huh. And did you tell anybody, any of the staff about it?

D: No, they didn't help me.

I: They knew but they didn't help you?

D: No.

I: Who did you try to talk to about it?

D: Talked to the, to the nurse and they, they said, "I can't help you, Dylan. I'm sorry." I was tied to the bed. They tied me with those strings, those ropes, but I got out of them with one hand.

I: Do you remember how long you were tied to the bed for?

D: For, for an hour.

I: For an hour?

D: Yes.

I: Did it happen often or just once?

D: Twice.

I: What was that experience like for you? How did that feel?

D: It was bad and upsetting.

Within this account, Dylan's suffering was apparent. Unable to connect with the people around him, he found himself very much alone and isolated within his psychic reality.

THE REVOLVING DOOR OF PSYCHIATRIC HOSPITALIZATION

Dylan described his first psychiatric hospitalization, which might have been around the age of seventeen, possibly earlier, and the sequelae of being started on neuroleptics:

D: It was back from 2006, January. I was in [Hospital] for fourteen days.

I: And what was the reason that you were in the hospital?

D: I was out of control.

I: Do you remember what you were diagnosed with?

D: Psychological voices, and stuff. I was there for fourteen days, and they made me, made me bloat my body like this.

I: The medications?

D: The Depakote, made my, my body gain weight, like this. I couldn't get out of it. I took those pills like fourteen times. And I couldn't stop taking it.

I: So you're still taking Depakote?

D: I stopped.

I: You stopped taking it?

D: Yes, 'cause it made me gain weight like this, after what happened. And I started, I started eating like a, like a dragon heir all the time.

I: So, you were able to switch your medication to something else or you're not taking medication at this point?

D: I am taking medication, at my house. I only take the four pills in the morning, the Haldol and the other pills, and I only take the Seroquel at nighttime and the Haldol.

I: But once you took the Depakote, it caused you to gain weight and you haven't been able to lose it?

D: No.

I: Has that been uncomfortable?

D: That was very uncomfortable. But I lost, uh, I lost a lot of weight and I, and I gained the weight back again, I'm going to try it again. I don't take the Seroquel no more, but I only take the Geodon, but I stopped taking that because I was, keep vomiting and vomiting although, um, in the bathroom.

I: So it made you sick?

D: I thought, yeah, it did, it made my, my stomach churn and it was upset, upsetting me.

Dylan's experience is not an uncommon one. An induction into the mental health system through hospitalization inevitably includes the initiation of psychotropic medication, and for psychosis, neuroleptics are the standard of care. While these medications arguably have their benefits, many also carry the risk of physiological harm (Breggin, 1991; Whitaker, 2001), significant weight gain being one common side effect. Dylan's psychic distress was alarming, however, and despite the potential risks, medication is thought to provide the most expedient form of relief. Dylan's account of his initial experience with medication reflects a downside of this kind of intervention, especially if not accompanied by psychosocial support and/or therapy:

D: They gave me Depakote because I got like this.

I: You mean it caused you to gain weight?

D: Yes, it made me like this. That's what happened.

I: Did it have any helpful benefits? Did the medication help you in any way?

D: No, it didn't help me. It just made me gain weight by eating a lot of food.

Even after his medications were changed, Dylan was prone to mood dysregulation, and his ability to function in the world remained significantly compromised. Sometime between the second and third interviews, Dylan returned to the hospital, this time reportedly for five weeks:

D: I been back to the hospital back in um June, June nineteenth.

I: This summer?

D: Yes.

I: How come you were in the hospital again?

D: I was still upset but um . . . I, I got the new medicine. It's called Lithium . . . Lithium, Haldol, and Propranolol.

Dylan's many hospitalizations reflects both the severity of his suffering as well as the mental health system's limited capacity to respond to it. His need to return to the hospital resulted from his persisting struggle to negotiate the chaos of his internal reality, particularly within the context of an already complex external world. His multiple stays on inpatient units represents what many others with similar vulnerabilities endure, as hospitals provide limited opportunity to access the kind of sustained support and holding that such vulnerabilities warrant.

GOOD VERSUS EVIL, AND THE HEROICS OF FORGING AN IDENTITY

Dylan's immersion in his fantasy-scape posed a challenge in our inquiry about the potential origins of his difficulties. His ability to access or articulate his early life was restricted. He mentioned his family infrequently and when prompted, only disclosed snippets of information about them. For example, during the first interview Dylan reported that he lived with his mother and younger sister. He stated that his parents had divorced when he was ten years old and that he had not seen his father "in a long time."

The couple of instances in which Dylan elaborated on his experiences with family were emotionally evocative and painful for him. For example, in the following exchange, Dylan's comments about his voice hearing quickly transitioned into anger toward his mother:

I: Have you ever been angry with your mom?

D: Yes, I have.

I: What have you been angry with her about?

D: She keeps telling me to stop, go, go to work, go to work, I didn't want, I don't want nothing to happen.

When asked about what he feared might happen, Dylan spoke of his grief over the loss of his beloved aunt:

I: What does that mean you didn't want anything to happen?

D: I don't want nothing to happen to my mother or my family.

I: Why would anything happen to your mother or your family?

D: Yes.

I: How come? Why would you think that anything would happen to them?

D: Just don't want to, I just don't want them, I don't want to lose them like I lost my, my, my Aunt Olivia.

I: Your aunt?

D: She, she died from cancer back from 2003.

I: So, about ten years ago?

D: Yes, it was.

I: Were you close with her?

D: Yes, when I was young, uh, she, she put me to sleep, we had, my cousin and I had fun together, she also gives me something to drink when I went to sleep, yeah.

I: It sounds like you really miss her.

D: Yeah, I did, but now she's gone and there's nothing that I can do. I won't see her for a long time.

Brought back to his anger toward his mother, Dylan responded:

I: But sometimes your mom talking about you going to work makes you angry?

D: Uh, yes.

I: How come?

D: She just, she wants me to move out of here for good and I told her, "I gotta pay money for that, for the apartment, money and everything, I gotta pay for." And she said, "I don't care, the, the people at um, Fountain House will pay for it for you." That's my mom, but I told her, "I gotta pay money for that."

These three excerpts offer hints of Dylan's fear of his own anger, in this case, toward his mother. The struggle to contain his anger can be interpreted both in the split represented by "General Blassord"—who might be seen as holding Dylan's destructive impulses—and in his deflection to a more tolerable emotion, sadness. The above exchanges might suggest one role that voices have played in Dylan's psyche, allowing him to split off and project out the thoughts and feelings he could not tolerate within himself.

The themes of being "out of control" and feeling both endangered and dangerous surfaced repeatedly throughout Dylan's interviews. His belief in the threat of dragons, demons, and ghosts suggests an attempt to symbolize the source of his felt danger. It is not uncommon for children's experience of vulnerability to crystallize in a villainous archetype. These characters are the stuff of children's books and fairy tales, as well as adult horror and fantasy genres. However, as children develop into adolescents and eventually into adults, the primal terror these figures evoke usually dissipates and is replaced by better-articulated responses to a more nuanced and abstract conception of the world and an integrated sense of self. Dylan's belief in literal monsters seems indicative of a need to externalize that he never outgrew. While this massive evacuation of internal "badness" allowed him to distance himself from his own destructive impulses, it also rendered him vulnerable to feeling out of control and at the mercy of external danger.

As a counterforce, superheroes symbolize Dylan's attempt to find refuge from these destructive forces. The presence of characters like MegaManX, the Musketeers, and Cyber 24 in Dylan's internal life reveal a desire to be rescued from inescapable threat. His stated goal to become a musketeer further captured his desire to be "good," to have control and feel empowered in this role as a force of good in the world.

Given the paucity of information about Dylan's early childhood, it is impossible to pinpoint any specific traumas as the context or precipitating events that might account for his flight into fantasy. It is possible, however, to draw inferences about potential aspects of his early development based upon his narrative. Dylan's expressed anger toward his mother, his apparently absent father, and his persecutory fears, rescue fantasies, and emotion dysregulation suggest difficulties early on. His flight into a world of fantasy indicates a need for protection from some unbearably painful aspect of his past.

From an object-relations perspective, Dylan's emotion dysregulation speaks to a failure of maternal function, particularly in relation to the essential provisions of soothing, mirroring, and containment. Dylan's struggle to translate his emotional experiences into words—illustrated by his recounted moments of explosive acting out—suggests a significant deficit in his ability to mentalize, a developmental achievement made possible by a caregiver's capacity to metabolize their child's negative feelings and return them in tolerable form. This is consistent with Fromm-Reichmann's (1954) assertion that early emotional deprivation sets the stage for a regressive preoccupation with the self's "badness" and fear of uncontainable aggression.

Dylan's need to reside in a world of fantasy suggests early environmental deficits in the arena of interpersonal safety. Both Sullivan (1956) and Fromm-Reichmann (1954) wrote about the drastic measures that a child's psyche might take to establish a sense of security, including sacrificing all other personal and interpersonal needs beyond this. The resulting loneliness can set the foundation for the construction of an elaborate fantasy in order to fulfill unmet intimacy needs. Dylan's immersion in a world of dragons and superheroes is an example of this kind of prosthetic use of fantasy to meet the essential need for relationships. While not all of the figures of Dylan's intrapsychic life nurture good or positive feelings, many others prove their loyalty through their protection of him from evil. Moreover, there is utility in the externalizing symbolization of that which is painful or taboo, accomplished through the villainous personas in Dylan's internal landscape. For one, projecting the bad or unwanted parts of the self allows for the preservation of that which is good. And secondly, there exists some degree of control over that which is wholly fantastical. As Dylan remarked regarding one such villainous character, "I got rid of him . . . I banished him for good."

Lacan's structural model also helps to elucidate aspects of Dylan's difficulties. From a Lacanian perspective, insufficient mirroring would have left Dylan vulnerable to the foreclosure of the paternal metaphor, barring his entrance into the Symbolic (Vanheule, 2014). This lack at the level of the Symbolic can be seen in Dylan's struggle to translate his experiences and sense of identity into words. For Lacan, what results from this foreclosure is an inability to move beyond an egocentric, concrete worldview in which the person imagines him or herself to be the central focal point and motivating force of the other. For Lacan, this foreclosure also denotes a deficit in a person's capacity to respond to questions about his or her own existence—including aspects of identity such as gender, sexuality, and life purpose. Dylan's narrative brings Lacan's idea of the stabilizing delusional structure (Vanheule, 2014, p. 121) to life. Dylan appeared to rely on his fantasy world to anchor his sense of himself in spite of the apparent gap in his self-concept. From this perspective, Dylan's fantasy-scape would provide him with a sense of self and life purpose that he could not construct for himself in the relational world.

During the conversations, Montana experienced Dylan as carrying a persistent yearning for recognition. At the end of the final interview, Dylan stated, "I'm just going to change my life and then see a girl and then meet her, take her on a date and then I'll marry her one day . . . the perfect girl . . . someone like you." After spending three hours together, Dylan had developed a positive transference. He had been deeply engaged throughout the interviews. While he struggled to put his life story into words, the intensity of his affect and his strong eye contact conveyed a desire to be seen and recognized. A prolonged narrative engagement in individual and/or group psychotherapy would probably be needed to help Dylan explore his fantasies so that he could understand their function and so that he could begin to develop an integrated sense of identity. His openness and apparent desire to be understood would certainly lend themselves to this kind of ongoing work.

Chapter Six

Terry

Holding On

Veronica Ozog, Michael O'Loughlin,
and Secil Arac-Orhun

Terry is an Afro-Caribbean woman in her early twenties. She was raised in the Caribbean and brought to the United States when she was eleven years old. The interviews offer a glimpse into the life of a young woman struggling to formulate her identity in a new country, with the added hardship of psychic distress. Although she said others view her as being of African descent, referring to her as "black," she said that she views herself as alienated from African-American culture to the extent that she has come to view herself as "Caucasian," describing herself as a white woman with light skin. Secil explored the meaning of this and other identity questions in three interviews that often challenged Terry's ability to structure her narrative. She approached each interview with a pleasant, yet distant stance, rarely showing emotion. Further, she struggled to share her thoughts and experiences. It seemed she had not yet had the opportunity to process her life and her confusion was at times palpable as she spoke in circles and tangents in an attempt to understand herself and to be understood by Secil. What emerged from their discussion was Terry's effort to understand her place in a world that she experienced as harsh and rejecting, as well as her tremendous and moving desire to find a place to belong.

MIGRATION

Born on a small island in the Caribbean to a close-knit family, Terry shared fond memories of her childhood, swimming in the ocean, going to theme parks, attending school, and spending time with her mother in the city during the school year, and with her father in the countryside in the summertime: "I had a good time when I was younger in the Caribbean," she stated, "but by the age of eleven, I was already going to be moving to America."

Terry's mother decided to move to the United States, bringing Terry with her, to join other family members already living in the United States, including Terry's grandmother:

> I: Do you remember how your family or you decided that you were going to move? Why did your family move?
>
> T: Well, my mom, uh, wanted to move because, uh, her family lives in America and they really wanted to spend some time with us and to let us live in America.

Although her mother and father were divorced, Terry described their relationship as civil, and the move did not prevent Terry from seeing both of her parents. Each June, Terry's mother accompanied Terry to her country of origin so that she could still spend her summers with her father, who would then accompany Terry back to the United States in August:

> T: I was living there and, uh . . . I usually would go, I had to go to school so they had to help me go to school and, um, after school, when school was out I would usually, uh, visit my [country of origin] again so I would have to come back on time to go back to school from the Caribbean to America, America to Caribbean, so I could still spend time with my mom and my dad.
>
> I: So, uh, your father stayed in the Caribbean or he moved with you to America too?
>
> T: Well, he stayed in the Caribbean. Just that when he had to carry me back to America to go back to school. He would usually, uh, get picked up by the airport and carry me straight home and then he would probably leave on his way to the next site back, uh, because he . . . right back to the Caribbean because he was living with, uh, they were, uh, they were together my mom and dad but they . . .
>
> I: They were together, you said?
>
> T: Yeah.
>
> I: So, they weren't divorced?

T: They, they were practically divorced by then by the time I was going to be eleven. By yeah, because I was really young and, uh, he was with, he hadn't had any wife. My mom was pretty much single so I, he would just bring me back to go to school and, uh, he would stay at the house for some time until it's time for him to go, to go get the next plane back to the Caribbean. Yup and um . . . well my mom actually would, uh, carry me to the Caribbean to meet my dad. I had to stay there and then go right back to America so I pretty much, when I was eleven I moved to, to America. I still had a lot of time to spend, time with my mother and father anyway, as I went to school and spent the vacation in the Caribbean. Yup.

Terry emphasized her delight in being able to spend time with both of her parents, as well as her siblings and extended family in the United States. When asked by Secil how she felt about moving to the United States, she shared:

T: It was nice because I . . . because I had a lot of family.

I: Mm-hm.

T: Uh, and I wasn't very, it didn't seem to be, um, like a handful or, uh, it was, it was just like being in the Caribbean. It was like you know I had a mixture of all the Caucasian and even African. So, I was just like practically having a very good time all the time, hanging out with my grandmother. I pretty much was, uh, very happy having a good time. I didn't have to miss anyone anywhere. I was just very happy 24/7 practically like having a good time, you know, like I would play sports, I would swim a lot in the Caribbean. I was playing a lot of sports in, uh, in America, in America because, uh, I used to go to the park and hang out.

Beyond her life at home, Terry described an enjoyable, active lifestyle in the United States:

I always liked playing sports in America. My like, my extra time from school after homework and even at school because I don't have any homework and I was pretty much going to the beach a lot in the Caribbean. I was having a good time. I was like practically like hyped about my good life and very active you know like, like practicing sports and I'll go to the school gym be in the school gym like play volleyball and stuff and like having a good time at the school play and everything. So, I was ecstatic. I was having a very good time. I was very pretty much like doing hyper-happy.

In idealizing terms, which may not reflect the reality of her lived experience, she described herself as a good student and a popular figure:

> It was that I had good grades. I had very high grades. I passed all my classes. I did all my homework. The lowest grade I ever got before was a 90 so I was getting like 90s or like the highest grade I ever got was like a hundred and then extra credit. So, I was getting like 98s and extra credits or practically, uh . . . a hundred extra credits because I . . . my failing grade was a 90. My practical lowest grade was a 90. I passed all my classes and I always passed all my classes and I was pretty much like, like a honors student, you know, and I was like pretty much even though I'll go out with my friends, getting all my classes done, and I was very intelligent, and cared about, and I was very popular and I had a lot of fun and everyone loved me and I was like-like-like perfect to everyone and I pretty much carried on my life correctly, you know, passing my classes.

While Terry shared idealized family and school memories, she avoided sharing about hardships she likely encountered in relocating to the United States as a child, leaving her childhood home in the Caribbean. Overall, Terry described her life before and after migration as idyllic. However, her current life difficulties suggest that the experience of migration was likely a profoundly difficult period for her. There is in fact an established relationship between the stress of migration, including social stress and isolation, and psychosis which dates back to the 1930s (Ødegaard, 1932). More recent research has found that with migration there is a risk factor for psychological development and identity formation (Garcia-Coll & Marks, 2012; Grinberg & Grinberg, 1989, 2004). With migration comes a need for acculturation: an often overwhelming experience of having to adapt to a new environment (Bustamante, Cerqueira, Leclerc, & Brietzke, 2017) with potential consequences such as depression, anxiety, and even psychosis (Foster, 2001).

EARLY ADOLESCENT STRUGGLES

Terry began to experience severe psychic distress around the age of sixteen, when she was beginning to contemplate going to college after high school. This transitional period between high school and college is a common age for psychic difficulties to emerge. For Terry, the first signs included racing thoughts, forgetfulness, and a hard time falling sleep. Her goal of attending college became less plausible and her new priority became reducing stress and taking care of her mental health, while seeking an alternative educational path. Terry left high school without a diploma and decided to get her general high school equivalency diploma (GED) instead. Here, using the terms "phobia" and "schizoaffective," she describes her struggles:

T: I was like, like I practically finished high school.

I: How did it feel to finish high school?

T: I felt ecstatic that I finished high school because I finished all those, those courses so quick and so brilliant so I was very ecstatic about going to college.

I: So, what does "ecstatic" mean for you? How does, what does it mean for you?

T: It means that I was like very . . . I had high self-confidence and high self-esteem and high self-es . . . enthusiasm and I was, I had high self, I was like myself was highly ecstatic about it all when I all went to college. I tried to go to college but that's when like my, that's when my phobia was like starting to get, to be like, like really weird. So, I was confused about how I was going to get through college but when I had my GED like that so quick I didn't need to go to college. I had all the education I needed to get a job and to start college later so I did but I . . . but I practically was starting to be schizoaffective. Having a mental problem, insomnia, amnesia, and racing thoughts being phobic so I type of started taking care of myself.

Terry had her first hospitalization at age sixteen. By her early twenties, Terry had been hospitalized three times in the United States, the last of which occurred the year before these interviews took place. Although Terry's explanation of why she had been hospitalized indicates possible feelings of being overwhelmed, and includes the fairly typical experience of an inability to sleep, it is unclear exactly why she was hospitalized. Terry had trouble reflecting on the onset of her difficulties, noting memory problems for this period of her life. She shared reasons that, while suggestive of her struggles, did not make her difficulties explicit:

I: Can you tell me a little bit about how you were feeling before getting into the hospitals? Like before being hospitalized and in what ways it helped?

T: Uh.

I: Or didn't?

T: Well, it really helped it, uh, it helped because I, uh, it helped me because I needed to be at the hospital to actually, um, like stay there because I was practically very tired, make my way home. And I felt as

> though I was gonna, I was feeling like I couldn't get any rest. When I went there it helped me to sleep. They helped me out with my meds and, uh, I was there for some time and they realized I was doing fine and that's when they let me leave actually, yep.
>
> I: Uh, you said like when you go there you would get rest. Was, prior to the hospitalization it was so like, you were very tired and there was a lot of things going through your mind? Was that . . .
>
> T: Uh, well there wasn't anything going through my mind but I was tired. So, I would get some rest. There's nothing going through my mind at all I wasn't stressed out thinking at all. I just went to the hospital so I like, recover.
>
> I: And what were you feeling before hospitalization?
>
> T: Uh, I was feeling tired and I was feeling as though that I might really soon forget things because of how tired I was.
>
> I: Sorry?
>
> T: I was feeling very tired and I was feeling as though I'm starting to forget things. Like I so, I realized I did forget a couple of things so that's what took me to the hospital.
>
> I: In all of the hospitalizations this was what happened?
>
> T: Yeah.
>
> I: So, you would get tired and start forgetting things?
>
> T: Yeah.

During her first hospitalization, she had a bad experience with her first therapist, who she believed did not understand the way she communicated, nor what she was experiencing:

> My first doctor really was a handful with all the therapy because I had like, I had like, uh, a weird therapist. It was, uh, the therapist was very white and didn't really understand my language and I got misdiagnosed with schizophrenia and so I had to like, uh, tell my mom about it and speak to my mom about like, uh, like how . . . how I was feeling and doing and with the doctor there and, uh, I stayed there for some time so when I did get out the hospital I had to like try to go to another clinic where I could declare myself formally diagnosed and try to take . . . and

try to take care of myself, uh, really quick and like help myself out with my schizoaffective disorder.

Terry was eventually discharged with a prescription for an antipsychotic medication. However, soon after, she was hospitalized for the second time. This time her condition, by her account, seems to have worsened. This is when she was given the diagnosis of "schizoaffective," which she embraced. She also embraced the concept of "phobia," which she felt was an accurate descriptor of her struggles. This time, she was held in the hospital for more than six months:

T: As I was trying to, uh, like, like finish off college with my phobia and, uh, schizoaffective disorder, the schizophrenia pills and the phobia I was going through. I did, uh, get out of the hospital and I was taking a very high dosage of schizophrenic pills but I got a little sick so I went back to the hospital. It was at a hospital and they really thought that I was practically that a slight bit schizophrenic but very schizoaffective, my phobia. So, I was like phobic, I was like phobic and I had secreting glands and I was not doing very well and I, I was taking antipsychotics so it was really affecting me. I was very moody and I had like mood swings and I was very tired. I was doing a lot of work and I was, I had no memory of what was really true so I . . .

I: What kind of memories did you have of that time?

T: I remember being at that hospital for like a couple of months at the beginning of the year, at the end of, uh, the begin . . . at the end of a year and, uh, it was November and September. It was like September going into November so at the end of the year practically December and I was there for like three months and I had to add on another three months and at the third . . . I had to add on another few months and then to add the third few months I had to stay there for three extra weeks before I'd leave the hospital.

She described her family's response during this time as worried but supportive. In particular, her mother made it a point to visit her often:

I: I wonder how you felt about it and how your mother felt about the hospitalizations?

T: My mother felt, uh, very worried.

I: Worried?

> T: Very, yeah, so she was like practically visiting the hospital a lot, like caring and like bringing me like meals and, uh, like ice cream and shakes, McDonald's and stuff because I really don't have the fast food there so she would visit like once every . . . once, once every like three days a week and she would bring me fast food and, uh, she knew I wasn't having much fast food so she brought me a lot of fast food and she thought that if she actually couldn't make it that she spent really enough time caring about me because it was like pretty much bothering her all that happened and at the place at the hospital.

Terry continued to reflect on her mother's experience coming to visit her in the hospital:

> She was feeling pretty friendless because there was actually no African Americans there really, just a bunch of Caucasian people at the clinic so she was doing fine. She just visited forever and at the last of the, the last of the three months where I had to spend three more weeks I pretty much, uh, knew I spent six months there. It was less than three months like five months and it was, I just had to stay there an extra three weeks, three weeks and she was there a lot. She was getting very tired working very hard.

Although the time line gets a bit confusing, at around the same time, or when Terry was almost seventeen years old, she was put into a special program for emotional support, where she worked on recovering her social skills and learned from others who were experiencing psychic distress. During this time, she describes attempting to embrace her new identity as someone who was, as she termed it, "schizoaffective":

> T: By the age of sixteen I was, uh, pretty much schizoaffective but I got better right away and I was a little phobic because of my schizo . . . , because of my schizoaffective disorder but I didn't have to take any medicine or any pills or anything. I am, was practically perfectly healthy and I should not, uh, I really should try to be in a phobic program and hang out in a, in a phobic society but I don't have to take any meds or worry about my health ever. There was definitely, uh, recommended to not take any meds or go to the hospital or take any treatment for phobia. Just go to, and if I was getting like, like that it would be nice to go to a phobic program.
>
> I: What is a "phobic program"?
>
> T: It's like when you go to school and you go to school and this, and you go to school in a special school, special schools where they have, uh,

phobic, phobia, uh, classes because you are, because if you're phobic you know like, you can't be in a crowd and you can't be crowded and stuff because of, uh, who you are and what's your heritage and whether you're Caucasian or not.

I: You talk about phobia. Was that an experience you are familiar with?

T: Well, I wasn't familiar with phobia at all but I, I actually got phobic one day and I . . . I couldn't believe it so I was just like rather in disbelief because it didn't seem like I was very sick. Like, I was sick at all. Living and believing that I was phobic I just ran away from school and went home and then my family took me back to school and lied to the school, then lied to my mom's house and went back and forth lying and just being weird.

I: Being weird?

T: Yeah.

I: What do you mean by that?

T: Because I was phobic.

I: How did it feel like to realize that you were phobic like to understand that you are phobic? How did it feel?

T: It felt like I decided to be responsible and understand I'm phobic and just be a phobic person.

I: Sorry?

T: I decided to make me understand that I'm phobic it made me want to be very responsible as a phobic person. So that's when I was in junior high school at sixteen and I was just about to go to, uh, I was just about to go to, uh, I practically didn't have to finish junior high school because I got all the books under control and everything so I was like living very weird and, uh, I finally went to, uh, high school at the age of sixteen going to be seventeen soon and, um, I practically went to summer vacations and it was like and it was nice there and I was in a different program there was a lot of kids just like me and I had a good time hanging out. It was such a nice environment to be phobic because, uh, I was in a phobic program with other phobic kids. And we were not really phobic, we didn't spend all our excess time because of our living standard. It was like money and being rich because you really don't spend like that it was a good time

> because I really appreciated my friends and I really understood the, the issue of being that phobic and I, uh, really, uh, understood when you're not phobic how you really care about your friends . . . I was hanging out with all the phobic friends and I was having a great time with my phobic friends. My friends were all phobic they really cared about me and I was having a wonderful time.

Terry described a place where she felt she belonged. Though with her tendency to idealize her experience, it is hard to be sure how she really felt. Spending time with other individuals facing similar life struggles provided psychosocial support that helped her to accept and incorporate her experience with psychosis into her identity. In the presence of others with similar distress, she described an atmosphere where her natural sociability came forth and to some degree she thrived.

HOLDING ON

Terry had difficulty broaching the topic of her psychic distress and discussing her experience of being hospitalized. Overall, she focused on the positive aspects of being hospitalized, those which, perhaps, allowed her some peace and distance from the distress she was experiencing leading up to the hospitalizations:

> I: Looking back at the hospitalization, what things do you remember like interactions with doctors? Therapy? Can you say a little bit more about how it felt like for you? What were your emotions at that time?
>
> T: Um, at the hospital, um I was practically, uh, I was practically like doing fine. Um, because it was like Christmas time being over there and I was there celebrating Christmas and, uh, I was like, I was doing fine. I was in a good mood I was playing the group games and, uh, going to all the different classes and programs they had. Like doing your nails, getting your nails done and all that. Brushing your hair. Doing like artwork with all the different classes and groups. Like Bingo and watching TV, listening to the radio, reading my magazine. And I was having a great time. And I didn't really see my doctor much. My doctor did come and see me a couple of times. And I was able to get rest if I was really tired in the day. And, uh, I was like, I would always get my meds and go to sleep on time. The medicine actually gets to work and I actually got to sleep. And, uh, that was practically it. That was all that was going on there. All that happened. I tried not to get in the way of other patients' like, mental illness either. And so, I was just like, I was just like, you know not getting into their way and not getting into my own way. I was just around there

eating breakfast, lunch, and dinner and watching TV. And, uh, all that stuff. Yep.

Terry's experiences surrounding hospitalization remain unprocessed. At this point she is very much immersed in them and not yet apparently able to look back and reflect on them, as she is currently working through her understanding of these experiences and still experiencing psychic distress. Perhaps delving into certain emotions at this point in time would be too difficult for her to bear. Or perhaps the hospital offered a place of respite, free from everyday stressors. In sharing her understanding of the purpose the hospitalizations served, Terry used definitions likely also used by clinicians in institutional settings to describe her experience:

T: I went to my therapist and they practically helped me.

I: And in what way did the hospital help? You said, like, it helped you to get rest . . .

T: Yep. It helped me get rest, it gave me meds. And, uh, I was, I practically. . . . Well, I usually go there for my mental health and it, it was like therapy and psychiatry and I was relaxed and I didn't have to worry about um, about forgetting things. You know my, I checked up with my doctor about my amnesia. When I was at the hospital it helped me to actually, uh, recover, and be able to remember things again because I seemed to be a wreck back then. That's why I was going to a program, at _____ working . . . my record with my mental illness it helped me to know what my illness is and how it works what I should do the side effects of my medicines and all that.

I: You said it helped you to get to know your mental illness?

T: Yeah.

I: Can you tell more, what is your understanding?

T: My understanding is that if I don't get rest at night it's because I'm having insomnia and if I have racing thoughts, it is because, uh, it's because I do have symptoms of racing thoughts. And if I have amnesia, if I keep forgetting things it means I'm having cases of amnesia. Yep.

Although Terry has taken on the label of "schizoaffective" as a part of her identity, she strongly minimized her struggles and the impact her experiences have had, and continue to have, on her life. Terry minimized her mental health issues in comparison to physical health problems, and found comfort in knowing that she was physically healthy. In fact, she shared that both she and her family were relieved to learn that she was "only schizoaffective":

I: What did it feel like for you to hear that (you were diagnosed as schizoaffective)?

T: Well, uh, I felt as though that I wasn't really living very hard or like having any really serious health problems at all. I didn't have a health problem. I felt as though I was happy that my life was so much better, it's so much better than it could have been.

I: What could it have been?

T: Well what could have been practically health problems like diabetes. Yeah. Or high blood pressure could have happened. Or any of those other diseases. And I was so happy that I was living like so much easier you know with such a nice life like I deserve you know. Like all my family has always wanted.

I: Sorry?

T: I was so happy that I was living a better life like I deserve. All my family was happy.

I: All of your, who was happy?

T: My family members. They always wanted me to live.

I: Your family?

T: Yeah, and with all of us, they always wanted me to live with hope that I would live with a not health problem like diabetes or high blood pressure. But something better than that because everybody gets sick now and then. I practically got, uh, a mental illness called schizoaffective. And it was very easy to live with a schizoaffective disorder and living life. If you're schizoaffective you don't have anything to worry about. They classify it as phobic and you might end up phobic. But, it's not much at all. It's nothing so, uh, so um I was practically like, like, like it was practically, uh, very nice that I was like actually living with such an easy, uh, mental problem with schizoaffective disorder. I was surprised that I was so happy just like everyone always wanted.

I: Sorry?

T: I was so happy that I was like surprisingly like, healthy. Just like my family members always wanted.

I: So, you felt healthy and it almost sounds lucky you didn't have other difficulties?

T: Yeah. Yup. That's practically it.

PLACES OF COMFORT

Terry described her hospitalizations as well as her time at Fountain House as places of respite. To Secil's question "How was your experience of being hospitalized?" she replied:

> It wasn't terrible. It was like very relaxing. It made me feel, uh, like I'm going to be doing well. Yeah, it was type of like, uh, like, like, like if I was like relieving stress. I felt like I was going to be better soon.

Referencing Fountain House specifically, she noted:

> It's relaxing. And it's easy to, uh, live about. And it's very nice. And it's, uh, it's like very relaxing and I don't get very tired, I don't have racing thoughts. The place is like, it's very nice. It's relaxing. Yup.

Hospitals were places of rest for Terry, places which, from her description, allowed her to, as Winnicott suggested to "become unintegrated, to flounder, to be in a state in which there is no orientation, to be able to exist for a time without being either a reactor to an external impingement or an active person with a direction of interest or movement" (Winnicott, 1958, p. 34). It is possible that her hospitalizations allowed her to begin to relax and connect to her internal environment and needs without the overwhelming distraction of the outside world, which she experiences as suffocating and crowded. These respite spaces also helped her to recognize her strength and ability to make it on the outside:

I: Uh, how do you understand your phobia?

T: Uh, I understand my phobia that I can't stay in crowds for too long. In a huge crowd for too long I just need to leave the crowd. And that I can't stay in an environment where I am never going to be in a crowd because I really gotta be in a crowd for some time so I am able to actually, uh, survive in a crowd and that I don't have any worries because I don't have any health problems. So, my phobia is just type of rapid where I feel as though if I spend thirty minutes in a crowd then I spent a year in a crowd

> so how I'm healthy and how I'm doing it doesn't matter I'm just going to be alright phobia wise.
>
> I: Uh, you said . . . you used the word "survive" in the crowds?
>
> T: Yeah.
>
> I: It's almost like you feel like you can survive?
>
> T: Yeah, I feel like I can't survive. *Can* survive.
>
> I: In the crowds?
>
> T: In the crowds, yeah, as long as I am type of not staying there for too long I feel as though I could survive in the crowds. That's amazing, 'cause if you really had serious health problems you know, you think that you can't be in a crowd ever but the truth is you have to try to be in crowds sometimes so when you are in crowds you won't get really sick so, uh, I was very happy that I thought that I could be in crowds and I was able to be in crowds and survive.

Terry described a place of solace away from the daily hassles of life that inevitably come with having to go to school, hassles that would become even more difficult to handle while dealing with psychic distress:

> Okay . . . Uh, I was here at Fountain House because, uh, I sort of, um, have schizoaffective disorder and I graduated from high school and I was very scared about going to college with being schizoaffective. I was worried about not getting enough rest, and forgetting my books, and being too tired because, to even care about school. And being too . . . like having racing thoughts and trying to actually get to class, there's the class and the books and the education done correctly. And so . . . I, uh, sort of . . . I sort of decided to not go to college but to go to Fountain House. I really wanted to just go to Fountain House instead of college also . . . And there was plenty of programs but the only one I decided was best for me was Fountain House, 'cause it's around my way, it's really close to my house, and it feels like home, and the, the setting is very different from the others 'cause the others they do serious therapy and it's too tiring, it's too much, and I'm schizoaffective and I forget, I forget very easily so it wasn't really helping me at all to be at any of the other programs but it was helping me to be at Fountain House. So, I came to Fountain House because of that and it was, I thought it was a very nice place and, uh, I kept coming back to Fountain House 'cause it's, it's very nice to be at . . . I came to Fountain House instead of college because I really didn't care

> about college at all, it was hectic, but Fountain House wasn't very hectic at all. And it was a very nice place and I was pretty much hooked on being at Fountain House it was like, it was something I had to do because it was, uh, bringing out a positive side of me.

Terry had difficulties explaining her rationale for choosing to go to Fountain House over other mental health care facilities:

> Yup and Fountain House is, uh, such a wonderful place you know, I focus my positive energy all the time and I feel as though my negative energy is focused that it's getting better its recovering, doing fine, and, uh, when I was living I kept coming here because I knew (inaudible) when you always radiate positive energy that, uh, you do (inaudible) it's not like everything's positive some things are negative and with all the other programs my negative energy was pretty much all, uh, pretty much all very, uh, busy so it was, uh, a natural desire to not be at a negative energy program becau . . . so but to be in a positive energy program because it was real tough to be at the other places with all that negative energy working so hard on positive energy. I thought that the negative energy was probably, uh, negative energy is to just force yourself to have positive energy and that I have got a positive energy and I, uh, need to relax my negative energy to keep my positive energy positive.
>
> When you think about all that work being schizoaffective, where you have to get some sleep or else you're very tired, you can't do things, you forget a lot, and you have racing thoughts, so it's, uh, it's so, um, so stressful to, uh, actually stay in a, in the world environment. I realized that that's a true story that that's actually real that if you're schizoaffective that you just got to, go to this positive energy place you know where you if where you don't have to waste that you can't be in a negative energy base surrounded when you have schizoaffective.

Although part of Terry's difficulty lies within her, she was able to reflect on the other piece of the puzzle: a difficult "world environment," one that encompasses many stressful expectations. A world which Terry has difficulty being in. Terry is clear that psychosocial stressors and the complexity of everyday living posed an extraordinary challenge for her.

STRUGGLE WITH BELONGING

Terry went from living on a Caribbean Island that is "very much grounded on race and social class" (Georgiana, 2013, p. 172), to living in the United States at age eleven. Georgiana notes that the Caribbean region's "national cultural identity is largely a hybrid of European, African, Amerindian and Asian cultures, in other words, essentially creole" (2013, p. 172), which leads to a hybrid identity for those living there. This struggle to formulate an identity as a little girl growing up in the Caribbean was likely further complicated by Terry's migration to the United States at a young age. In the United States, others viewed her as being "black" and of African-American origin. However, this is not a culture with which she identified and she experienced severe dissonance when confronted with working-class African-American culture.

The interviews were very much framed by Terry's imagining herself as a Caucasian woman, one who felt like she did not belong when in the company of African-American individuals as she could not relate to them as people and did not understand their discourse. Ultimately, not being able to relate to African Americans, whose culture differed significantly from her culture of origin, she developed a counter-identification to American blackness and embraced a Caucasian identity:

> I: What about it was tough for you there [psychiatric hospital]?
>
> T: It was tough for me there because I'm schizoaffective and since I'm schizoaffective being so tired and all that negative energy and I'm all the way Caucasian I don't have any African in me. All that stuff . . .
>
> I: Sorry, can you repeat?
>
> T: Since I was, it was, uh, not good for me schizoaffective to be there, amnesia racing thoughts the insomnia and stuff. It was terrible for me to be over there. Because I couldn't remember anything everybody said and they were really African Americans there and they were terribly like saying so much I was terribly, uh, feeling left different feeling like I don't belong because I have no African in my family. And it was real different and it was very negative . . . positive became negative and so I just couldn't stay in a program like that anymore. I just had to search for a program that's totally different. Because it was a lot of pressure, it's always been a lot of pressure for me to hang out with African Americans. I tried to be racist and to feel because I don't feel as though I belong, you know, I found something Caucasians do feel. And I tried to, uh, get away from African Americans and not stay there not be around them anymore. I feel left out. I feel like I don't belong, like I am not even somebody that they even accepted to feel left out though, I just don't want to be there.
>
> I: You didn't feel like you were at home?

T: Yeah, I didn't feel like I was at home. It made me homesick, very homesick.

Terry spoke about African Americans as people alien to her, people she struggled to understand and connect to while in a psychiatric setting:

T: Yeah, because yeah, I didn't feel very, uh, safe mental health wise because I'm in this program and if I'm working with the Caucasian, um the Caucasian employees that I understand and I get the picture and I'm speaking my language, all the Caucasian languages, and I'm really getting a good idea. But the fact that the African Americans were speaking, I never really heard a damn thing or understood a damn thing they had to say and I was very confused you know. They try to be English, you know after slavery how it was and how they learned to speak English, try to learn how to act or how to be because of their heritage. And that's where I was at and that's how it is to be Caucasian with sitting there and you're trying to understand an African person. And it was very weird I felt as though my mental health was in danger.

I: So, for you it almost wasn't like they were speaking the same language with those people that you didn't feel safe with?

T: Yeah because I didn't really get to understand their language and they were being very weird.

I: By weird what do you mean?

T: They were pretty much putting themselves through a lot.

I: Sorry?

T: They were pretty much putting themselves through a lot. They were they were very, very angry and grumpy and they seem to be, they seem to be not be able to take care of themselves. That was very weird because when you're grumpy or angry and you can't take care of yourself. It's sad. I mean being Caucasian that makes you feel depressed that's why people have depression and stuff you know? And they can't seem to do well when they have their health problems that's what health is about if they were African American, so they don't really care and that was, what was a lot of pressure because I really, really just had to sit there and understand everything that was going on. So, I really didn't like the fact that I had to be there for the rest of my life because I can't do college.

Terry offered a description of herself as a slender, brilliant white woman:

> T: I was just a beautiful, vibrant, very pretty long headed white girl with such white skin being all Caucasian with such nice nails and I would get pedicures and manicures and grow my nails, keep my body like very thin and I would, I was modeling so I was like practically trying to like be ecstatic. I was trying to be like thin like slender. I was trying to be like a twig. I was trying to be a like bony, a bony twig skeleton figure girl and I was exaggerating about my vanity and who I am and how I live, and my IQ. I was like a friggin' genius. I was a generic genius.
>
> I: You were a generic genius?
>
> T: Yeah. A Caucasian genius.
>
> I: What does it mean?
>
> T: I was like practically . . .
>
> I: You say "Caucasian" a lot. What does it mean to be Caucasian for you?
>
> T: Well, it means that I like go to school.
>
> I: Mm-hm.
>
> T: And that I um, I'm more Caucasian so I'm not very comfortable around, uh, Africans and African Americans . . .

Terry's idea that she is a white woman, and her counter-identification with White American culture, was deeply felt and likely served a powerful protective function, keeping her insulated from realities perhaps she is not yet ready to tolerate.

AN UNSETTLED LIFE

In speaking of her childhood and current family relations, much as she spoke of her time being hospitalized, Terry spoke mostly in idyllic terms. However, her strong desire to support, provide for, and do right by her family also became evident. In response to "How was your relationship with your mother since childhood?" Terry spoke of halcyon days, stating:

> T: Well, my relationship with my mother was very acceptable. It was like, uh, particularly a lot of fun. She was very, very loved, and cherished, and cared about and I would like, uh, try to save my allowance to buy her birthday presents, Christmas presents, uh, and my dad, Father's Day presents, Christmas presents you know and help her out around, uh, the

> times because I was very young, growing up, trying to learn my books. I do Mother's Day, Father's Day, Christmas and, uh, I tried my best and if I learned anything else I would be able to support my mom and dad with, like, presents and whatever that matters. And it is also because I was very young and I had a good time with my mother and my father and I was very happy with such high grades and such a nice life and such a nice dad, such a nice vacation and such a nice mom and such a nice time and so I pretty much was very, a very happy kid. I had a lot of time in the crowds and I was very popular. I was very happy with all my family members 24/7 visiting. I was doing fine. I was doing so well. I was like A-Okay. I was like doing particularly very happy, you know, at school and life for what it truly is and I truly really truly care and truly spent a lot of time growing up, being a kid, having all that ice cream and spending all that time in the beach water. It's really cold and um, like going to sleep very warm. If I, it's like any type of chilly in the nighttime and I had a great time.

In a regretful tone, Terry shared a concern about possibly failing her family and not being able to support them in the same way they supported her. She lamented the loss of how she used to be, including having "high self-esteem" and "confidence" and being "thin":

> T: I really like needed to be there for them because they really supported me and I really couldn't be cranky and not be able to not like be there for too long but I tried so hard to support them when I don't, being so young, and I'm quite new to this stuff and I'm not going to be happy about the fact that I failed them if anything else.
>
> I: Failed them?
>
> T: Yeah. If anything, else with Mother's Day, Father's Day, Christmas and holiday season so I went to winter vacation in schools. I wasn't going to be happy as an eleven-year-old or as a nine-year-old or eight-year-old going to be ten. I wouldn't be very happy like if I learned anything else at, uh, twelve or thirteen and I couldn't support them so I was like very like ecstatic spending time with my mother and father, my good grades, having a great vacation like, like practically ecstatically. I always had very high self-esteem and very high confidence and self-enthusiasm, very high self-enthusiasm and I was very ecstatic with confidence. So, I was doing great in life, very well all my life so when I did pa- graduate from high school go to college for some time like that I had a lot of self-esteem. I was doing fine. I never was heavyset and I was just like very thin and I was very like happy and everything.

Later on in the interview, Terry went on to share additional thoughts about her body image, speaking of herself as underweight when in fact this was evidently not true:

> T: It's practically like insulting that I'm under ninety pounds.
>
> I: Sorry?
>
> T: I said it's practically insulting that I'm under ninety pounds and I'm twenty-four.
>
> I: Well, how, how is it insulting to be under ninety pounds and what does it mean to be ninety pounds for you, like what does it bring with it, being ninety pounds?
>
> T: Well, being ninety pounds is that I've been ninety pounds for a while now so when I do start gaining weight being older I'm practically going to start being very skinny with all them pounds on, I'm going to end up being eighty pounds and then I'm going to be very scrawny and I'm like living, doing a lot of work, taking care of a lot of kids [referring to sister's children] so . . .
>
> I: So, it's, it's a lot of responsibility for you.
>
> T: It's a lot of responsibility for me. I handle a lot. I handle plenty. Yeah and I'm eating like crazy, vomiting all the time so if I'm a little anorexic here or there anyway it's just like . . . scary when I'm so tiny.
>
> I: You were vomiting?
>
> T: Yeah.
>
> I: At that time?
>
> T: So, I just quit eating. I wasn't eating at all. It was all about my books and I didn't care. See I didn't need to eat. I need to like stay thin so I could eat and not be that anorexic, just a little anorexia is a lot. It's very important, you know, because you're going to- when you get older, you're getting older and you're Caucasian and you're like small, you're eating like that and you're putting on the pounds and you're not, you're not (inaudible) African, you get really pretty and you start to like hate your body because you got to go to the beach, you have to be a cheerleader and it's annoying that you're so terrible figured so that's when you

really start caring about being anorexic so I tried real hard to be anorexic . . .

Reflecting on her relationship with her father, Terry further spoke about the desire to be beautiful and slender:

> (*sighs*) My relationship was very nice with my dad because I'm like daddy's little princess and I'm like, I have the royal, I have such a royal name and such a royal life. It's a royal pain, you know, because I'm just like, I'm like ecstatically a lot of fun. I would enter beauty competitions a lot and I've won a lot of beauty competitions in elementary school and in junior high school and in high school and going through college I also entered a lot of beauty competitions too and I went through a lot of beauty competitions and I was very beautiful and I was very pretty and I was very thin and I felt very . . . I felt like a had very high self-esteem with such a thin body and being so young and so underweight that I would 24/7 go like try to like, like perfect my image to have a slender figure so I could really waste my time in my bikinis freely and so I was just . . . like over-exaggerating about everything.

Eventually, Terry shared that her father had passed away, sharing that she did not know exactly when or why he passed away:

> T: . . . but my dad did pass away.
>
> I: When?
>
> T: Uh . . . I think, uh, that I, he probably passed away because my mom was like thirty-three because she's a grandmother now. She's a grandma and my dad is a grandfather.
>
> I: So, when did your father pass away?
>
> T: Well, my father passed away because he had another wife and he, he was a grandfather, and he had, uh, two sons and one daughter and the son had a child with his wife and the girl was getting older and she also had a child and my sister had a child and, uh, they were getting old. My father was forty. My dad was like going to be fifty. My mom was going to be fifty soon and my dad was going to be sixty soon and they, my dad had two kids, two grandkids. My mom had one grandkid and, uh, well, being at the age of twenty-four going on twenty-five, I didn't have any kids and I didn't really have any time to date at all to even have a boyfriend being so sick so I pretty much spent a lot of time with my mother and father

trying to get better and my dad he passed away but I didn't even know at what age he passed away anymore or what time because . . .

I: How did you feel when you . . .

T: Because it was my, my mother and my father were grandparents and I was so young and I was practically the youngest but the oldest, I still didn't get, I'm still the oldest in the middle child, and I had a grandfather and a grandmother and I was twenty-four by then and I was, uh, practically living in a house with, uh, a mother on my mother's side and a father and two mothers on my dad's side and, uh, and, uh, I . . . practically became an auntie so I'm practically an aunt, an aunt.

With pride, Terry continued on to speak of her role as an aunt, stating "My role in life is practically that I have a lot of family members and I'm an auntie" sharing that she is "living a role model life" to set an example for her sister's children. In reference to this role she concluded: "I need to be the best. That's my role. I have to be the best, better than the best."

CONCLUDING THOUGHTS

Throughout the interviews, Terry's struggle to narrate her life experiences was unmistakable as she worked hard to understand herself and to be understood by the interviewer. What emerged from these interviews was a glimpse into a life filled with un-metabolized, complex issues, including migration at a young age, racial identity confusion, psychiatric hospitalizations, and a deeply touching need to belong. In speaking of her experiences in relation to other people, Terry often used race as a baseline for understanding herself and others, suggesting an enduring sense of inadequacy and a struggle to experience a sense of belonging.

Terry has faced multiple life disruptions. Yet, her strength and resilience is evident as she continues to seek and take advantage of therapeutic services, and to make the best of her life circumstances through putting herself out in the world despite often feeling tired and overwhelmed. She continues to have the motivating support and love of her family, who she cherishes, and she takes her role as an aunt, sister, and daughter very seriously. She has taken it upon herself to take care of her well-being in an effort to be the best she can be for both herself and her family. Despite various obstacles, Terry continues to hold on and persist.

Chapter Seven

Teresa

Looking for Love

Montana Queler and Michael O'Loughlin

Teresa was an endearing fifty-seven-year-old African-American woman who was born and raised in a large city in the Northeastern United States. She reported that she had been a member of Fountain House for fifteen years but had begun experiencing psychic distress long before this, dating back to her college years. She seemed comfortable and aware of what we were to discuss as we began the interviews, though it soon became apparent that she had her own ideas for how we should spend our time. For instance, Teresa's response to a question about the circumstances leading to her membership at the clubhouse consisted of a description of her love affair with the son of a famous American real estate mogul, "E," and the international work that she believed he was doing in collaboration with Fountain House:

> I: If it's okay with you, I wonder if we could begin by talking about your life, beginning perhaps with why you are here at the clubhouse.
>
> T: Well, it is it was such a big surprise. I've been here at the clubhouse for the past fifteen years and I never thought it would happen, but the big surprise has been I've met my honey bun, my soul mate, my godsend. And he is now in Australia, with the Australian clubhouse in Queensboro heading up a clubhouse there in Australia. So I am very proud of him that he takes such an interest in my affairs. And my affairs is to build fifty-four Helen Keller international institutes in the fifty-four capitals of Africa right next door to fifty-four clubhouses in the fifty-four capitals of Africa. So I am just so blessed to have one of the [Name] family members

> on my side, to see that those two things two . . . houses . . . two clubhouses are done . . . and um, what else?

This kind of disjuncture between interview questions and Teresa's responses occurred repeatedly. The fantasy of this love affair, to which Teresa returned often, appeared to be a safe and happy place for her, perhaps a respite from other subjects that evoked discomfort. However, there were also moments in which Teresa was able to reflect in a grounded way on truly upsetting experiences, such as moments of personal oppression and racism, the onset of her depression, and the physical and emotional abuse perpetrated by her mother. Montanta's initial impression was that although Teresa could discuss these aspects of her life, many unresolved conflicts remained. It seemed that these internal conflicts were somehow being resolved through her fantasy relationship with this famous man. In an effort to make sense of what these conflicts might be, we attended closely to the losses and disappointments Teresa articulated during the interviews.

FIRST BREAK

When asked about the initial onset of her depression, Teresa immediately referred to the loss of her relationship with her close friend Jane. A friend from high school, Jane seemed to have been Teresa's most intimate confidante throughout adolescence. During the interview, Teresa referred to her love of her blind girlfriend who, in the transition to college, became increasingly independent, leading to her detachment from Teresa. Teresa spoke of their simultaneous move from their mutual home city to another major city as if she had expected that their relationship would continue to thrive. From Teresa's perspective, their matriculation at separate colleges—though in the same city—would not affect their ability to remain close. However, the distance their move created proved to be devastating for Teresa:

> T: Yes. My girlfriend Jane, Irish Catholic, blind since birth. I was her eyesight and she was my, how can I say it? I was her eyesight, and she was my, was my . . . mouthpiece. We went through high school together, we went through Spain together, through France together. My mother and father put nine hundred dollars in my pocket and Jane's mother put nine hundred dollars in her pocket. And they said, "Teresa, Jane, go to France" (laughs). And we went to France and ended up at the University of Madrid. So, Jane, my love of Jane. And . . . when we graduated together from high school, she went to college in [City] and I went to [same city]. And (shrugs), just naturally that seemed to be the best route to take. To channel my love of Jane. And one thing that didn't go too well was . . . the winding away of Jane and I for Jane's seeing-eye dog, Luna, a golden

Labrador Retriever, Luna Tuna Fish to me, Luna to Jane. I got so sick when I was in [City] going to college and Jane was in [City]. They didn't wean me away from Jane, and . . .

I: What do you mean by that?

T: Jane's independence from me onto Jane's dependence on her seeing-eye dog. No one weaned me off. No one told me I would feel this way . . .

I: It sounds to me like you were mourning a loss, and that's what the depression came from. Is that your understanding?

T: Yes, yes. Jane and I parting ways. Deep.

Describing the onset of her depression at eighteen, Teresa recounted:

> Sleeping, sleeping, and not getting out of my bed. It was the most God-awful feeling I've ever felt in my life. Not wanting to dress, not wanting to take a shower, not wanting to brush my teeth, not wanting to braid my hair. You know what I mean? Just so, depressed. It was more than just . . . it's like something I've never felt before.

Further, Teresa went on to recount her mother's inability to recognize and respond empathically to her pain; "She was very violent toward me. And although she was a nurse, she still didn't understand what was going on in my life." Bollas (2013) posits that psychic breakdown is frequently engendered by a significant rupture or interpersonal loss that echoes an unresolved childhood trauma. Teresa's account of her initial psychological impasse captured both interpersonal loss—her loss of Jane—as well as clues to what might have been the original trauma, illustrated in her mother's response to her suffering. When asked about how it felt to receive support from other figures in her life—her sisters, aunts, and another friend—Teresa's persistent need for her mother's love rang loud:

> It hurt. It still hurt because it was my mother. It still hurt, pained my heart . . . the pain was still agonizing because I needed it from my mother—not my girlfriend, not my father, not my sisters, but from my mother, who threw water at me, wet up my bed, hit me, slapped me around. Not good, not good, not good, no . . .

During the interview, Teresa repeatedly alluded to an unmet yearning for love and recognition. While the first and primary loss seemed to be that of her mother, and subsequently her loss of Jane, Teresa spoke about her alienation from other friends as well. For example, she cited strained ties with friends in her African-American college advocacy group. She reported that they spoke disparagingly about her relationship with Jane, who was white:

> T: And I was called by my black friends, a Negro.
>
> I: By your black friends in high school or college?
>
> T: College.
>
> I: Uhuh, and what was that about?
>
> T: Having Jane so close to me.

When asked about the collapse of her social support network, Teresa explained:

> To hold on so tightly, to need so sincerely. I was a very needy person. When I got sick, I wanted to hold on to my friends so close, and that made my friends turn away from me . . . they couldn't deal with that feeling that I have. They didn't know what to say or what to do with my mental illness because mental illness is so very misunderstood . . .

Concerned about her, Teresa's sister Linda convinced Teresa to take a medical leave from college. However, this resulted in Teresa living with her mother, who did not seem to apprehend her condition:

> She [Linda] said, "Teresa, come home." I was staying in bed for the entire day and night. She said, "Teresa, come home, let me take care of you." She studied to be a nurse. Just like my mother, my mother was an RN. And I said, "Okay, Linda, I'll come home." I was so very depressed. She said, "I'll take care of you." So when I went home with this depression, my mother did not understand. I couldn't brush my teeth, comb my hair, take a shower. My mother would have fights with me. I cried, and I cried, and I cried.

Soon after returning home, Teresa reported that she felt a sense of urgency to reunite with a former college love interest:

> T: I went, I went, wanted to see one gentleman who I had a longing to see.
>
> I: Somebody at school?
>
> T: Right, so what I did was, I went to the store, and I stole money from the bakery shop in my neighborhood. I jumped over the counter with my pajamas on. I jumped over the counter, stole twenty dollars, jumped back

over the counter, and went to . . . went to . . . Amtrak, with my pajamas on. The police picked me up. This stranger picked me up, because I had on slippers, I had on a nightgown, and I had only twenty dollars to my name because I stole twenty dollars from the bakery . . . that was really a downer for me, stealing that money from the bakery.

I: You were at a really low place when you did that . . .

T: Wow, whoa.

I: Were you feeling depressed at the time?

T: Oh yes, I wanted to see this man so much.

I: Was he one of the men that you had been in a relationship with?

T: Yes . . . yes, yes I was.

I: And were you talking to him at all while you were home?

T: No, not at all. I wasn't talking to anybody, I wasn't talking to my friends, I wasn't talking to my psychiatrist, I was just crying, crying, crying.

I: Hmm . . .

T: The police picked me up, brought me back home in handcuffs, and they threw me down on the couch. That was really, really bad, Montana, the worst.

I: It must have been scary.

T: Yes. Man, man, oh man, oh man . . .

I: So they entered your house, and they threw you down on the couch?

T: Yes, yes.

I: In front of your family?

T: In front of my mother, in front of my sister, who I, who was in charge of watching me twenty-four seven . . . my sister Linda was in charge of watching me. I took my sister Linda, shook her, shook her, shook her, and punched her out. Punched the living breath out of my sister Linda. She fell on the floor with no breath left in her. That was another downer . . .

I: This was a time after the incident with the police?

T: Yes, that um she was in charge of watching me, and I fought with her. I not only fought with her, I punched her out, then I went to the second story, the third story, in my parents' brownstone house, the third story, and I jumped out of the window. My-oh-my-oh-my, people watched me jump (sighs) . . . what can I say? I fell on my knees, and bruised my knees.

I: Mmm . . . did you break any bones?

T: No, just bruised them, just bruised my knees.

I: Had you intended to hurt yourself?

T: No.

I: What was your thought process going into that?

T: In any way possible, I wanted to get to this man. It was just a terrible, terrible, terrible thought, thinking that I was in love, ugh.

I: Did you feel he would sort of maybe rescue you from your depression?

T: Yes, yes, yes . . .

Within this, Teresa's subjection to perpetual surveillance is juxtaposed with her aching for love and recognition. She believed that if only this ache would be fulfilled, her depression would lift. Building on Winnicott's notion of mirroring and on the trauma of misrecognition, Charles (2014) writes,

> The child who fails to find herself in the gleam in her parent's eyes is a lost soul. This child can spend her life looking in all the wrong places for that gleam she sensed she needed, even though she may have lost touch with any idea of what is being sought. The deficit, then, is experienced as a painful absence that cannot be relieved. Because the gleam is linked with the parents, we can spend our lives seeking out exactly the types of disappointments that are all too familiar. (Charles, 2014, p. 72)

FANTASY AS FULFILLMENT

It is within Teresa's elaborately conceived fantasy of her love affair with a prominent mogul that her need for this kind of profound validation emerged in its most crystallized form. During the course of the interviews, Teresa repeatedly referred back to their relationship, depicting an almost Disney-like romance with projections of perfection insinuated into each detailed facet. Teresa delineated their plans for their future in the following excerpts:

> T: I just can't wait for my Tiffany ring and for E to genuflect on his knee and for making me a bride, his bride, to get married with a caravan leaving from here, New York, to DC . . . to get married in the Immaculate Conception Cathedral in DC, to have four hundred people as guests and then for my house to be built with my swimming pool and my golf course in the backyard . . . What else? Four hundred people as guests at my wedding, the cake, the black cake for four hundred guests, is now being made as gifts for every family member and friends who come to my wedding, that's all.

Later in the interview, she related:

> T: God bless Africa, God bless Haiti. I would love to pick up a baby, and two babies, after nine months of being married to E, to pick up E Junior II, and nine months after the baby boy is with us, to pick up Mary Teresa, our pair, our boy and girl, playmates, with a lot, a lot a lot of African baby clothes.
>
> I: Nine months seems like a significant number . . .
>
> T: Yeah, nine months (patting her stomach). Nine months being pregnant, nine months carrying the baby . . .
>
> I: So it's symbolic?
>
> T: Yup, yup . . . And I intend to have a trip celebrating my job as Vatican Ambassador, Ambassador to the Vatican. I hope and pray that I can also bring my family to Rome to celebrate my job with me. So, that's what I want E to do with my family, so we can celebrate my job soon. Another thing is, to keep it in the family, I don't know if you know of Victoria Five Movie Theater that's been closed now for about thirty years, down the street from, down the block from the Apollo Theater. You've probably heard of the Apollo Theater. Right down the block, about five doors away from the Apollo Theater, is the Victoria Five Movie Theater. E and his father will give the keys to the Victoria Five Theater, to be the healthy and happy competition for the Apollo Theater, so that's what my brother-in-law, my sister's husband, that will be his keys to keep the job in the family. E's relationship with Harlem. And to keep it all in the family, my sister J and her husband, to open up my restaurant, The Ambassador, and also for my father, bar and grill of the . . . the bar and grill of the restaurant The Ambassador. And also, my girlfriend, my best friend . . .

> Oprah Winfrey, to Gayle King, as Teresa to my best friend from college, ever since then, to have her . . . to have her . . . just be by my side, just to be there, close to me. Oh, my brother-in-law . . . to produce, be the executive producer of movies, to bring in millions of dollars, to produce movies, to make movies, and that will pay for the fifty-four Helen Keller internationals, to bring in the millions of dollars to make movies.

Teresa's stories were replete with features illustrating her fantasy lover's staunch devotion toward her, indications of a vested interest in knowing and attending to the things that matter to her. The content of these stories highlight Teresa's wants and needs—the need to feel at the center of another's universe, to constitute their primary motivating force, and her passion for charitable service. Her fantasies seemed to represent an attempt to counter her profound sense of emotional deprivation and loneliness.

At the manifest level, Teresa's romantic fantasies were not only a stand-in for the love she was unable to garner from her mother. Her fantasies also merged with her yearning for communion with the person who first served as a fantasied maternal surrogate—her best friend Jane. During the interview, Teresa's expressed desire for connection with Jane manifested in stories that suggested a psychic merger between Jane and Teresa's beloved E:

> I: Did you and Jane have a romantic relationship?
>
> T: No, that's what the doctors included did not understand.
>
> I: Okay . . .
>
> T: This lesbian relationship, the doctors wanted to know more about it. And that's what I struggled with in public and in private. Jane holding my arm, me holding her arm, to walk. That's it. Me teaching her how to cook. Me teaching her how to dance . . . because she asked, "Teresa, teach me, teach me how to dance." Hey, what can I do? Put your feet, your left foot on my left foot, put your right foot on my right foot, turn on Motown. Taught her how to dance. She met her man. My mother said, "Teresa, all you need to do is ask E, 'E, close your eyes and turn around.' You don't have to say anything else, just do your dance." That's what my mother taught me. "Teresa, tell E to close his eyes and turn around, and knock him down on the bed." And it worked.
>
> I: It worked?
>
> T: It worked. So we'll be going on our cruise soon. My mother says, "Teresa, you don't need a chaperone like you needed in your prom, a chaperone. You don't need a chaperone." So we'll be going on our cruise

> to the Caribbean, we'll be going on our cruise in Hawaii, we'll be going on our cruise in Greece. Three cruises to go on before we get married. It's just the most beautiful way to get to know somebody. To travel, experience.
>
> I: Mhm, and that's what you had mentioned doing with Jane as well, right? The two of you went on a trip together?
>
> T: Uh, yes. Paris and Spain.

In this latter passage, Teresa's comments seemed to capture the desire for interpersonal connection, and yet they also expose a need to do this within the circumscribed space of fantasy. True intimacy is messy, and for Teresa, interpersonal connection often proved at best disappointing and at moments shattering.

FANTASY AS REFUGE

Teresa was ultimately able to return to college. She described her graduation as her greatest accomplishment: "It took me five years to graduate, and that was my proudest moment . . . that was my proudest moment that I've ever had in the world for myself." Within the context of this achievement, Teresa again conjured her relationship with Jane:

> I missed Jane's graduation. She received a five-minute standing ovation. I received a two-minute standing ovation. My father cried when I graduated. My friends told me that my father left the auditorium because he didn't want anybody to see him crying. My sister and I graduated on the same day, the same time. So I understand who enjoyed who more.

In both references—to Jane and to her sister—Teresa's comments seemed to reflect her competitiveness and a need to see herself as desired, lauded, and loved. Teresa's tendency to characterize her life story in such comparative terms suggests a deeper sense of insecurity and loneliness that her grandiose fantasies could serve to quell and conceal.

After graduating, Teresa channeled her activist aspirations into the pursuit of a graduate degree in fundraising:

> I: And what led you to that decision?
>
> T: Mm . . . because of the poverty and hunger in the world. I wanted to work with organizations such as UNICEF, work for the United Nations, work for the Peace Corps, mm . . .

> I: And what turned you on to that while you were in school? Or was it the time that you took off from school? Because you said that you had gone to school thinking that you wanted to work in the theater . . .
>
> T: Right.
>
> I: So what changed your mind?
>
> T: Mm, I couldn't act. I was so very stage, suffered from stage fright.
>
> I: It made you anxious or nervous?
>
> T: Yeah, yeah, too upset, too nerve wracking. I mean, I couldn't work as an actress. So I says, well what would I do then? What would I do? And what was open for me was Africare. I read an article, about Africare. And Africare was one of the organizations that came from the Peace Corps—African-American graduates from the Peace Corps started Africare because they did not like the way the Peace Corps members treated Africans. I said, well let me look into this.

However, soon after pursuing this path, Teresa's initial difficulties resurfaced, leading to another impasse:

> T: . . . starting the New York City chapter of Africare, didn't work. I became too engrossed in the suffering and um feelings, hurt feelings of, here it goes again—black and white and white and black people. So, I figure, I'm gonna have to do something like, about this. So I went into Harlem . . . and I lived in the black nun's convent for three months, trying to figure it out in my head, what is it that I'm going to do with my life? Three months in the black nun's convent will help me . . . I also, um, I also joined the choir at my Baptist church in Harlem, so that helped. But um, it was me getting all sick again.
>
> I: While you were living there?
>
> T: Yes, yes.
>
> I: What kinds of things were you experiencing?
>
> T: Mm, hunger and poverty, and I needed help, I wanted help badly. So I was just praying to Jesus, "Oh help me, help me, help me."

Teresa's narrative suggests a relational sensitivity, which she alluded to throughout the interview. It was the hunger and poverty of those she aimed to help that she felt so keenly. And yet, this was not simply an empathic reaction; her answer to the question reflected a merger in which the boundary between her and the world had dissolved. From an observer's perspective, Teresa had financial resources and sufficient food. From an intrapsychic perspective, however, Teresa was deprived and starving. This can be interpreted in terms of the erasure of a boundary that would have allowed her to feel contained—literally, bounded—and therefore psychically protected from the plight of the external world. It can also be interpreted in terms of Teresa's interpersonal longing, a felt need to be fully bonded with others. These interpretations are complementary. The yearning for a kind of preverbal love, in essence boundaryless, is rooted in the kind of connection that in ideal circumstances occurs in infancy with a primary caregiver. Unmet, this yearning persists and manifests and presses for fulfillment through connection in similar form (i.e., without boundaries). For Teresa, such fulfillment was met through fantasy, through her sense of unity with an anonymous group of others whom she imagined shared her pain, thus providing a kind of imaginative solution to her need for recognition.

Teresa's portrayal of what followed from this subsequent breakdown was consistent with the pattern previously delineated; she found solace and refuge in the love of another. Also consistent with her prior account of romantic dalliances, this love was grand and, although potentially based in some tangible experience, it had the flavor of fairy tale:

> And He [God] helped me. He, and Jesus, introduced me to Mamadou Johnny Blue Jay Sekka Cordobez. Johnny Sekka, I knew Johnny Sekka. Man-oh-man. Senegalese ambassador, Senegalese African actor. Millionaire actor. African actor. Tall, dark, and handsome. I loved him, and he loved me.

Almost seamlessly, Teresa's narrative transitioned from this into her current love affair with "E":

> He died and I was so, oh I was so sad when he passed away. I was so proud to say I knew Johnny Sekka. And I miss him so much. But you know what? I asked Jesus for another millionaire, and Jesus gave me a billionaire philanthropist, and then Jesus gave me another millionaire, in the E family, Montana. There it is, now we're up to date.

This last statement seemed to indicate a vested interest in glossing over the years in question. Teresa was content to luxuriate in the realm of her fantasied present reality, in which she could be the recipient of abounding love and affection.

Acquiescing to continue the interview, Teresa spoke about past difficulties related to her sexual development:

I: So, we're back at the convent.

T: Yes . . .

I: You lived there for three months and . . .

T: Yes . . .

I: . . . said you got sick again. Does that mean that you were depressed?

T: (sighs) I was a Catholic in the Baptist Church in Harlem. Harlem Baptist Church. The Baptist Church in Harlem. Wow, what an experience. And I was trim and slim and sexy and wanted and loved. Whew, nice, dynamite. But, here I was again, going out with men, going out with men that didn't understand me, or I didn't understand them. I didn't understand my feelings all the way back to my prom. I, I just didn't understand my feelings as a young black woman, mmm . . .

I: What feelings didn't you understand?

T: Sexual feelings. Being so tight with my boyfriend, wanted to be married first before I had sex, to be special, in that way. My mother says, "Teresa, you don't need a chaperone," like I had a chaperone when we were at the prom. I didn't need a chaperone anymore.

I: Did you need a chaperone?

T: (laughs)

I: Did you feel you needed a chaperone?

T: No (laughs and pauses) . . .

I: Where is your mind going? What were you just thinking about?

T: I don't know. Special, special, absolutely, positively, out of this world. Out of this world like astronauts, out of this world.

I: Did you know you were special at the time?

T: No, not really, not until now, not until E has come into my life.

Toward the beginning of this exchange, Teresa spoke to a kind of relational difficulty in which at some point, navigating her own feelings and the feelings of another became overly stimulating and taxing. Within this excerpt, her transition to the fantasy of her marriage to her beloved E appears to represent what emerged as a compromise between wanting to feel romantically loved and not knowing how to negotiate the complexity of intimacy in order to bring such a union to fruition. Teresa could imagine the ultimate conclusion represented in marriage, but the multiple ruptures and repairs through which intimacy builds remained unfathomed.

Teresa described her inability to maintain relationships with college friends and partners as well:

> T: The loss of love, the loss of love. When I was sexually intimate, with men, and just losing that friendship, that bond that's so close, so very tight, that's so very special . . . that can't be replaced . . .
>
> I: What do you think it was that caused you to lose those bonds?
>
> T: (shrugs) To . . . to hold on so tightly, to need, so sincerely . . . I was a very needy person. When I got sick, I wanted to hold on to my friends so close, and that turned away, that made my friends turn away from me, so I thought.
>
> I: Because they were scared of how much you needed them?
>
> T: (sighs) Yeah, they couldn't deal with that feeling that I have. They didn't know what to say or what to do with my mental illness because mental illness is so very misunderstood.
>
> I: How do you feel it's misunderstood in your case? How did you feel misunderstood?
>
> T: Mm, my wants, my desires . . .

Here again, the intensity of Teresa's interpersonal needs was apparent. It was both the misrecognition of her experience by others, and also the essence of Teresa's need—for a complete, unbounded kind of connection—that perpetuated her alienation. Teresa's abiding longing exposed a vulnerability to continual disappointment and loneliness.

For example, Teresa described the despair that ensued when she discovered that one man's interest in her did not match her own:

> T: . . . and what he wanted from me was to be his secretary, receptionist, and manager. Afterwards, after we made love together, he wanted a receptionist, secretary, and manager. Montana, I didn't want to be his secretary, receptionist, and manager, I've been there, done that.

> I: You mean you didn't want to be his employee after you had just slept together . . .
>
> T: Yes (laughs) . . .
>
> I: Right.
>
> T: Yes.
>
> I: That sounds understandable to me.
>
> T: I wanted to be his wife, I didn't want to be his employee . . . I wanted to be his wife, so, I wanted a bodyguard too!
>
> I: Did that end up leaving you feeling really upset? Was that one of the things that . . .
>
> T: Sad . . .
>
> I: . . . triggered a depression?
>
> T: Yeah, another depression . . .

There was an exaggerated quality to the adult relationships Teresa described. There appeared to be an absence of depth despite Teresa's apparent creativity and poetic sensibility. In addition, her repetition of the statement "I didn't need a chaperone" and the idea that she too would like a bodyguard suggests some worry about her own vulnerability and doubt in her ability to adequately protect herself. Teresa's sensitivity, both to disappointments in her personal relationships as well as to larger forces in the world around her—a landscape of racism, inequality, aggression, and sexuality—became especially activated as she began to develop into an adult and take on a role of subject and agent. Serious in her commitment to activism and philanthropy, Teresa made efforts toward pursuing these interests professionally but lacked sufficient support and the internal resources to become effective. Her relationship with E not only seemed to represent her desire to be loved and feel "special," but also to facilitate the kinds of social change that once fueled her passion and life purpose:

> So I'm like, "Damn this is a good life, I want a big part of it." So I said, "Jesus, I want a millionaire," and Jesus showed me a billionaire philanthropist, and then he showed me a millionaire in E . . . and he showed me a billionaire philanthropist . . . so I'm doin' okay, A-okay, I'm doin' fine. All this fame and popularity, I said, "Jesus, use my fame and popularity to

> end hunger and poverty in the world"; jobs, jobs, and more employment, that's my goal, that's my prayer, to have E and Teresa, use our fame and popularity to end hunger and poverty in the world, amen.

Within this, Teresa's attempt to address her felt sense of lack, both in love and work, is well captured. Her fantasy aptly encompasses fulfillment of her need for love and recognition by another person and by people more globally, while also allowing her to see herself as an effective change agent for good in the world.

ENCOUNTERS WITH PSYCHIATRY

Teresa's initial encounter with the mental health system occurred in the context of her first depressive impasse. She reported a mixed experience, in which she felt both helped, but also at times misunderstood, by her psychiatrists. Regarding her first experience with psychiatry, she recounted:

> T: And I went to see a psychiatrist in [City], and he said, "Teresa, all you need is, you don't need any . . . you don't need any . . . um, medication, you just need to quit the relationships with these men." I said, "Please, doctor, please put me on some kind of med." He said, "No."
>
> I: How come you wanted medication at the time?
>
> T: Because I got depressed, I got so very depressed. I was suffering from depression.
>
> I: And it sounds like your doctor felt that your depression was being caused by or made worse by the relationships . . .
>
> T: Yes . . .
>
> I: . . . that you were having with these men?
>
> T: Yes.
>
> I: Do you have a sense of why that was? Looking back do you agree with him? Were those relationships not healthy for you?
>
> T: Uh, no, I still believe in what I thought was causing my depression, um . . .
>
> I: Which was?

T: The anxiety with my courses of study, and the negative relationships that I had with these gentlemen, and like I said before, the torn relationship I had with my girlfriend.

I: Yeah . . .

T: Jane.

In the face of her psychiatrist's misrecognition, Teresa's depression deepened, ultimately leading her to take leave from college and return home. There she began seeing another psychiatrist who recommended electroconvulsive therapy (ECT):

T: Oh, that's when I was going to see Dr. G, a Trinidadian doctor . . . and he asked me, "Teresa, what was it, what is it that you would like to do?" I said, "Dr. G, I would like to graduate from college." He said, "Okay, keep me in your hands." Shock treatment. And it worked. I spent one year and a half, a year and a half without medication, and going to my last year, my senior year in college. It worked.

I: When you say, "it worked," what do you feel it did for you?

T: I was off of all medication, and I did not have to go to any psychiatrist. He was in [City], I was in [another city]. If I needed somebody, he would turn me on to a doctor [in my city] . . .

Teresa related that she agreed with the decision for ECT, particularly favoring this option over chemical intervention:

T: I didn't care for it [medication].

I: The idea of it, or the way it made you feel?

T: The idea of taking meds . . . I didn't care for it at all, Montana . . .

I: What did you think it said about you?

T: That I was sick, mentally sick. It was terrible to feel that way, that I was "sick," mental case, dirt . . .

I: Did that come from the outside? Is that like a message that you heard from other people?

T: (sighs) Yeah, from inside and outside.

The lack of helpful psychotherapeutic options that might have framed Teresa's suffering in terms of psychosocial stress and relational loss left Teresa with the ambivalence of accepting the "fact" that she had a biologically based mental illness. While from Teresa's account it seemed that one or more of her early psychiatrists viewed her difficulties within the context of psychosocial stressors, Teresa's portrayal of this experience suggested an overarching sense of invalidation. At some point in the interview, Teresa also alluded to feeling misunderstood, and possibly even being judged homophobically for suspected sexual interest in her female friend Jane:

> T: Right. They [psychiatrists] says, "Just get over it. You're a beautiful young lady, and you could have as many men in your life as you possibly can, so just get over this Jane thing, and get into a man thing in your life."
>
> I: Mhm, did you and Jane have a romantic relationship?
>
> T: No, that's what the doctors included did not understand.
>
> I: Okay.
>
> T: This lesbian relationship, the doctors wanted to know more about it.

While it was unclear whether Teresa's interest in Jane may have had an erotic component, what was clear is that Teresa's feelings were minimized and dismissed. Both medical and psychosocial intervention failed her. Shamed and stigmatized, Teresa was left to grapple with her feelings—about her relationships, losses, and about her depression and whether to take medication—largely on her own. This is an extraordinarily tall order for someone who is already mired in psychic collapse.

Teresa's resistance to medication continued to play out over the course of her adult years. She recounted multiple periods during which she rejected the medication she was given. For example:

> I remember throwing out my medication in the toilet over and over and over again, at least three times because I wanted the high, I wanted the mania, so what I did was threw out my meds three different times during my illness . . . throwing it down the toilet . . .

And later she recounted:

> When I had to be put on, back on the hospital, I said I took the wrong attitude. I says, "I don't need this. I don't need this hosp, this medication." (sighs) That was a terrible, terrible attitude I took from my doctors, my nurses, from my parents, from my sisters and brother. When I was in

prison, for six weeks, I didn't take one um, bipolar medication. That was an awful, awful thing.

These memories were untethered from any particular period in Teresa's narrative. Rather, they surfaced as part of a blurred timeline that Teresa conjured for the sake of the interview. Asked about when she received a diagnosis of bipolar disorder, she related, "I don't remember the time, I don't remember the day, all I remember was the experiences." This statement seemed to capture a broader trend in Teresa's presentation. The timeline between Teresa's graduation from college and the time of the interviews took on a kind of amorphous structure. The years were glossed over, eclipsed by fantasies of the present and future, emerging only in fragments. The moments during Teresa's interviews in which she took flight into her fantasied love affair with E represented some of the most coherent parts of her narrative, perhaps reflecting where her mind preferred to dwell.

Unfortunately, Teresa's encounters with the mental health system seemed to reinforce the misrecognition she had experienced in her early relationships:

> T: Uh, running around the hospital, so many hospitals, um . . . so many times being . . . held by the police, mmm . . . so very many hospitals that I was in [Hospital 1, Hospital 2, Hospital 3, Hospital 4], a lot, and they had like given me needles, putting me in the isolation unit, the isolation room, that wasn't good, wasn't good at all. They wouldn't explain to me . . . they said, "Teresa, you're smart enough to know what's going on with you," but I wasn't smart enough to know.
>
> I: Or maybe it didn't have anything to do with intelligence?
>
> T: (nods head) Yup, because if someone took the time to explain to me what was going on in my life at these times, maybe I would get better sooner.
>
> I: So, if you could talk to those people who were supposed to be helping you at the time in the hospital settings, if you could tell them what might have been helpful for you to hear, during those periods of your life, what would you tell them?
>
> T: Help me. I was just so afraid, so ashamed to say, "Help me," to ask for help, just a matter of, "Help me, would you please help me, whatever you could say or do to help me, please help me do it."
>
> I: What would have helped?

T: Taking time out . . . the doctors in the, in prison just say, "Take your meds" (gestures to mimic writing notes), "Teresa B took her meds," "Take your med," "Teresa B took her med" . . . I didn't even take my med.

I: So their responsibility was more . . .

T: Just their job . . .

I: . . . to the documentation end, you know, to document that they had done their job in observing you taking your medication, but . . .

T: . . . and that was it.

It is not difficult to imagine Teresa having many misgivings about the course her life took, including unprocessed feelings toward her family, friends, past romantic partners, and the mental health system. Unable to actualize the many hopes and dreams she had for her future, Teresa ultimately conformed to a lifestyle that fit within the ideology our society deems appropriate for a person diagnosed with what hospitals call a "serious and persistent mental illness." At the time of our conversations, she reported adhering to a medication regimen for her diagnosis of bipolar disorder, living in a residence with others similarly diagnosed, and participating daily at the clubhouse. She talked about having a positive relationship with her family members now that she had accepted her own culpability for their prior conflicts. Her other main source of support came through her participation in a "Clozaril Believers Group" which she attended weekly. Whatever personal sacrifices she made with respect to her feelings and desires, many were most likely unconscious decisions made to maintain ties to the important people in her life. Meanwhile, her fantasies about her love affair with E and their plans for the future can be seen as representing a compromise between living for herself and living according to others' expectations. In this way, she could have the life she wanted (at least psychically), while also having the security of family and a community.

Teresa's resilience and her charming disposition, friendliness, and naiveté were heartwarming and made her feel relatable, even while her tendency to live in a personal fantasy was at times distancing. Interpersonal relationships were traumatic and at their worst shattering for her, and her deep longing to connect and be the center of someone's universe spoke to this early trauma along with her desire to transcend it. Through her ability to establish affable rapport, she seemed capable of eliciting the love and adoration she yearned for, and hence creating a social support network for herself. Teresa's narrative, especially in those moments in which she articulated her desire to be heard by psychiatrists and other medical field staff, exposed her need for receptive therapeutic services that would allow her to make sense of her trauma and build vital internal resources. Provided with the opportunity to get the therapeutic help she needed, she may have been better equipped to navigate the challenging yet rewarding landscape of interpersonal love and to pursue her passion for social justice.

Chapter Eight

Kyle

A Conflicted Life

Secil Arac-Orhun and Michael O'Loughlin

Kyle, a Caucasian man in his fifties, was born and raised in a suburban US town. He held a college degree and was looking for a job at the time of the interview. Kyle has been struggling with psychiatric difficulties since his teens. At the time of the interview, he was living alone in the Fountain House housing program and supporting himself through disability payments. Although he had an education, as well as financial resources through his family, he reported his psychiatric difficulties as being too difficult to manage and he struggled with basic living skills, such as motivating himself, having friends, maintaining a job, and feeling safe. He had felt like an outsider since his teens. Kyle stated that he felt more connected to nature and animals than to people, as he found interpersonal relationships too complicated. He stated that he had disappointed the expectations of others, along with his own expectations for himself. Throughout the interview, Kyle frequently voiced his concern that he might not have much to offer for the interview, saying, for example: "I just hope I have enough to say, I don't know if I have much to say . . . I don't know if I have much to say . . . I just hope I can explain. I mean, I hope I have something to explain." In many ways, this paralleled his subjective experience that he did not have much to offer others in his interpersonal relationships.

THE BEGINNING OF KYLE'S DIFFICULTIES

Kyle reported that his difficulties began in the ninth grade. He elaborated on the difficulty he encountered navigating the social dimension of high school:

> I would say, like, um, uh, that around ninth grade . . . a little late in ninth grade is when I started not feeling well . . . I've been ill for, like, since high school, maybe. I have, I've been on medications since, since, early college, since early college, yeah, yeah. I, I really, I can't say that I was ill. I think I just . . . I just felt very isolated in high school, and I never, had—I felt like I just couldn't make any choices . . . I felt I had disappointed some people in high school. I just started going downhill, and, and, I liked this one girl, I think, in ninth grade, I, something, I was just too shy to, to fulfill, to help anybody out or anything. I just was too shy, and then I couldn't, I just couldn't navigate all these friends and people. And I have two older brothers, and they went through the same high school, and it's just so much pressure. It's just so much pressure.

Kyle could not pinpoint any one event that might have caused his past and ongoing psychic struggles. When asked about the difficulties that brought him to the situation in which he was living at the time of the interview, Kyle spoke primarily about his challenges with activities of daily living:

> I live, I live alone, in Fountain House housing . . . and, it—I used to have two roommates . . . I had that . . . them for nine years. For nine years I lived with roommates, and then I graduated to the, um, level one housing . . . and that gave me the opportunity to try to live alone, and it's, it's, it's fine living alone, but it's um, it's . . . I gotta say it's a little more disturbing than living with roommates (laughs). In some sense, uh, 'cause it's more chaotic, I, I can't . . . it's hard for me to plan my . . . hard for me to plan, hard for me to keep order in my apartment, and um, and motivation is like, uh, like, is, is pretty tough for me. It's like, today I just—uh . . . I'm lucky I got here (laughs). Um, but anyway, um, so I currently, um, I'm doing okay. I'm a little nervous that my niece might be moving in with me, and um . . . I'm a little nervous, I can't, I'm in a conflict. I really don't know what to do. I feel in some ways it would be good for me if she was there, uh, in—though it's just a one-bedroom apartment, I could give her a room, you know, but . . . it's, um, at the same time I'm very, um . . . ashamed sort of, of myself . . . in my current state. Um, like no one in the four years in my apartment, no one really has visited me there. . . . it's just hard for me to get along with people that are . . . it, it, it, that says something to me, it's kind of, that it's um . . . that something's not right . . .

ROLE OF ATTACHMENTS

Both intrapsychic and environmental factors seemed to have contributed to Kyle's suffering. Kyle was born into a family that was unable to meet his needs for recognition and attachment (Fonagy & Target, 2000a, 2000b; Kohut, 1977). A close look at his family dynamics and social isolation points to possible difficulties with temperament, attachment, and mirroring (Fonagy & Target, 2000a; Kohut & Wolf, 1978; Winnicott, 1971/1982, 1960).

Kyle was the third of three brothers and two sisters. His mother had an artistic profession, while his father worked in the legal field. Both of his brothers had been very successful; one of his sisters had been hospitalized several times due to psychiatric difficulties. Kyle explained: "There's a lot of pressure, especially if your brothers are doing well, and I have two brothers and two sisters, and, and my father, my mom were successful people." Kyle mentioned how he felt isolated from his family and noted his sense of being different. He had never been comfortable socializing for as long as he could remember:

> I guess I, I think I feel like I was afraid from the outside world, of the outside world of people when I was a young age . . . like, but my brother and I, we, if the doorbell rang, we'd run and hide. Uh, that was, we always did that, we did it jokingly, I think . . . My brother, yeah, we, we . . . if, if the doorbell rang or if the phone rang, we'd run . . . and we didn't enjoy talking to anybody outside the family or anything like that. I don't know if that's normal or what . . . but I continued that, I think.

Kyle reported that his brother was eventually able to step away from the cocoon of the family and could face the outside world. Kyle, however, continued to struggle with this. As a result, both at school and at home, he had a strong sense of being different than others. This became a source of narcissistic injury for Kyle, which further exacerbated his difficulties.

For Kyle, his house and being with his family felt somewhat safe, while he had difficulty tolerating the social arena outside his home. The mother–child relationship is important for children who struggle with temperamental vulnerabilities, attachment, and socialization, and may be a containing experience that can facilitate the child's growth (Grotstein, 1995; Klein, 1946). When parent-child attachment—which is crucial for emotional regulation—fails, the child may become vulnerable to psychiatric difficulties (Aulagnier, 2001). Kyle suggested just such difficulties in his early maternal relationship during his initial therapy experience when he was in college:

> K: Like, my mom, like I said, she was more gregarious. . . . It's possible she was . . . she wasn't—she's not a very strong person. Like, in some sense, my mom, and, and . . . I mean, I, she's a very generous person . . . She's a very generous person, but . . . but she, um, uh . . . and I don't know exactly what I mean by not being a very strong person.

I: Can you, like, try to, like, say a little bit more? Or what made you get that impression?

K: Well, like . . . I'm not sure it's my own impression. Like, I remember one time I had to go to see . . . I had to see, um, a therapist. Like, I had to see a therapist when I got back from college. It was the first therapist that I saw, and, um . . . she made the statement, the therapist . . . she, uh, to try to get a reaction out of me, she said, "Your mom is not a very strong person, is she?" And, and, and, I didn't know what to say, I didn't know what to say. It made me, it made me start thinking a little bit, but she—might not be . . . she, in other words, she might not be very well-read.

Perhaps Kyle's therapist intuited difficulties in their mother-son relationship. Mother-child bonding depends on mirroring and containment, which allow a child to learn to regulate her emotions. When the mother-child bonding fails, the child cannot build the internal mechanisms necessary to navigate interpersonal demands, leaving susceptibility to psychosis, psychiatric difficulties, and unbearable anxiety (Aulagnier, 2001; Lacan, 2002; Winnicott, 1982).

Kyle explained that if he were to be in a romantic relationship, he could have another person—a girlfriend—outside of the family to attach to, he would not have to be in the role of a referee between his parents. However, he had difficulty separating from his family and felt pulled into the parental conflict. A parental figure who will serve as a container for the child's anxieties is crucial for emotional regulation and the formation of the self. However, in Kyle's case, his parents were unable to attune to him to facilitate further development. Kyle appeared to have an enmeshed relationship with his mother, adopting a parentified stance, rescuing her at times when he felt that she was unable to protect herself. He remembered his anger toward his father for cheating on and eventually leaving his mother, and also his sense of responsibility for not having better extricated himself from the dynamic:

It was a real tough thing. I would have rather . . . but it was my—I considered it being my own fault, being a referee, because . . . I mean, it was basically, I could . . . if I had a girlfriend or something like that, or serious relationship outside the family, there's no reason I would have had to really care about this situation that much, you know. They could do it themselves, you know . . . But I, I think, um, I lacked the skills to, to really . . . not only social skills, but possibly the courage to really get into another relationship with somebody outside the family, you know, so . . . so it's . . . I don't blame, really, my parents or anything for what . . . for what, what happened. I mean, I sorta . . . I'm mad at my dad . . . (laughs). Let me tell you. I'm kinda mad at him, and, you know, it's horrible. One

> time, I—just, like, about five, six years ago, you know—it wasn't clear where my dad was going, and I went down to his office, and, and, for some reason, I said I better follow him. So I followed, and sure enough, he winds up at this woman's house. I was, I was extremely angry (laughs).

There were several reasons predating the affair that contributed to the strain in Kyle's relationship with his father. Kyle shared that he and his father had little in common and that his father was emotionally removed:

> My dad basically didn't talk. He never talked, for instance, about girlfriends, or he never talked about girls, me and girlfriends, or me and friends, or, me, uh, we would never have a conversation like that, you know. . . . He, he, my dad was probably a very shy person as well . . . I think my, my dad's a good person, a decent person and everything, and, but he, uh, he j-just, you just, you just couldn't talk to him about personal problems or anything like that.

Kyle felt as though his father did not understand him. His father's cheating created further stress on Kyle. It is not a coincidence that Kyle first initiated therapy during college, around the time that he discovered his father's infidelity. Kyle was emotionally unequipped to manage his feelings about the affair and his parents' conflict and he felt torn between them. Kyle entered college without having developed a foundation for effective self-containment, individuation, and emotional regulation.

NAVIGATING SOCIAL RELATIONSHIPS

Throughout the interviews, Kyle was sensitive to what the interviewer might ask and frequently voiced his concern that he might not have adequate information. This seemed consistent with his felt sense of needing to accommodate the needs of others, reflecting concerns about his own dependency needs and the self-sacrifice required to have those needs met. Kyle reported that he struggled with being different and with feeling that he was less than others for as long as he could remember; however, he recalled that his difficulties started in high school, when the demands of socialization placed more pressure on him. As social demands escalated, Kyle became increasingly withdrawn. Moreover, his brothers' relative success reinforced his sense of failure. During the interviews Kyle frequently recounted the pressure he felt to be like his brothers. His inability to keep up with them became a reminder of his inherent difficulties. Kyle felt that the expectations and perceptions of others defined him. As he struggled with his own identity, external social pressures became ways in which Kyle tried to measure himself. "To be more like a man," meant that he needed to smoke marijuana or become sexually active. At times the boundaries of whose expectations he was fulfilling became murky. Even as an eight-year-old, the messages he received about what it meant to be a man were shaping Kyle's perception of who he should be:

> It's funny, it's embarrassing, but I, I remember like, in the second grade, like, I went over to some friend's house, and, and the mother of my friend, or . . . they asked me a strange—not a strange, an embarrassing question: "Does your mom kiss you goodnight at night?" (Laughs). And I lied. I said, I said, "No, she doesn't." You know? A-a-and like, that, I think that, that was, um . . . sort of like, um, I think being a man was more like, that, um . . . you don't need your mom that much, or anything like that.

Kyle's interaction with his friend's mother reflects some feeling he had early on that his attachment to his mother was not age appropriate in the eyes of others. While he had to evolve socially, he could not navigate the demands and expectations of individuation. The demands of growing up caused tremendous difficulty and struggle. He recounted the trajectory of his isolation and depression during the course of his school years as follows:

> I had a lot of friends, I think. Had a lot of friends and was optimistic about, uh, things, um, didn't know what was gonna . . . the future would bring, and things of that sort. And, um, but was optimistic that there was something good about, um, maybe what was gonna happen about having a girlfriend, or just life had something good to offer. And, um, I sorta changed into this, um, thing where things became pretty dark. Became pretty dark. Life became pretty dark for me. And, uh, I didn't, I ended up . . . I decided to graduate early from high school, and, uh, that means I, so I took, I took classes, um, in tenth grade and I also took classes in eleventh grade when I was in tenth grade. So I tried to bunch up my classes, determining that I just wanna get out of here. That was my, that was my philosophy. My philosophy changed, and I was embarrassed in high school. I just wanted to get out of there. Everything changed.

Although Kyle had the intellectual capacity to complete school earlier than he was supposed to, the interpersonal demands were too much for him. Without the structure that high school provided, Kyle found himself floundering, ill-equipped to navigate college on his own. The expected transition to adulthood was too high a hurdle. Reflecting on his attempted foray into romantic and sexual relations, Kyle recounted:

> Socially, I never had a girlfriend in high school. It's disappointing. And college, really. I mean . . . college, I had one girlfriend but it didn't work

out either, you know, so . . . Um . . . I guess I . . . I just . . . I guess I thought she-she-she, um, she-she-she really wasn't, uh . . . I-I-I-I really don't know, I guess . . . it just . . . I didn't know why she wanted to be my friend, really. I don't know why. Uh, I, it-it-it seemed like there was some other reason besides me, some other reason besides me. I wasn't, I wasn't sure . . . she was a very popular person on . . . in college, on campus there. But, like, her name was [B]. She was, she was nice, very intelligent person, and uh, I . . . but I don't know. I just . . . I didn't feel too close to her or something like that, and if you don't mind me saying so, I know one time we slept together . . . and like, um . . . and I didn't do . . . I just like, um . . . I just smoked some grass, and grass didn't have a good effect on me. I wanted to be alone. I wanted to be alone, and so I just lied in bed and, just, that's it . . . You know, um . . . (quietly) . . . But I-I-I-I-I didn't . . . um, I-I-I-I didn't do anything. You know, like I just lied in bed there and, uh, and, uh . . . after that, everything went downhill.

During the interview, Kyle articulated the tendency toward dissociation he experiences when faced with interpersonal interaction. This vulnerability would inevitably be heightened by the intimacy demands of a romantic relationship. Describing his experience within the context of more superficial interaction, Kyle related:

K: It's like, day to day, I, I get the feeling that people, I mean, uh, I think they feel that I'm a phony. It's kinda painful, like, and like, the painful part is I might agree with them (laughs) . . . For instance, I'm afraid to take out my garbage in my apartment building, and I have to do it at night or something like that, you know, late at night. And, I'm afraid that people will see me and stuff like that.

I: What do you mean by phony?

K: That I might say things that are, have nothing, that just, that are not heartfelt, that are not heartfelt. For instance, today I was coming down the stairs, and I, I, this woman was coming up, and she had two bags. I said, "Do you need any help?" You know? And she said, "Oh, no thanks. My apartment's just right over there, just one more floor there," and I said, I said, "Oh, okay, fine." And then, for some reason, I said, "Oh, mighty cold outside, it's really cold outside," and she didn't answer back, and I, it just seemed like, why did I say that, you know? Like, I feel like I'm not grounded in this world, un-unfortunately. I-I-I-I, unfortunately, I've never really had a, um, had a girlfriend or anything of this sort, and um, that's, I think unfortunately might be the roots of my problem. I don't mean to say that but it's, I feel like, alienated and not true to what's really going . . .

Kyle's past was filled with regrets about his perceived deficits, most of which coincided with interpersonal encounters that were opaque for him. Kyle seemed to know that something was wrong, but he was unable to discern what it was. Kyle cited various interpersonal encounters as signifiers of his failure. He reported that he was unable to recover after these events, which included moments within his family, his school and friendships, his professional relationships, and finally his romantic relationships. During the interview, he shared his sense of failure about not having been able to achieve the developmental milestones that others around him had mastered:

> K: I don't feel very smart person, you know, I don't know, right now.
>
> I: R-right. Is there any way that people make you feel that way? Like, a way that they react, or the way they do something, that makes you feel like, um . . . that?
>
> K: W-well I . . . not in terms of the way they react to me but in terms . . . from my perception, it seems that people handle their life pretty well. Th-that's, that's all I can say. It seems people are accomplished. My brothers, they seem like accomplished people. They know how to talk to people. They know, they, um, they know how to, um . . . raise a family, maybe, or something like that, raise kids. A-and, um, p-people—everybody, they s-seem pretty good at life. People seem pretty good at life. I don't, I don't, I don't feel like I'm that good at it.

Consistent with his difficulty transitioning into adulthood, after graduating from college, Kyle also struggled to maintain employment. He remembered:

> I got a very good job at a museum. And, um, that job, um . . . became very difficult over about a year. And, um . . . it's just, there's just so much pressure and I just . . . it was a good job. I could have really made something of myself, I feel . . . um, in my field. I was working as a printer in the, um, basement of a museum in [a city], and just printing out business cards, and uh, film schedules, and things of that sort, with two other, um, colleagues, like, and . . . uh, also doing some photography, darkroom photography. But, um, I may—I don't know if it's a nervous breakdown or something but I, I, I reached some sort of like, um . . . like, climax or whatever. I don't know w-what it was but I, it's just like, I had to decide whether to stay or to go, and, um, I, I decided I better go, and so I left the job and, and after that I just sort of went downhill.

While both external and internal factors can affect self-esteem, at times internal attacks may be more powerful than external sources; this can culminate in depression (Mendelson, 1997). Kyle's inner critic frequently attacked his self-esteem and appeared to be much more powerful than the feedback others provided. For people struggling with self-esteem, having a capacity to love and work is challenging, and this challenge, in return, can further diminish their self-esteem (Mendelson, 1997).

AN UNSAFE WORLD

At some points in his life, Kyle's ability to make sense of his experiences became impaired and he felt unsafe. For example, he recounted a time during college—though he had similar instances in high school as well—when he became acutely anxious while under the influence of marijuana:

> And I really don't, as far as symptoms and, um, things of this sort, all I can say is that, like, sometimes I remember one of the bad symptoms was I smoked some marijuana in those days [in college] and whatever. And, um, actually we grew some or something. And, and there was a lot of pressure. My brother went to a big, uh, uh . . . went to a very good school, went to [prestigious] University, or whatever . . . My oldest brother was very smart. And he invited us up there. And, um, I remember, I just had like a nervous, sort like nervous breakdown. Smoking some reefer, I just could, I couldn't move. I couldn't move. And people were . . . I was paranoid, some sort of paranoid incident. I felt that I went to the bathroom in my pants. But I couldn't understand if I did or if I didn't. I just felt terrible, and um . . . it was excruciating. And so, um, I, that happened a couple times . . . Yeah, anxiety. Mostly just anxiety, and I just couldn't handle it. And, um, uh . . . so eventually, I went to college and then I got, I went to see a counselor at college, and, and the counselor said, "You might be ill," or something like that, and they gave me some, some medications and stuff . . .

Kyle recalled that these instances in college were not the only time when he struggled with feelings of intense fear and paranoia. Kyle's sense of feeling weak, intruded upon, and defenseless continued into his adult life. At times of intense fear and negative emotions, the boundaries of what and who is safe became indistinct for Kyle. He described how his first hospitalization resulted from a period in which he became consumed with thoughts about the government's involvement in the 9-11 attack and other domestic terrorism:

> K: Yeah. It was traumatic. It was pretty traumatic . . . because I was just going to the movies. And, and somehow I got into the hospital. I landed in a hospital, and I tried . . . but when I was there, like 9/11 was kind of, the city then, everyone was walking around with machine guns down in the subway . . . And it was, like, really, it was a bad scene.

> I: Yeah, very anxiety provoking.
>
> K: A lot of anxiety, but at the same time, in my head, I'm thinking, you know, this thing was sort of designed, in some way, I felt . . . desig—that 9-11 was designed. In particular, I thought these, these letters that contained anthrax, there were some letters that were sent that contained anthrax . . . Which is, um, uh, a powerful, um, um, chemical. Which if you open a letter y-you get killed, you're dead, or something. But I thought that our government was sending out those letters, and I made that point at the [hospital], at that some of these things are being designed, are, are designed, that the government is behind some of these things, and I think they took it, they took it like way too seriously or something like that. Um, but uh, anyway, um, I, I thought I was wrongfully put in the hospital then, but nevertheless I, um, I didn't, um, I didn't feel too good about things, about politics, and about illness. I got into a mess in a bad way, during that period . . . And so I don't know if it was anger . . . Or whatever, but it was something not too good.

Kyle's concern about the safety of presiding authority figures—expressed in his preoccupation with government terrorist plots—manifested in the hospital setting. He felt himself wrongly confined and was mistrustful of the medical staff. Furthermore, his persecutory thinking and its projection into his external world continued even when he tried to isolate himself and flee from society:

> I kinda went up to that cabin that my parents have . . . I went up there, and I started planting some apple trees, and . . . And I tried to make a go out of farming, and I also was doing some landscaping on the side for this, um . . . then things were going okay. And then I got a job, like, in this yoga place, um, that was like, um, a retreat, a yoga retreat center. And, um, that went pretty well because I could identify with people in-in there, and I was of course living alone in, in the woods, kind of in a dirt road, and um, it was good to have a job. I was lucky to have a job. And I had the job for about two years, and then, like, um, I'm not positive, but like I wasn't, I didn't really hear any voices or anything like that but it was just, like, I thought like, some people in [a city], like, like I thought an old therapist that I'd seen was making some—was sort of directing some people at the job . . . I didn't know what she was planning. And, um, so I—ultimately I made a mistake on the job, and they s—and I'm not sure if I left or they let me go, I'm not sure, I think I just left, um, and um, and then I got very upset and I—was at the cabin, and um, I believe I might have tried to hurt myself. I did hurt myself a little bit, and I, I felt—I better drive myself to the hospital, or something like that. And so that's

> what I tried to do—uh, and, uh, and I—from what I remember (laughs), the guy was just like, he was just like, really mad at me, the doctor, um, and—and just like making fun of me or something, and—and, like, I . . . so he put some stitches on me and—and stuff like that, and sent me back.

Kyle also suffered from tremendous persecutory feelings toward himself. After losing his job, his anger, humiliation, and desperation became overwhelming. Furthermore, with such a sense of loneliness, Kyle found himself frequently questioning his purpose in life:

> I: What keeps you trying?
>
> K: Well, um . . . I, I, I, I don't think it comes from inside me. I don't think there's anything inside me (laughs). You know? I think it's really, unfortunately, I think it's, um . . . which is not a good answer, not a good answer, but I, I think that it's, it's mostly, um, peer pressure (laughs) that keeps me trying, y-you know? It's like, um, and plus it's, I, I mean, it's . . . I'm afraid. I'm afraid of, of, of, of-of, of death and things of that sort. Uh, or, pain, fear of hurting myself, you know. I, um . . . used to, maybe, did some damage to my arms and stuff like that.

CRITICAL FAMILY, CRITICAL SOCIETY

Throughout the interviews, Kyle expressed anxiety about how people would perceive him and specifically that his struggles would be misunderstood. This concern perhaps stemmed from the kinds of responses he received within his family. Kyle reported that his sister was diagnosed with bipolar disorder and had been hospitalized on several occasions, but that this was not discussed in the family. Kyle could not pinpoint the source of his discomfort but noted some concern about being judged by his family:

> I: Was your family judgmental of you?
>
> K: Um . . . I, I, I, I think a li . . . i-i-i-it, um . . . i-i-i-it seems like, it seems like they are, but I'm not positive. I'm not positive.
>
> I: Yeah . . . In what ways did you understand their judgments?
>
> K: Well, like right now. I mean, for instance, I can't ask my brothers over to my, to my, I've never really told my brothers that I was on benefits, that I had an illness.

As a result, Kyle felt more comfortable in nature, as he did not perceive judgment in nature:

> Basically, it, it made me want to be alone more because, um, there was less people around, less people would j-judge you . . . And nature, uh, I became much more fond of being in nature . . . 'cause there's no judgment in trees and mountains and things of that sort. But people . . . I don't know. It just . . . yeah, I guess I really don't have much to say.

Kyle did not feel like his family understood his distress; he reported that his father had even told Kyle that therapy was a waste of money, despite the fact that Kyle needed therapeutic support to survive. This view reflected the prevailing perspective of the family:

> I think, people in the family believe that it's a weakness to have to go to see a th—psychotherapist . . . I did seem incredibly weak, uh, during the process, uh, you know, so I can't really, I agree . . . (laughs). I mean, I don't agree with them, I just, all I know is I felt like a weak, I mean very, defenseless.

At a certain point, however, Kyle's mother did support Kyle seeing a therapist. Her approach changed when, during college, his psychiatric struggles became too severe to deny. Still, Kyle seemed to hold an idealized view of his family, leaving him inadequate in his failure to fulfill their expectations. His attempts to keep his psychiatric difficulties a secret likely contributed to him feeling "phony." Kyle stated that he had not told his family about the extent of his psychic distress. As much as Kyle related that he did not want to judge his family's approach to his psychic struggles, it left an indelible impact. For Kyle, his family's view of therapy as a waste of money was a reason for embarrassment, humiliation, and further alienation from his own family, even though it was something he truly needed. One tragic effect of his family's stance was the way Kyle internalized the necessity that he circumvent psychiatric hospitalization—even when he needed it—out of concern that it would be funded by taxpayer money. He came to see his own needs as burdensome to society, which inhibited him from receiving the care he needed:

> K: I . . . there's been times where I very much wanted to go into the hospital, but um . . . I tried to, um, hold back, uh, from going in because it's expensive (laughs). And, like, um, that's the main reason I try to hold back: it's, it costs money. Not . . . I mean, for the taxpayer. For the taxpayer. I wouldn't have to pay, but y-you know, somebody's gotta pay, I guess, and so I-I don't even feel comfortable, even though, like, about, like, [the] last couple years I had to struggle for about six months to stay out of the hospital, I would say. It was a, it was a big struggle to stay out, um . . .

> I: So you mentioned, eh, the taxpayers and mentioned that you had to struggle, but you didn't go to the hospital, in part, because it would be a burden on the taxpayers?

> K: That's part of my reasoning . . . for not to go, not to go. It's like, it's . . . I guess I also, I didn't want it to get into a pattern that, that if I start feeling really bad that I should go into the hospital, a-and maybe that was, I always thought I could, could bear the anxiety a little, little bit more. So, um, I, uh . . . I don't know if it was the right choice or not, you know?

Kyle's shame about the course his life had taken came through in the interviews time and time again. He worried about being a burden to his family and to society and felt ashamed for needing the supports he received:

> I can't, I can't, I haven't been able to make money. I, there's a lot—when you're on benefits, I just wanna say that, uh, there's a lot of pressure. There's a lot of pressure, especially if your brothers are doing well, and I have two brothers and two sisters, and, and my broth—my father, my mom were successful people. And if you're on benefits, it's, it's just a lot of pressure. It comes from everywhere. You just go to the—food stamps, and the cash register. It's like, you know, y-y-y . . . I live in a fairly poor neighborhood in _____, and gosh, other people are paying money, and I, I have, I'm like, uh . . . blond hair, blue eyes, and I'm, I have food stamps or something. And it's just like, uh, it-it's kinda like, there's just not enough to go around, and-and-and, um, I mean that-that's one pressure, that's one pressure, maybe just at the cash register, uh, um . . . of, with food stamps. Um, the other pressure is, um . . . w—I mean, my, all my social activities, everybody says, "What do you do?" You know, that's the first question, "What are you doing right now?" What can I say? I'm struggling with some vague illness . . . And I'm not even sure I do have an illness, but some vague illness, and I'm on benefits? You know, that's like . . . basically I've been on unemployment, unemployment benefits for fourteen years now, and it's very, it's tough—it's degrading, it can be degrading to you.

Kyle's difficulties in connecting with others extended beyond his family and early peer relationships. He reported some feeling of dissonance about his belonging to Fountain House, reflecting internalized shame about his failure to live up to his family's standards for success:

> K: I would never invite my brothers here or anything like that, but that's just my own personal thing . . .

> I: If you invited your brothers here, what would they think? Or feel, for you?
>
> K: Um, they would just say, "You can do better than here. You can do better. You can do better" (laughs). You know, I think they would just say, "You're not that, you're not that ill. Why are you here? Why, wh-get moving," you know? . . . it's hard—there's high standards in the family, and I don't know if I'd live up to them. You know? Too high. Too high for me.

Kyle's words illustrate a painful sense of not belonging. He feels that there is no place for him in his family, social circle, or neighborhood, nor is there even a place for him in the clubhouse to which he belongs.

NAVIGATING LIFE

The demands of college life became too much for Kyle, so he dropped out of the university he had initially attended. After a brief recovery period, he completed his bachelor's degree at another university. Still, his struggles continued. His passion for nature led him to aspire to earn a master's in environmental science; however, he reported being unable to meet his research advisor's expectations, so he left the program. Afterwards, Kyle worked at a variety of jobs but usually quit them as a result of interpersonal difficulties, the demands of the work, or the paranoia he experienced from time to time. These kinds of difficulties emerged in his pursuit of creative opportunities as well:

> Sometimes, peoples' expectations, or I believe, maybe, the perception I have of peoples' expectations, I just—sometimes I—it's just too much. And I feel people were asking for an awful lot after the exhibition. They wanted more drawings, more things, and it was just, like, I don't know. I couldn't handle the pressure of it; it's as simple as that. I'm not enough of an artist. I didn't have enough skill and, and, um . . . confidence in myself to really give them what they wanted, and uh . . . so that's the way I feel. That's what happened. If anything happened, I felt I just didn't have enough confidence in myself . . . and that kinda goes back to the idea of me being a phony. Uh, me being a phony, because, remember, I went to a school which was pass/fail and did visual arts. I just, very easy.

When all of his family and some family friends came to the exhibition, the occasion became a source of shame for Kyle, rather than an opportunity for him to be proud of his accomplishments:

> I would have preferred to go into the hospital rather than, than go to that exhibit, but-but I did. I forced myself to go . . . I felt extremely anxious, and . . . Most of all, the worst part about it was that, um . . . like, when I go outside, there's no, there's, I guess I mentioned, not having a girlfriend is like, it's not just, like, I think, like, a lot of people, like, they may get married, and they sort of are able to hide, in some sense, about, you know, you don't have to expose yourself so much if you have either a girlfriend, or . . . so I just appeared alone. And uh, I had no friends, and um . . . and everyone else came to the openings.

Kyle's profound sense of loneliness and tenuous self-worth emerged as major themes over the course of the interviews. As the conversation progressed, his mood appeared to grow increasingly morose. Experiencing unbearable isolation, Kyle questioned the purpose of his life and perhaps thought about giving up:

> It's possible. But, when I say "give up," it's just like, it's sort of like saying, well, I'm-I'm-I'm-I'm so old, I'm this amount of years, and . . . um, you know, I'm not gonna get married, I'm not gonna have a family, and I'm not gonna be a wealthy person. I'm not gonna be a very skilled person. And so, basically—when I was up at my mom's place, I just felt so, you know, I mean I'm feeling so depressed that I, that I, I felt like, I don't mean to say this but I feel like I want to just crawl into a coffin. Crawl into my grave . . . When I tried to clean up my room this morning, I noticed some things—the coffee has been there for months . . . And, like, there's, um, there's only a plate in my apartment for me . . . So I don't know, you know? Like, I'm buried under ten feet of snow, or twenty feet of snow, or mud, and I just can't get out, and it's just overwhelming, and there's no place to start. I can't dig myself out, you know? It's just, it's like, um . . . and so, um, uh . . . but the pain is really in trying.

As Kyle talked about giving up and about his deep depression, his feelings fluctuated between darkness and hope:

> And, but that's beside the point. The point is that, yeah, th-there's pain. I've tried many times, it's a battle, it's a battle to, you know, I haven't completely given up. If I had, I w-would, I probably wouldn't be here now. Or I wouldn't, I wouldn't have bothered to come to the interview, maybe (laughs). You know, or something like that, maybe. I don't know. So I haven't completely given up, I might say, or I might think to myself that I have. But I don't, I don't, I, I guess I haven't, so I keep on trying. I keep on trying, you know to um, uh . . . put on and wash, put on and wash my clothes, and take a shower maybe, and-and hopefully.

Although Kyle did not feel comfortable defining himself by his creative talent, at the end of the interview, he gifted Secil a souvenir that he had handcrafted, which was how he wanted her to remember him.

CONCLUSION

Kyle's difficulties appear to result from deficits in environmental provision in his family which left him lacking in confidence and quite resourceless in interpersonal situations. Despite his endearing presence and his motivation, sadly Kyle has had major struggles in the core areas of love and work and he experiences considerable loneliness, sadness, and some shame. Kyle's sense of isolation and longing for connection were palpable. He stated that he had been attending the same clinic for the last thirteen years and had felt that the staff had given up on him. Kyle has not had the opportunity to benefit from insight-oriented therapy, which would have the potential to give meaning to his struggles and help him find the motivation to move forward and live a more fully engaged life.

Chapter Nine

Courtney

A Misrecognized Woman

Secil Arac-Orhun and Michael O'Loughlin

Courtney was a smart, funny, insightful, thirty-four-year-old, Caucasian woman. She spoke of her life story with frequent pauses, which pointed to the difficulties and struggles she had both in her past, and while retelling it. As she struggled, she was insightful at moments, and confused at other times. She used self-deprecating laughter and she often gazed to the side while recounting her experiences. She also appeared fragile and vulnerable. She frequently lost her train of thought, perhaps a manifestation of her tendency to dissociate as a way of coping with difficult, unbearable emotions which understandably were stirred up by the interviews. Courtney's life story was marked by trauma, including sexual abuse by her father and denial by her mother and sister. Courtney's core struggles revealed recurrent violation of her physical and emotional boundaries by caregivers and authority figures, misrecognition and invalidation of her struggles, and emotional isolation. Her narrative also shows the ways she dealt with multiple levels of trauma, the complex system of coping mechanisms she employed, and the intricacy of her psychic structure.

ABUSE

Courtney grew up in a chaotic family. Her family consisted of her mother, a former nun who started working after Courtney turned four; her father, who also worked, and her sister, eighteen months younger. Her parents were married until she was in her teens, and then got divorced. The family dynamics were complex with a shared pattern of secrecy and denial. For example,

Courtney's father was an alcoholic, but her mother did not acknowledge to Courtney either his addiction or the abuse that Courtney was enduring. When he behaved inappropriately, the family did not talk about it. Courtney explained:

> If he came, if he showed up to a school play or something, he would come late, he would interrupt, he would . . . like, fall, he was very clumsy, and my mom was under the impression that that's just the kind of person he is, he's just a clumsy person. But I know that he used to drink, so I'm guessing that when he was in the bedroom, he was drinking, and then—you know, the reason he's forgetting things all the time and showing up late is 'cause he's drinking. I don't know, but I'm guessing that that's really what was going on . . .
>
> He used to bring strange women to the apartment and he would do nude photography, in the apartment, and my mom would take us out of the apartment, we would go to the park or the museum; and then they were all over the wall, so I grew up with, like, seeing nude strange women, like, photos all over the apartment. And they took them down after the, uh, supermarket delivery guy, like, he saw them, and he made—and my—when mom went to the supermarket, she heard, they were Haitians, so she heard them talking in French, she understood what they were saying, they were talking about it, so she, they took them down.

Thus, unless there was an outsider to witness the inappropriate behavior, no one acknowledged it. Her description depicts how odd her environment was for Courtney growing up. As a child, Courtney was made uncomfortable by the nude pictures and her father's behavior, but only as an adult was she able to acknowledge that it was problematic:

> Now it makes me uncomfortable, to think of it happening, because it's so obviously inappropriate, like so obviously inappropriate, um, I just remember kind of like, well, people have photos of their family on the wall, they don't have photos of like, strange, black-and-white pictures, of people they don't know. Especially people they don't know without clothes. I remember the women not looking that happy, which is a little disturbing. Um, like very awkward, like maybe . . . so I guess that's really, I just thought it was strange. But . . . I didn't understand it, but I didn't ask.

Courtney was a victim of recurrent sexual abuse by her father, and her story is also marked by misrecognition of her struggles by her family who could have been a source of support for her. Courtney recounted the abuse this way:

I: Can you say, what—like what was your take on what was going on?

C: Well, my father was sexually abusing me, from when I was very young. And I was very scared. And I didn't tell anybody. And, he threatened to kill me and . . . so that was really hard for, since like, I mean, believe it or not, I know it's hard to believe that I remember, but since I was like three or four.

Courtney's father perpetually violated her boundaries, often in an egregiously coercive manner. For example, he gave her alcohol and possibly other substances when she was a child to render her defenseless:

C: I know that uhm, when he was abusing me he, he would give me alcohol. And ah . . .

I: Do you remember?

C: I, what?

I: Do you remember that? The taste? How you felt?

C: I remember laughing, but I don't . . . it was when I was very young. And he put it in chocolate milk, and it was like this is special chocolate milk, you get to drink it only in Daddy's room, and I got to blow, like, the um, the bubbles in the chocolate milk, with the straw, which my mom hated, you know, blow so many bubbles that I, that they ah, came out of the glass. But . . . when I was older, and I would try to fight him off, he would . . . I don't think it was alcohol, I think he gave me drugs, honestly. I think he gave me drugs because he would hold my nose and make me drink it . . . I don't think it was alcohol.

The effects of these traumatic experiences surfaced in different facets of Courtney's life. She felt depressed from very early on. Courtney recounted how her suicide attempt, at age eleven, was her way of trying to escape:

I was in Girl Scout camp. I was away for two weeks. And I knew I was counting the days to go back. And I didn't want to go back. And then when I got back, I tried again, I tried to hang myself but it didn't work. I didn't know how to kill . . . [laughs] I mean, it's not funny. I didn't know how to do it effectively 'cause I was a kid, like, I didn't think to take pills, you know. I just knew, like, from the movies, if I jump off some place, or if I try to hang myself, but it didn't work. I fell, like [laughs] I, like, I hooked up the jump rope to the door and I shut the door, but you know, I didn't know how to hang myself, you know, I just didn't know.

Afterwards, she related that she was trying everything to avoid her father, because she thought that if she did not kill herself, he was going to kill her. Escape in any possible way appeared to be a good idea to Courtney's eleven-year-old self. She spoke of her attempt to self-regulate unbearable affects:

> [S]elf-injury from like fourteen, I mean a lot a lot, I mean, trying to run away, how I was, you know . . . self-esteem . . . I was fifteen, but I was like, taking my mom's liquor so I could go to sleep. So I would just, after she went to bed I'd have a little drink and I'd go to sleep. And then when I was seventeen, I started drinking every day. I stopped going to school . . . I was just numbing myself.

Courtney started to have a crisis (e.g., drinking, running away) in middle school and high school.

> And then when I was fifteen, I—I guess I kind of snapped. And that's when I stopped showering and I stopped brushing my hair I stopped. I was cutting school I didn't go over there anymore. . . . School, wanting people to even hug me, not making friends, not doing good in school, self-injury from like fourteen, I mean a lot a lot, I mean—trying to run away, how I was you know—self-esteem.

The isolating and painful impact of abuse made Courtney feel lonely and separated from her surroundings and her peers:

> I hated everybody, I didn't . . . I didn't, I had maybe a couple of friends, but I didn't really; I just wanted to be alone. Also, I was in physical pain from being abused so I didn't really, I just wanted nobody to touch me, I didn't really . . . I started drawing a lot, you know, I didn't, I just didn't really, I didn't understand like playing sports or games, like, I just really was by myself a lot.

Eventually her parents got divorced, after which her father usually did not spend time with the family. However, Courtney visited him at his home and the abuse continued. Courtney was now left unprotected, and she lived in a state of terror, fearing for her own life:

> I: Uh, you mentioned uhm, feeling scared. Both as a child and then like for example, you trying to jump off the tree, and feeling scared to tell anyone. Yeah a lot of things you were holding in.
>
> C: Yeah, I was too scared. Because I had tried . . . I was going to his house after school, and he told me that if I said anything, he would tell my

> mom that I ran away, but he would really kill me and hide me somewhere. So I really thought that he would do that.

Egregious examples of her father's abuse will be revealed later in the chapter during the discussion of the return of Courtney's repressed memories.

Ferenczi (1988) noted that after experiencing sexual abuse children often felt confused and split. He theorized that this split feeling was a consequence of identifying with the aggressor and that when the abused child introjects the aggressor, "he [*sic*] disappears as part of the external reality, and becomes intra- instead of extra-psychic" (Ferenczi, 1988, p. 228). Afterwards, when the external threat ends, the child feels confused about the nature of the threat, as the aggressor has been introjected (Ferenczi, 1988). In this vein Courtney recalled:

> [W]hen I was younger, I knew something was wrong, but I didn't know what to say. And then I wouldn't know how to say it. And ah, then I was afraid he was going to kill me so I didn't say anything. But again it's confusing 'cause my, I don't remember so much of my life. It really depends, like, which part remembers it. So I don't know. I remember feeling like I was bad. It was me. Well, I just felt I was the one causing all the trouble. You know, and to be told when I'm growing up, you're just too sensitive, you have a big imagination, you know, and then later on, you know, you have mental illness, you—you know to just be dis—disregarded is really hard because I did it to myself. I learned how to do that to myself. I mean that basically taught me not to believe my own eyes.

Several other important figures in Courtney's life were emotionally unavailable, behaved inappropriately, or were abusive. Many who could have provided safety and emotional support also betrayed Courtney's trust. This list included her mother, sister, stepfather, school counselor, and some of her therapists. Courtney recalled her mother and sister denying her experiences. For example, when Courtney talked about a difficult day at school, her mother would change the topic, and when she was going through a difficult time, her mother sent Courtney to live with her father. Courtney's school counselor, rather than providing safety, also crossed important boundaries, "he [school counselor] would talk about sex but he never touched me, but he uhm, he was very un- it was just very unprofessional." In fact, most of the channels that Courtney approached for help were denied and closed to her. During high school, she began drinking and using drugs to numb her pain. She recounted:

I: What was going on in high school; do you remember what were you feeling?

C: I was very angry, I was very depressed, and I didn't know why. I wasn't doing well in school, and I was doing things, like I was yelling at teachers, and I didn't have any friends and—I was just—I wasn't showering, I mean I really was not—I mean I would stink so bad kids wouldn't sit next to me. Like it was really . . . they sent me to the guidance counselor in high school, who ended up being abusive, so it was really a bad [laughs], it was a very . . . not sexually but, um, like he would talk about sex but he never touched me, but he was very un-it was just very unprofessional . . . I did end up going to see a therapist at a youth clinic while I was in high school but not for a long time. So, but basically my mom, she, she kicked me out of the house, and she sent me to live with my father who had been abusive. But I hadn't told anybody so it was just a mess. And then I started doing drugs, so I didn't and, I didn't get the help that I, that I could have.

RE-EXPERIENCING THE TRAUMA: "THE REPORTER"

Years after the trauma, after Courtney had moved away from her mother's house, and after many years of therapy, Courtney was able to recall her repressed child self and remember the significant abuse she endured. Before making sense of her dissociation, as a young adult, Courtney was sexually involved with men who either violated her boundaries or were abusive. Courtney appeared to be reenacting the trauma through this behavior. In many instances of chronic abuse, dissociation is the only way victims can endure the mental pain engendered (Garland, 1998). For Courtney, dissociating allowed her to function. As an adult, having had some distance from her father, Courtney was eventually able to feel safe enough to process some of her early experiences with her therapist, displaying the catastrophic split behind her dissociative response. Through this she discovered child versions of herself that communicated repressed memories with her adult self. This connected Courtney to a time in her childhood when she had endured unspeakable abuse, the child versions of Courtney were communicating with the adult Courtney about the trauma she endured as a child. Courtney referred to her dissociated selves as "they" or "she" or "the reporter." She did not fully recollect the sexual abuse until a few years ago when one of her younger selves began "talking" to her:

I: How did you feel? At that time?

C: I didn't remember what happened with him, so . . . as I was living there I started to remember some weird things, which is like when I was talking about the writing, the writing, the one who writes to me, I remember more, but . . . uh, you know like the pieces she remembers of when things were happening connects with the pieces I remembered when I was fifteen . . . he had like a storage bed, and it had a door under the mattress, and he would put me in there. And um, he would uh . . . he threw a box of tissues, 'cause I wouldn't stop crying, so he threw a box of tissues at me, and a red towel to clean up, because we, he had just had sex with me, and I was bleeding . . . and um, so I was down under this be . . . you know I was short, and the bed is like maybe this high, so it was like a good, like six . . . like a coffin, basically. But wide, you know it was like a king-size bed, that's like this high, and um . . . so I guess he left the tissues and the towel in there, for years, because when I was helping him pack up his apartment to move into the two bedroom where I was going to live with him, he told me "can you go in and get the videotapes out of there to pack up?" So I said okay, and he must have forgotten, and there were all the tissues, and I remember seeing what is all these tissue, what is all this, this is gross! Why'd you have this in here? And I remember he got very quiet, and he just wouldn't look at me, and he would just turn his back, and I was like "Dad, like, what is all, what is this? Get me a garbage bag, this is gross!" And um, he got me a garbage bag, and uh . . . so I remember . . . that happened when I was fifteen. But I didn't remember that I was the one who was in the bed. I didn't remember where that stuff came from. And then when the Reporter was writing to me, she wrote out the memory, so now I know how it got that way . . .

After years of therapy, Courtney started to experience alters that were different personality states that relate in different ways to the environment and self. At one point in the interview, she recalled the first time she came into contact with one of the split selves she had been protecting:

I: You said, you talked about escape and also about having different sides to your identity. Parts to your identity, yeah. And, I wonder how—when did you first realize that and how did that come about? What do you make of it?

C: When did I realize that's what was happening?

I: Mmhmm

C: Last April, I hallucinated myself talking to myself. But it was like me when I was, it was me when I was eleven, and so she was sitting on my chair and talking to me. And I got very scared, and I called my therapist.

> And she, she didn't really know what was happening at first, but then, she [the split self] was telling me things that I didn't want to hear, like she wouldn't leave me alone, like she was following me all the, all day and, talking, you know, talking to me, and then she was making me write. Like, she's called "the reporter," she was making me write; basically she was talking to me through writing, and um, so I told my therapist more about that, and then we started to figure out what was going on. 'Cause I didn't have memories of, at all, for . . . for many . . . most of my childhood.

The repressed and dissociated memories made Courtney feel out of control. Recalling the painful memories was scary and difficult for her. Yet, as she started to make sense of her memories, that process gave her a measure of control.

The capacity to symbolize depends on a properly functioning internal container, which develops through internalization of a containing object. In trauma, this internal container is either lost or damaged (Garland, 1998). In Courtney's case, her mother and sister were not available to hear her trauma and act as allies. This lack of support and containment left Courtney with experiences that were too anxiety provoking to hold in mind. As a result, although she was able to recognize that something was troubling her, she was unable to discern what it was:

> I didn't really know what was happening. I didn't know, like, I didn't see the bigger picture because I, each part was, different parts were going into therapy so I didn't . . . [laughs] they didn't really know about each other. You know, but they . . . but I always kind of knew something was wrong. That's what I mean, I mean, I knew, like, I wasn't functioning good at work, I was having a lot of trouble holding a job or focusing or going to school or making friends or getting in bad relationships, like, I knew stuff was wrong, but I didn't know how to get better. Like, I didn't know what was going on.

On several occasions during the interview, Courtney forgot what she was talking about or got lost while talking about painful things, which may have been Courtney's way of dealing with emotionally difficult memories and thoughts. She at times asked, "I don't, was that your question? How did I . . . when was something wrong?" or "What did you ask me?"

Reflecting on the roots of this dissociative process, Courtney related:

> I think that's when I started to develop different parts; I remember one was a protector and she would have a sword, and she would, like, do magic spells, you know, like thinking, I . . . I made ways to deal with it,

> with kind of protect, like for me . . . you know. I, I didn't have any power but I made different parts to protect myself from him.

As Courtney's mother and sister were not allies, and the caregivers responsible for her safety were either abusive or dismissive of her abuse, she developed a "protector" self that attempted to care for her and protect her from harm.

A FAMILY IN DENIAL, A TRAUMATIZED MOTHER

Courtney's mother's and sister's indifference and denial compounded her confusion and suffering. Implicitly, Courtney understood that denial and repression were required. When she talked about her trauma, she was punished by being ignored and abandoned. She described her mother as unavailable and overwhelmed:

> I was very scared to, to say anything. And my mom was very overwhelmed, so I think really just . . . kind of fell through. I mean, she just didn't know how to help me, and I don't come from a big family and it . . . also very isolated family, and but, I mean I . . . you know it's those things, like when family is so close they don't want to see what's going on but, you know if there had, I just was very isolated even as a kid and even in my family. So, but there was things wrong going on for a very long time.

Mirroring of a child's experiences is essential to the wholeness and unity of the child's self-concept (Lacan, 1977), but Courtney did not receive the validation she needed. Further, she was criticized for her reactions. Courtney's mother's inability to accept and reflect Courtney's experience back to her in a helpful way was experienced by her as a betrayal. At the same time, Courtney started to doubt her own experiences. Although Courtney tried to elicit empathy, understanding, and validation from her mother, the way her mother rejected her left Courtney feeling abandoned. She explained, for example, how her mother denied the abuse when Courtney first attempted to tell her about it:

> I told my mom when I was eighteen. I remembered part of it, but not a lot, and I told her. And I was like, "Did you ever leave me alone with him?" You know, I just didn't remember like how it would happen, but I remembered part of it. And she said no. She was like, "You're very sick." She's like, "I'm sorry you, I believe you believe this happened, but it didn't happen, and you know, you need to go see a doctor," and that was it, basically. That's what, and I tried to talk to her about it many times.

Courtney was denied her own experience by her mother and sister employing a form of abuse known as gaslighting:

> I confront them and . . . my mom and my sister, about it now, and they don't believe me. So that's a whole other thing, like when I was eighteen, I confronted them but, and I tried a couple more times, but they don't believe me . . . basically it colored every, everything . . . Some of them I remembered and then, but I must have tried at least five or six times and I even went so far as one time, I just couldn't take it, and I stopped talking to her. And I moved away, and I didn't tell her where I was going, I just couldn't handle that she wasn't believing me.
>
> And then, when I remembered more . . . she was always, like, "Well, if it really happened, you would know details." So then when I told her the entire incident, I told her over the phone and she was crying, and I was crying, and I thought well maybe she believes me, and then she left me a message on my phone saying how sick I was and you know, the, how could I do this? How could I make something like that up, and my sister, I asked her, I don't know how old I was, because I asked her again when I was like in my late twenties, I asked her, and she said "No." She said, "You already asked me that." And I said "Really? I don't remember."

Courtney's mother's inability to tolerate her daughter's suffering had a profound impact. Her relationship with her mother was filled with conflicting feelings of being loved and having fun with her mother on one hand, and feeling like her mother had betrayed her on the other. Courtney talked about her mother not having the capacity to tolerate her struggles:

> She seems to think that I was kind of just born with mental illness; she doesn't believe anything [laughs]. I mean, she just thinks I was born this way, which I mean . . . if she can't deal with all this stuff, it would make sense if someone can't deal with this happening—they don't want to accept they had a part in it—then it makes sense that she would be in denial. And yes, it's been happening since I was so small that it wouldn't maybe look like it's been happening my whole life, maybe I was born that . . . she thinks I'm like, very oversensitive, or like, I'm disturbed.

After a while, Courtney gave up any hope of trying to convince her mother. She explained the way her mother not only denied but also rationalized her father's behavior. As she reflected on her father's drinking and how the whole family including herself failed to see it, Courtney noted:

> I didn't really put it together. Because I figured, that's such an obvious thing, like . . . wouldn't you put it together? [laughs] But if my mom, my

> whole life is saying well he's just—that's just the way he is, he's just clumsy. He really loves you in his own way, like all this stuff it was like, I never . . . no one in my immediate family was an alcoholic, so I didn't witness the results of it.

The way her family dealt with her father's behavior was through denial. Denial by the figures responsible for Courtney's safety did not give her any choice but to maintain the collective silence. Courtney appeared to deal with the abuse, along with her mother's and sister's misrecognition, through dissociation and conviction in her own badness and this eventually led to her psyche being exposed to external stressors.

INTERNALIZED BLAME: "I REALLY THOUGHT I WAS A BAD PERSON."

After Courtney's mother and father divorced, when Courtney was a teenager, her mother married another man who turned out to be hostile toward Courtney. He used to enter her bedroom while she was asleep, reactivating Courtney's memories of traumatic boundary violations:

> C: But she didn't date a lot. She just like dated this one guy and then they got married.
>
> I: How did this affect you?
>
> C: Well, he . . . I guess technically he's, he, he died, but technically he's . . . he was a little bit kinder, like he never . . . physically did any, anything . . . but . . . he was just not a nice person and I had moved back because I had had like, I had a breakdown where I tried to move out, and then I stopped taking my medication, and then I just lost my job, and I . . . it was just, I, couldn't take care of myself. I finally ran out of money, and I moved back . . . So, she didn't really want me there long term, but it ended up being long term, and he didn't really like me being there. He didn't respect privacy . . . They didn't have a laptop, but there was a computer in the room where I was sleeping, and he would come in while I was sleeping to use the computer. It was very awkward.

Courtney's narrative included several elements related to internalizing the trauma and taking responsibility for the things that happened, such as believing that she was a bad person, which she thought explained why she was chosen for the abuse, rather than her sister. She believed she did not deserve a future of her own:

> I really thought I was a bad person, like, I really thought I was just a . . . that some people were bad and some people were good, and I was bad, so I didn't think about having a fam . . . definitely not having a family or kids of my own, I didn't, like, have dreams about being something as I grew up. I just wanted to escape.

The belief that she was a bad person emerged to try to preserve the image of her parent as loving. Courtney explained that the only way to survive was through escape, whether through using alcohol and drugs, running away, or dissociating.

Courtney's tendency to take responsibility for the trauma she survived was revealed on several occasions in the way she described the things that happened to her. For example, when she was raped by a stranger as an adult, Courtney blamed herself and her drinking for it:

> When I got raped, I had been drinking. And I blamed it on the drinking I sai . . . I told myself, "Well it was my fault because if I wasn't drinking, I would have had the judgment, and then I wouldn't have gone somewhere with this person."

Another important figure in Courtney's life, especially while she was growing up, was her younger sister. Her sister's response to Courtney's abuse was similar to that of their mother. As Courtney explained, her sister could not "deal with it." Courtney said, "I don't tell her, like, what I'm telling you, like, she doesn't want to hear it:"

> She really kept her distance she—I'm not close with her, like we don't talk about feelings. But I, you know, I love her, like I tell her I love her and I see her, I only see her maybe once a month, which is kind of hard. But I know that she doesn't really want, um, like, this is as much as she can do.

Courtney frequently compared herself to her sister. Their differences, especially Courtney's belief that her sister was not sexually abused by their father, were confirmation of Courtney's "innate badness." The impact of the abuse was so isolating that it created vast differences between the siblings' life experiences. Her sister's ability to keep her distance from the abuse and from Courtney left Courtney feeling different and "less than" her sister. Courtney had conflicting ideas about her sister; for example, at one point, she reported thinking that her sister, who has experienced professional success, was smarter than she; she characterized her sister's choices in life as "smart moves." At another point, however, she reported that she, herself, was just as smart but was held back due to the effects of her traumatized past:

> I don't think she's any more smart than me. I used to think maybe intellectually she was, but . . . I don't think so. I think that we just had different things happen to us, so . . . because she wasn't abused, as far as I know, and as far as she's told me, and as far as what I can see . . . that things just went different . . . like it just went very different. You know?
>
> And she went away to school; it was very smart, because she was able to get out, and when I was struggling to be in college, and you know, leave, you know . . . if maybe, if I had been away, it would have been like more—I would have been more stable. 'Cause, I didn't build a support system. Like my sister, from a young age, had friends, she was friends with people's families. I don't think my dad molested her. I mean, she doesn't believe me . . . I don't know if she repressed something so deep that she doesn't remember it at all, but she . . . it didn't happen. So this whole time she didn't have any experience of that . . . like of any of that. And she was—my mom didn't ever kick her out for any reason, you know? She didn't have to live with him.

When asked what she thought about her sister's experience compared to her own, Courtney related:

> Well, I mean, I'm very angry that he did it at all. Um, I kind of can't imagine what it would be like, like that's kind of where I get angry . . . like, I can't . . . like what would have happened if I, if that stuff didn't happen to me? Like what would I, what could I have done? Because I'm just as smart as her.

Her sister's different life, confidence, and success were reminders of the effects of the abuse Courtney had endured and how it marked so many aspects of her life.

LOOKING FOR MEANING

Courtney's story revealed a deep desire to search for meaning and help. Apart from the general isolation and helplessness that resulted from the trauma, Courtney also felt helpless with doctors and therapists. Nevertheless, she did not give up looking for the right kind of help and treatment:

> [The illness] got misdiagnosed a couple times. You know, just from general anxiety disorder, depression, dysthymia, then bipolar; then they would say bipolar I, bipolar II, and, then psychotic featu . . . depression with psychotic features. I mean, they really just, they just threw a lot of

names at what was going on. But I didn't remember what was going on, so it was really hard to figure out.

Courtney continued to feel unsettled by the nature of her troubles until she found a therapist who helped her understand. However, when she first heard the diagnosis of dissociative identity disorder, she resisted it:

> I didn't understand what, he, you know, he showed me the book, the *DSM* book, and all the . . . and some of it fit, but I didn't really understand, and I thought he was crazy. I'm like, "I don't have multiple personality disorder. What are you talk," but I, he must have been hypnotizing me because . . . I remember he said . . . "I want to speak to [name] now," and I was, I was like, "Dr. P., I don't have multiple personality [laughs] disorder." And he laughed and I laughed . . . I just remember that one, like, moment of [laughs] like him showing me, being like, "This is ridiculous." Like no, this is not, I'm bipolar, this is not, no, you know. And then I remember just being like, okay, well, maybe you shouldn't look at this [laughs] right now. Yeah. Yeah, I dropped out of therapy after that.

After some time, Courtney reported that the diagnosis helped clarify some of her internal experience:

> Well, I think it's important to get the right label [laughs]. Because the treatment is different . . . labels can be good because if, if I know more about the symptoms of something, I can look out for it, because sometimes it's so common, I don't even realize it's a symptom. I didn't realize not everybody hears, I mean, I know it sounds ridiculous, like voices in their, I didn't realize that.

A therapeutic relationship is important for the processing of trauma, and yet there is the possibility of trauma being enacted in the therapeutic space (Gartner, 2001; Herman, 1997; McWilliams, 2011). For example, Courtney experienced boundary violations from therapists. Further, similar to the way her mother and her sister denied her experiences, some therapists were dismissive. Courtney reported encountering therapists who over-simplified her diagnosis or tried to see her experience as only symptoms that needed to be removed:

> But I think it's, it is dismissive, like it is very dismissive to have somebody say, "Oh, well, you just have general anxiety disorder." I mean really, like, general anxiety disorder, PTSD, depression, major depression, dysthymia, bipolar II, borderline personality disorder, then, back to depression, then DID, I mean it's like, wow, can you people, what is your problem [laughs]?

Through treatment Courtney tried to reframe her struggles, view her experience from different angles, and assimilate these insights into her self-concept. She developed a more accepting attitude toward herself, her experiences, and her struggles. She felt that unless she tried to listen to what her voices and the dissociated portions of herself were saying, she would not heal: "I think it's really important that, um, like they don't feel like they're gonna be killed. You know? 'Cause that was an issue. You can't just make them go away. That's not gonna work." She elaborated on the importance of this aspect of her healing by displaying remarkable self-insight:

> So there's funny stuff, but then there's stuff, like things that . . . memories, like whole memories they'll tell me and I'll write it down. Um . . . some of them are just trying to keep me safe, like they're very critical, 'cause they just want me to be safe . . . it's like, almost like . . . they're not gonna go away 'til I listen. I think eventually they'll calm down. And I know during stress it's more, but they're just trying to keep me safe. But I think that they know things I don't know, consciously, so, I don't really want to just get rid of them . . .
>
> I didn't know what was going on for years and years of my life. I'm not just suddenly going to give that up. This is the only way I can figure out the puzzle pieces. If I just block this, then what? Then I'm just switching throughout my whole damn life, not having any stable relationship or even, maybe a job, or anything, no stability because I'm always switching and dumping people and finding new people and acting different, and so, like, that's a nightmare I don't want to go . . . there's, I don't want to go back to that . . . No. I can't. I don't feel like it's an option. I feel like if I do that, I'm kind of killing myself. Because that's years of my life that I'm not gonna remember now? I mean years, like I've got over ten years where I just, I mean, and the years I do remember, it's like one day of the year or two days or one week or . . . so I really, I think it's really important. This new therapist, I think she thinks it's important. I don't think she's trying to make them go away.

At the time of our interview, Courtney was trying to pay attention to her dissociated experiences to manage them as best as she could. That was one of the reasons she found it helpful to write the stories of her childhood selves. The writing process helped her feel more in control. Further, the way she tried to protect all her selves reflects her attempt to construct her narrative in a more integrated and complete way. Courtney spoke to her difficulty of managing the conversation between her multiple selves:

C: I don't want to get rid of anybody [different selves]. But they need to start behaving . . . I'm not gonna . . . let, like, my eight-year-old [self], pick a boyfriend. Like, that's not happening again . . . Five [year-old self] doesn't get to decide what I do with my day. I'm not just gonna be playing with playdough all day. That's not okay.

I: How do you negotiate things with different selves?

C: I don't really know how. Honestly, I've been telling everyone, just hold on. We're gonna find a good therapist. But, I just try to ignore them; I tell them to go to bed. Or like, go to the corner. But sometimes it doesn't work. And then I have a bad day . . . But it gets tricky, too, because if I let someone take over, and I paint something disturbing, I can't ignore it. And then it's, like, very upsetting. Because I realize what I just painted. Or I'd be painting something grown up, and then the, like, a little kid, and then I have like a cat drawing in the middle, I'm like, what did you do? [laughs] Why did you do [laughs] this to me? I'm trying to do, you know I'm trying, so I mean, I try to have a sense [laughs] of humor about it. You know, so far nobody's mean up there . . . Some are mad, but not like malicious.

One way to think about Courtney's struggle is through the lens of self-states. From this perspective, personality can be understood as "a set of multiple self-states" that stem from normative dissociative tendencies (Gartner, 2001, p. 179). Courtney tried to give meaning and life to her multiple self-states by actively listening to them. She also sought the help of a therapist who was willing to accept her and help her make connections between these self-states.

As the trauma and recurrent betrayal left permanent marks on Courtney and impacted her ability to form relationships and trust people, she was able to find help and meaningful relationships through friends at Fountain House and at Alcoholics Anonymous. She explained:

C: Uhm, but then when I was in the woman's shelter and I was being stalked. I started to feel hopeless, so I was worried that I would start drinking again, like I knew it was going to happen. Uhm, so I started going to AA. So now I've been in AA a little over two years. So that's how. That's how.

I: Did you find AA supportive, helpful?

C: Yeah. I think really for me AA really worked because I . . . nobody told me to leave, you know I was very awkward. People . . . gave me their phone numbers, uhm, I had to, I made a deal to check in with somebody

> every day, so even though I didn't have a therapist, uhm, I was checking in with somebody every d- I was- you know, not just like did I drink but like did anything upsetting happen? How am I feeling? And I had to do that every day . . . so I would check in with someone every day. I went to a meeting every day. So . . . that was good because I was around people and it wasn't, didn't let myself isolate. I was around people a lot of times it was the same people, people in AA are used to other people coming in completely scraggly and, beaten down you know. Everyone is welcome. So, uhm, people interacted with me and I, uhm, took me a very long time to trust people and I still have like my reservations, but uhm . . . it took a long time.

In addition, Courtney spoke of using art to express her emotional and sexual trauma. She viewed her art as an attempt to symbolize previously unspeakable experiences. At the time of the interview, although her diagnosis served as a defining feature of her self-concept, she also identified herself as an artist, indicating her readiness to change her narrative and restore her experience. She exhibited an understanding and acceptance of her condition, and she was developing the belief that she could gain something from her experience and forge a new life narrative (Frank, 1995, p. 115).

CONCLUSION

Trauma, denial, and abuse have left profound scars on Courtney. The prolonged trauma, betrayal of trust, and emotional deprivation that she experienced, prepared the stage for traumatic dissociative processes. Only years later was she finally able to understand the things that had happened to her. However, as a resilient young woman, Courtney did not give up, and after difficult teenage years of alcohol abuse and other forms of self-harm, she appears to have found meaning in her life through her artistic expression and, through utilizing people who support her in her recovery process. Her resilience appears to be growing as her survival skills have developed. Although at the time of the interviews she did not have an intimate relationship nor did she hold a job, she has a strong desire to form meaningful relationships, and this is hopeful, because in spite of her trauma, she had not lost all her hope, trust, and willingness to form attachments. At one point, Courtney remembered that, although her mother and sister failed to believe in her, her friends at Alcoholics Anonymous and her program at Fountain House supported her and encouraged her to seek treatment. She has learned to seek out helpful people in her life. Courtney is seeking to build a network in order to create a new, more integrated and self-affirming life story. Her narrative highlights the role of trauma in producing what are commonly called symptoms of psychosis, and the importance of psychotherapy for processing trauma. She appeares to have insight into her difficulties, and she is working at telling her story in ways previously foreclosed by her family. Her story offers a reminder to clinicians to be mindful of the way diagnosis can both anchor and undermine a person: that it can both clarify and also serve to foreclose potential meaning-making. As much as diagnosis can provide a name and an understanding for the individual's struggles, it is also important that therapy focuses on moving beyond diagnostic criteria into understanding the person behind the symptoms.

Chapter Ten

Eliza

No Place to Call Home

Montana Queler and Michael O'Loughlin

Eliza was the first participant that Montana interviewed. A fifty-year-old Latina woman, Eliza's life contained unspeakable horrors that she courageously recounted in the three hours shared. She had endured tremendous trauma and parental violence, growing up with a father who struggled with alcoholism and who physically abused her and her siblings, as well as abusing their mother. During the interviews she impressed as fragile, frightened, and eager to please. Underneath her preparedness—evidenced by a notebook filled with ideas she brought to the interviews—her presence conjured the image of a child, cowering in the corner, rocking herself into a protective trance. Despite her seeming fear of the world, Eliza appeared earnest in her attempts to make contact.

Eliza's style of narration was comparatively fragmented and externally focused, which we came to understand as markers of a life marred by significant, and at times unspeakable, trauma. In addition to loose thinking, Eliza spoke with a speech impediment, compounding the communication barrier. The lack of cohesion in Eliza's telling of her life story might reflect what Frank (1995) has referred to as a "chaos narrative," a narrative style marked by the collapse of a coherent articulation—or understanding—of sense of self as the person surrenders to illness or crisis. Eliza's surrender may be understood as an adaptive response to a life ravaged by abject suffering.

CHILDHOOD SCARS

> Um, I grew up in [Suburb] . . . I grew up with my mother, father. They lived together when I was one to five years old. I went to kindergarten. I went to pre-kindergarten, first grade, and I attempted to go to second grade. Then my mother and father had a terrible mishap, and um, they had plenty of fights with each other and with my older brothers and sisters. So we had to move away and my mother was sure he would kill us. So we moved to [City].
>
> I: Mhm. Um, do you feel comfortable talking about what the mishap was between your mom and your dad?
>
> E: Um, my father used to beat her up because he used to come home drunk. He said he had a hard day's work and he needed a drink.
>
> I: Mhm. And do you remember seeing this as a child?
>
> E: Um, he used to drink at parties. I don't know why he was drinking during work hours.
>
> I: Mhm. And did you see the two of them fighting with each other when you were a little kid?
>
> E: Um, I had seen him hit her and yell at her, and she spent a lot of time hiding from him. Even from us, but we don't know about it. And he took us to buy guns, rifles. So she was scared he might kill us . . .
>
> I: Do you remember how you felt at the time?
>
> E: Um, I told him, "What are you going to shoot?" He said, "You, if I want to." But he would never shoot me. I thought he was gonna kill us all.

As Eliza continued to narrate her early childhood, her fear and conflicted feelings toward her father emerged:

> I: Did he ever hurt you physically in other ways?
>
> E: Um, when I come home from school late he would give me a spanking. Um, he was very nice to us around the holidays. He would buy us Christmas presents, birthday presents, Mother's Day, his birthday we would celebrate.
>
> I: Mhm, but on other days he wasn't as nice.

E: He would take us shopping a lot. It was nice going shopping with him.

I: Mhm, do you remember whether you were afraid of him?

E: No, um, mostly I was scared that he didn't love us. That's why he used to hit us.

I: Mhm, did you see him hitting your mom and your siblings as well?

E: Um, just me, I don't know about my sisters.

I: Mhm, and did you see him hurt your mom?

E: Um, he had a big fight with my mother one day and he said he was gonna really hurt her if she wouldn't listen to him.

I: Mhm, and what happened?

E: Um, she called and my sisters came and picked us up in a U-Haul van, and we moved to [City].

Not unlike many children who find themselves victims of parental abuse, Eliza interpreted her father's abuse as deserved punishment. This impulse to take responsibility for pain inflicted allows children to feel some sense of control over an environment that can be unpredictable and harshly punitive. In addition, the above exchange captures Eliza's need to see her father as good, as she abruptly undid his cruelty by listing the many ways in which he was "nice." Eliza would not have experienced these two conflicting sides of her father—the abuser and bearer of gifts—as ambivalence, an emotional experience predicated on the capacity to integrate good and bad. This ability can only be achieved in an environment where "badness" is tolerated and metabolized. Rather than promote this kind of integration, the abuse and violence of Eliza's early environment nurtured a deep and irreconcilable split between good and bad, badness becoming the proverbial hot potato that would be alternately internalized as a way of managing negative feelings toward the other, and then projected out as they proved intolerable.

Eliza was five years old when she and her mother fled from her father. Eliza and her mother subsequently moved in with Eliza's older sisters who had previously left the family home. Eliza never saw her father again. However, the fear that had fueled this severing of physical ties remained a constituent of Eliza's psychic life:

I: How did you feel about not seeing him?

E: Um, I missed him . . . Sometimes you try to look around the house when we move across the, across the street and think that he will park and do something for us, but he never did.

I: So you expected him to come visit you?

E: Yeah, nobody in the family really knew about my father . . . I lived with my older sisters, and my mother, and my younger sisters . . . I never thought my sisters would talk about him and say, "Oh that's him." And I've done it. I've looked at cars, "Doesn't that look like Daddy?"

I: How did your siblings respond to you when you said that?

E: She said, "You might be the one looking for the problem. You shouldn't say he's looking, he's there and he's not. 'Cause you know he's a problem." And then I didn't look for him anymore.

I: So it was something that you really weren't supposed to talk about?

E: Yes.

I: That must have been really confusing for you?

E: Yes, well my mother said stay away from people that would pick me up and just park their cars . . . She said, "'Cause you don't know if your father will come and kill you."

These seeds of doubt about the safety of the outside world—which perhaps began as a reasonable concern—flourished within a crucible of neglect and profound vulnerability as Eliza developed into an adolescent and young adult. During the latter years of her childhood and emerging adulthood, Eliza found herself very much alone with a mother who herself struggled with significant psychic difficulties, and then with men who seemed to have little concern for her welfare. Unexplained and irreparable rupture in early attachment relationships set the stage for fear of abandonment and the threat of loneliness. As a result, Eliza's psyche took flight into fantasy, finding alternative outlets to satisfy her need for play, stimulation, and soothing. This flight created a giant chasm between herself and the material world, rendering her disconnected and increasingly unable to navigate the complex world around her.

VOICE HEARING

In her flight from material reality, Eliza began hearing voices. Eliza reported that this started at some point in her early childhood:

> E: Um, I used to listen to, television, and as I stood in front of the television I talked back to the television and thought the voices came from, to me that way.
>
> I: From the TV?
>
> E: Yes, they used to talk back to me.
>
> I: And how old were you then?
>
> E: I was five years old.
>
> I: Around five years old?
>
> E: Even younger than that, but I really . . . most of the time I was just playing around with my toys and hiding out, then I'd hear voices.

Five years and younger placed Eliza within the reach of her unpredictable, contemptuous father. Around this age, Eliza's father also noticed Eliza's voice hearing. In response, he warned her against exposing this aspect of her internal experience to other people:

> E: My father said he was going to play a trick. He said never tell anyone that you are hearing voices and um . . .
>
> I: So your father knew that you were hearing voices when you were five?
>
> E: I don't know why, but I think he thought it was like imagination. (inaudible) that was pretty bad . . . "You're talking to yourself. Don't tell anyone you're hearing voices."
>
> I: Why did he tell you that?
>
> E: He spoiled me so much with food and toys . . .
>
> I: But why do you think he didn't want you to tell anyone that you were hearing voices?
>
> E: He says you shouldn't tell anyone that.

I: Because why?

E: He, he said you won't like what they'll think of you.

I: What they'll think of you?

E: Yes, he said they'll be naughty to you.

Lacking guidance, the vulnerable five-year-old Eliza was left to make meaning of her own now seemingly strange internal world. The threat that others would be "naughty" to her if they knew the truth of her voice hearing might have understandably engendered confusion, fear, and shame in little Eliza. It might have also encouraged Eliza to regard her inner world as alien and dangerous, a staging ground for reliance on projection to maintain a sense of goodness inside.

Eliza's description of her early voice hearing suggests that at times the voices served a vital function, allowing her refuge from a dangerous world while satisfying basic needs for creativity and play:

E: See the clouds, and oh that looks like a piggy pig and that looks like a reindeer . . . While I'm walking up the stairs on her apartment, or out the patio, or in the front playing with the children. I would talk to myself and say, "You can hear it too, I'm not just talking to myself. You can hear it."

I: Who was it that was telling you that you shouldn't talk to yourself anymore?

E: My sister that lived upstairs.

I: So you thought that she could hear the voices, too?

E: Yes, and I told her, "Well, you can hear what I'm saying," and she's like, "But who are you talking to?" I said, "To my phone." She said "Well, no talking to yourself or you can have no, um, togetherness with the others, because they think you're sick or crazy. So don't talk to yourself."

Eliza's account suggests that she took for granted that the voices or characters she imagined were a part of her external world. It was only through the critique of others like her father and sister that she came to see these as either anomalous or particular to her own experience. Her comments also suggest that these characters were constructed from facets of her external surroundings, perhaps used as a means of countering unresolved fear and mistrust of her environment. In the absence of a stable, loving attachment figure, Eliza's psyche erected in fantasy that which she was sorely lacking—love and a sense of security.

After some period of separation, Eliza eventually returned to live in an apartment with her mother. However, soon after this move, Eliza's voices began to interfere with her performance in school. Further, during the interview Eliza abruptly shared that she became pregnant and gave birth while in middle school, suggesting that her troubles also extended well beyond her functioning at school:

> E: In another apartment, I went to six, fifth grade, and I didn't do good but I graduated 'cause of my age. And six, seven, and eight, I graduated, but at eighth grade I had a baby . . . eight pounds, twenty-two inches, and I named my baby (inaudible), and she's a girl. And I went to high school. I couldn't do good in high school; too many voices.
>
> I: You had more voices when you were in high school?
>
> E: Yes, and the teacher said, "You're not allowed to do that in my classroom, say voices. It's bothering you."
>
> I: Were they bothering you, the voices?
>
> E: It was bothering everyone in the room, the voices.
>
> I: Because you were talking.
>
> E: Yes, and this test, and I'm talking at this . . . "Just get up and get out if you can't participate."
>
> I: What would the voices talk to you about?
>
> E: Um, whose seat is this? And I would say, "This is someone's seat," and "Well, I'm sitting here now, and it's time for a test." I said, "If I don't get (inaudible) how will I know what I learned?" I studied, and it didn't really sink in. So, "She's not really understanding, this is not the place for you" . . . So, I left school, but I didn't really leave school. I just went home and I told my mother, um, "High school is not working for me, can I go to someplace where it's less hours? Maybe I could spend time by myself and read," which sometimes I can and I can't. I need glasses. I have reading glasses at home. Sometimes I use them, and sometimes I don't. So, I went to another school . . . I went for three years, and I was slowly learning with the voices, very terribly, the voices. I said, "Come on, I want to be there from nine to twelve, twelve to three, do the whole

> six hours." And sometimes I did, and I graduated from basic, intermediate, and advanced classes.

During the interview, Eliza repeatedly emphasized the importance she placed on completing her education and obtaining employment despite the challenges. She related that she did not want to be like her mother who, according to Eliza, depended on welfare and had never been able to work outside the home. However, Eliza's struggle to navigate external reality continued to impede her ability to progress in the manner she wished. The responsibility of caring for a newborn and the increasing academic rigor of junior high school, compounded with Eliza's circumstances of abject trauma, poverty, and limited support from her mother, who herself was impaired by significant psychic difficulties, made her odds even grimmer.

Within the above narrative, there is evidence of a marked shift in Eliza's experience of voice hearing. There is not a modicum of pleasure to be found in these moments of struggle and frustration. The voices had become critical and judgmental in nature, in contrast to a modicum of companionship they had brought her earlier on:

> E: I turn the music on and I keep busy when I'm hearing voices, but um it comes through this explosion, I feel. When I've had enough, I just say, "*Leave. Me. Alone!*"
>
> I: When they get too noisy?
>
> E: They'll even speak outside of my mouth because they're noisy.

When Eliza was fourteen, her mother chaperoned her to a psychiatrist for the first time. This was when Eliza began taking psychotropic medication:

> Um, I was seeing a psychiatrist since I was fourteen years old. . . . And my mother really didn't know anything better than you tell the doctor you have problems, the doctor will give you medication . . .

Unfortunately, the medication was no match for the distress Eliza's voice hearing caused her. This initial encounter with the mental health system was to be the first of many.

INTERGENERATIONAL COLLAPSE

Later in the interview, Eliza disclosed that her mother also struggled with voice hearing and had been hospitalized when Eliza was fifteen. She reported that she had been unaware of her mother's affliction:

> I: Do you know whether your difficulties were similar to those of your mother? Do you know what she had been experiencing and why she was on medication?
>
> E: Well, my mother had hearing voices and she was saying that, they were, just wanted to drug her and don't want to listen to what they say and, "I'll be home," and "I want to come home." . . . She was going crazy. Her hair was a mess, um, she used to walk back and forth, she used to kneel to us, it was, like, it was scary. When my mother was sick, I was worried about her and us, because she used to not be herself.

Eliza's mother was later able to return home, though, by Eliza's account she never fully recovered. There was a repetition in psychic collapse as it emerged for both mother and daughter. Beset with her own severe psychic struggles, Eliza's mother lacked the internal resources to provide adequate containment for her suffering daughter. Eliza later commented on her own need to return to the hospital:

> E: And I had some . . . problems with my older brother, and my older sisters had convinced the doctors that they should keep me, and I was against it, but they kept me in the hospital.
>
> I: How old were you at the time?
>
> E: I was, after I had my daughter, I was about fifteen.
>
> I: That was the first time you were hospitalized?
>
> E: Yes, fourteen or fifteen. And I was hospitalized, and my mother was taking care of me. And she pressed the nurse, "Maybe she should be admitted," and they took me upstairs to the third floor. I spent like four weeks and a day or two. They gave me medication and an injection.

Still in the thick of a breakdown, Eliza soon returned to the hospital after being discharged:

> E: Then um the doctors prescribed me Haldol when I left, and then I was on it again on my own, and my mother came and she talked to me. She sat down. She said, "If you didn't need it the first time, you should have stayed in the hospital and this way you wouldn't have had to be admitted again." I went two times, three months, three weeks apart . . . I stayed for four weeks and a few days, and I was . . . I signed a permission slip to leave. And I had to sign myself out. I think I was hearing voices. It was very upsetting. I thought the world was coming down on me. It was like,

do you know what you're doing? Are you doing (inaudible)? Everything is turning out wrong.

I: Is that what the voices were saying?

E: Um, I wouldn't listen to them. They were screaming out of my mouth and I told, I told my mother that I want to readmit myself, and I did. So I stayed in a hospital when I was fifteen, well, um that time I stayed for two months. And I started to GED school, and I went to GED school for three years, and I graduated, and I didn't get a therapist. I got, uh, just a medical doctor.

Eliza's account of both her and her mother's experiences with the revolving door of psychiatric institutionalization was harrowing. Within her account there is certainly room for critique of the mental health system, for example, regarding the need for care or treatment that sets patients up for healthier outcomes. There are also insights to be gleaned about the role of the intergenerational transmission of trauma and how this crucial aspect of a person's life experience is categorically overlooked by the system. If we view the attempt to understand that which is essentially unspeakable to be one of our tasks as mental health professionals, there is necessarily an imaginative journey and re-construction that is involved in understanding Eliza. There is a matrix of intergenerational and sociopolitical influences that might have converged to shape Eliza's psyche. For example, during the interview Eliza noted that her father and mother's family had been born in a very poor region of Latin America. It is reasonable to imagine Eliza's family moving to the United States with hopes of making good on the promise of improved economic circumstances. However, if this had been their motivation, it never came to fruition. Further, in contrast to the envisioned opportunities that lay before them, Eliza's family found a country—and economy—fraught with racial divisions and oppression, creating significant vulnerability to emotional and psychological suffering.

SELF-MEDICATING AS AN ACT OF SELF-SOOTHING

Compounding the aforementioned factors, Eliza's adolescence coincided with the introduction of crack cocaine onto urban streets. After returning from the hospital, Eliza reported that she obtained a job as a clerk, allowing her to help support herself, her daughter, and her mother. However, soon after her release from the hospital, Eliza began using marijuana and crack cocaine:

E: And at sixteen, I started using drugs before I got my job. Then I started working.

I: What kinds of drugs did you start using?

E: I also used the crack cocaine. I used it quite often, but I didn't travel with it, you know, I would use it in the house, in the hallways, and um, I never ever had someone to use it with.

I: You used it only by yourself?

E: No, my brother used to say, if I'm doing it to tell him, and I never used to like telling him.

I: How come?

E: 'Cause I would have to get him some too.

Eliza's drug use can be understood at the intersection of the historical moment in which she was growing up, in an urban environment when crack cocaine's availability was widespread, and a psychological moment for her in which she experienced an urgency to escape the pain of her situation. In this moment, the desperate need for soothing would have trumped whatever awareness Eliza may have had of the drug's dangers.

Eliza's decision to keep her baby, despite her mother's expressed disapproval, might also be understood within the context of her emotional deprivation:

E: And I went to high school, and I had a daughter before I went to high school.

I: How did that come about? Did you plan to have a child, or was it a surprise to you?

E: It was a surprise to me. My mother was against it, but I want to have the baby, and I had a baby.

Despite having become pregnant accidentally, the prospect of a baby might have sparked a fantasy of unconditional love and the imagined emotional safety that its dependence on her would have offered. Further, a baby might have engendered some hope of gaining access to her own mother's maternal resources from which she had been cut off so early on:

I: Did you feel you had enough help at that time, 'cause it's a lot of responsibility, right, to take care of a baby? Did you feel like you had other people around you who were helping you through the process?

E: Yes.

I: Who was helping you primarily?

E: Um, my mother and my sisters. They helped me buy things. Before I had the baby, they helped me out when I went to the hospital when I had the baby. They helped me. . . .

I: And how was your mom with the baby?

E: Okay, she liked the baby. She helped me take care of her.

Initially, Eliza's mother helped her care for her newborn; however, with limited access to resources, Eliza and her mother struggled. Ultimately Eliza left her mother's home with her daughter in order to live with her child's father. It was around this decision that Eliza first gave voice to her conflicted feelings toward her mother:

E: My mother was very strict, it hurt me when I was growing up, she said that I was having sex too much, but I did get pregnant at a young age, at fourteen I had a baby girl, and . . .

I: What was that experience like for you?

E: It wasn't a very nice experience. I was hungry the whole pregnancy, but I did get something to eat, and someone else raised her.

I: Did you feel emotionally ready?

E: My mother potty trained her. I wasn't emotional, I was getting my mother's help, but the man said that he would take her away. My mother had the mentally ill. No excuse, I have no excuse my mother not knowing anything about it. Or I can say she's really sick and put me out . . . But my mother said I was eating out of her house and home with her boyfriend, so we moved away . . .

Eliza had difficulty discerning the meaning behind her mother's actions. This excerpt captures Eliza's unresolved questions regarding whether her mother was authoritarian or protective; neglectful or helpful; entitled to her own life; rejecting and abandoning; or too ill to see how much Eliza needed her. Given this, drugs would have provided a kind of salve for the aches of unresolvable inner and interpersonal conflict.

CYCLE OF EXPLOITATION

Unfortunately, Eliza's move to live with her boyfriend's family led to a repetition of her childhood experience, marked by further neglect and exploitation:

> [A]nd I tried to stay in his house, which I did, and they were very big with voices and food. They wouldn't feed me. And my money, they went out with it to parties, on flea markets, and travel to [Place], and I never spent my money like that, me have the job, why can't I go to [Place]? And I wasn't invited so I broke up . . . I would give them something and then I would give them it all.

Eliza felt isolated and vulnerable. Deficits in her ability to care for herself and establish and maintain healthy relationships emerged in this description. Ultimately, Eliza and her boyfriend broke up. Their daughter stayed with her father, and Eliza returned home to live with her mother. Eliza then lost her job, leaving her with no financial resources to attend to her basic needs. Her lack of psychosocial support sent her spiraling. Although Eliza was unable to articulate her devastation at the loss of her relationship, child, and job, her long-term return to the hospital during this period overtly reflects the impact of these stressors. Compounding these multiple losses, Eliza soon discovered that she was HIV positive.

The deterioration of Eliza's physical and psychological health rendered her defenseless against further exploitation and abuse. In a sense, her early abuse and neglect planted the roots from which later traumas could take hold. Throughout the interviews, Eliza seemed preoccupied with the theme of others taking advantage of her. For example:

> E: And I started taking it [medication] while I was work, at work, and, at home, but, I felt the cold shoulder from everyone they would (inaudible) for me, and they pay me in bottle.
>
> I: So you didn't feel people were on your side?
>
> E: Even my bank account, and my bank account, and my (inaudible) and they just took advantage of me.
>
> I: Who's "they"? Who took advantage?

> E: The people that come over and have my home, they steal my cigarettes and my clothes, my money. They stole my boyfriend away from me, and he said it's my own fault. I went out with this man and with that man, and I shouldn't have. I should've been alone.

Later in the interview, Eliza shared that she subsequently had two more children, though she presented this without context or elaboration. After reporting that both infants had been taken from her by the authorities at their time of birth, Eliza began to free associate on the subject of loss and mistrust:

> E: . . . I have this, I'm gonna take this from you. I stop that person right there.
>
> I: You feel that people are always taking things from you?
>
> E: No, I won't let them. They might steal it right out of my pocket and then they start talking about it, and I said well next time I won't have no money. I just won't have any money if you wanna steal it or try to get past me to take it from me for what you need it. I need it myself (inaudible) soap, shampoo, clean towel. I need things, too.
>
> I: Mhm . . .
>
> E: I don't bother you when you get your forty percent off your money. I don't, they cut my check, and I got a job, trying to save, and I get fifty dollars every month, and I still, my friends want me for my money.
>
> I: Your friends want you for your money?
>
> E: Um, people at the residence. I don't mention no problem (inaudible) . . .
>
> I: They what?
>
> E: I don't give them a problem, they shouldn't have to ask me for fifty cents, five dollars, ten dollars, anything. I can go to them for anything, and I don't have a boyfriend that's coming over, to hurt me or lay in bed with me, all that has stopped.

Eliza's concern about others taking advantage of her was an important theme that surfaced throughout her interviews. It is unclear how much her anxiety about others' intentions stemmed from actual experiences of exploitation, and to what extent her worry emanated from intra-psychic conflict. Regarding the specific content of Eliza's remarks, her comments were elicited in the context of a discussion about her babies being removed from her care, a profound trauma that clearly left enduring scars on her psyche and echoed the abrupt severing of ties she herself had experienced as a child vis-à-vis her father. Sexuality and motherhood are potentially evocative subjects for any woman, and were likely especially so for Eliza, tarnished by the terror and deprivation of her own childhood and also in her having become a mother while still a child.

The connection between external stressors and intrapsychic difficulties was reflected in Eliza's unconscious association between her experience with voices and with her mother's voice:

> I: One is bad? One of the voices is bad?
>
> E: 'Cause I talk back to them, and it comes right out of my mouth. It's bad.
>
> I: Yeah, that voice doesn't like to be spoken back to?
>
> E: Yes.
>
> I: But there's a reason you're talking back to it, right? It's saying something to you that isn't nice?
>
> E: Yes, my mother was very strict when I was a kid. She wouldn't let me be with other people in bed, or girls in bed with me. She wouldn't allow that and . . .
>
> I: You mean like sleepovers?
>
> E: Um, yeah, or go to their house (inaudible). But she found out and she said she was sick because of me.

In the above passage, Eliza's "bad" voice reflected an internalized persecutor, which bore a kind of resemblance to her mother's "strict" persona. Within this exchange as well as the one that follows, Eliza loosely transitioned from talking about her voices to her relationship with her mother, illustrating that the two subjects had an assumed, or perhaps unconscious, link for her:

> E: Yes, I had a nightmare the other night that someone was putting up chicken, and ate the chicken, and put it in between their legs, and I tried to run away from it in my sleep.
>
> I: So this, you were watching this other woman do this and you were trying . . .

E: No they were trying to do it to me.

I: They were trying to do it to you?

E: Yes.

I: Have you ever had a dream like that before?

E: No, and I didn't like it. It was very dark, and someone was there, but I don't know who. And I found my mother, she says, "You think I could do that with you?" And I said, "No, I don't do that with girls and boys, have sex. I'm older, I have (inaudible), I don't need sex" . . . And it was very dark. Like, my mother said, "I'm gonna put you in the dark," and I says, "Don't do that to me."

I: Had she ever done that before?

E: Yes, she's done it before to me . . .

I: She put you in the dark?

E: Yes, in my sleep . . .

These excerpts display the porousness of the boundary dividing Eliza's internal and external world, contributing to her sense of extreme vulnerability as well as the cognitive confusion that pervaded her narrative. There was no safety on the inside or outside of her, no corner of her mind stood protected. Even in her sleep, malevolent forces abounded.

THE INSTITUTIONAL REVOLVING DOOR

During the interviews it became clear that Eliza's adult life had been marked by a cycle of institutional transience. Periods of hospitalization and incarceration had consumed large chunks of her adulthood: "[W]hen I wasn't admitted to the hospital, I was being put in jail." During a period of homelessness, Eliza was arrested for selling drugs to someone who turned out to be an undercover police officer, leading to a four-year prison sentence. During her time in prison, Eliza continued to feel very much alone and abandoned by her family:

E: I did my time writing to my family, writing to my mother, writing to my brothers and sisters, and had no answer. I wrote to my daughter, [Name], I had no answer.

I: Nobody wrote back to you?

E: No. So, I was living in the dark in jail.

I: That must've been a really hard time for you.

E: Yes, and it was very cheap because everybody was getting a, a package and seeing people. So, I was by myself, and they shared with me, all wrote to their family could you gave me a package they can share with her, and they shared with me while I was in jail . . .

During her incarceration, Eliza's only psychiatric care came in the form of medication. Emphasis on psychotropic medication ran throughout Eliza's narrative, beginning when she was a teenager seeking a medical consult:

E: I was like thirteen years old, and I went to a small clinic and they said, "We're not trying to say you're crazy, but you're thirteen years old and having your baby at fourteen. Maybe you should talk to a mental health doctor about your condition." And they offered me medication when I was pregnant, and I went to them like four or five times. They were always checking. They was checking me for my feet, my breasts, my lungs. They was checking me with x-rays. Did a little pregnancy test on me. And since I was so young they said I should—having a baby—they said I should see a psychiatrist. "It's not, nothing against you but it's good to let out, it, you just don't know anything else about yourself. It's a good place to learn about yourself. Open up your feelings."

I: How did that make you feel when they told you that you should see a . . .

E: I got very upset . . . Yes, because I was pregnant and I didn't want to see a psychiatrist. I didn't want to tell someone my problems.

I: How come?

E: Because I wanted to go to school, and since I had to go to the doctor and do as I dropped out of school, but I graduated in three years. By the time I was eighteen, I had a diploma.

I: So you felt that because you were going to see a psychiatrist and getting mental health care you wouldn't be able to finish school? You thought it would get in the way?

> E: And I wouldn't be able to spend much time at home with my mother. I had other things to do. I didn't need it, but it turned out that I did because I accepted that they were there to help me and listen to my problems, and they said there will be medication for me. I was very against that. The first medication they gave me was Prylexolin, and they moved it to Haldol, and now I started taking Zyprexin. Once in the night and once in the day and Zoloft once in, three at night, one in the morning, one Zoloft in the morning . . . They said, "We'll try and see how it goes. If you really think you're okay and want to be on the street and be a bum. Well, do that if you want. Our, our door is open to you." So I took the help.

From this first encounter with the mental health system, medication was the main approach used to address Eliza's suffering. Whatever positive or regulating effects the medications may have provided, the potential for their effectiveness was no match for the scars left by Eliza's early traumas.

LONGING FOR LOVE

Over the course of the interviews, Eliza repeatedly spoke of her longing for love and connection. For example, Eliza spoke about her yearning to know her children who had been taken from her at birth:

> E: I have born two other children. A boy and a girl . . . and they were taken away from me, but they say if you can't (inaudible) a child, don't have a child.
>
> I: If what?
>
> E: 'Cause they didn't, it didn't cut. I just had two other children. I have three: [Name], [Name], and I call the little girl Princess, and they're missing. And I see people on the street and I don't know if that's my child, and I don't see them no more, and I wonder what happened to them.

There is a kind of parallel here between Eliza's relationship to her children and to her father. Just as she expressed yearning to know her children, as a child she wanted to know her father and scanned her neighborhood streets to find him. These separations were abrupt and psychically shattering. Having her children taken was a tremendous loss for Eliza, a repetition and reminder of the lack of control she has had over her identity as a mother and over her life overall.

During the second part of the interview, Eliza conveyed a longing and affection for her father that coexisted with her fear of his rage:

> I: How did you feel about not seeing him?
>
> E: Um, I missed him . . . Sometimes you try to look around the house when we move across the, across the street and think that he will park and do something for us, but he never did.

At the outset of the third part of the interview, Eliza related:

> E: I miss my mother. (inaudible) told you about my mother, but he told me I could visit her any time I felt. The nursing home she is in is for mental health which is in [City], and I could go there on my own. I don't mind looking it up. I miss my mother.
>
> I: You miss her.
>
> E: She raised me, and I miss her.
>
> I: What do you miss about her?
>
> E: Well, I miss the good times that she takes me shopping, treats me to a good dinner, breakfast, lunch. I love her dinner.

These comments point to the culmination of her feelings of longing and desire for connection. However, beyond the geographic distance between them, Eliza's disconnection from her family seemed to be in part a consequence of unresolved conflict, which Eliza alluded to only briefly:

> E: And my sister was having a cookout. Her birthday was the eighth. We went for the fourth of July. They had the cake . . . the invitation, but I didn't want to stay over. It was a crowded apartment—my daughter, my nieces, my sisters. They were all there with their children and their husbands, and it was just me and my daughter and my grandchildren and her husband, my sister's husband. We had a big outing. They did talk to me about mental health. She says, my sister, the youngest from the oldest, she asked me, "Are you still mental health? Do you have anything you want to tell me? Oh, don't be nervous. I'm not a bad person, but are you a bad person?" I'm not a bad person, she asked . . .
>
> I: She asked you whether you were a bad person?
>
> E: Yes, because she, she said, "Oh, I'm going to give you a hand, and you're not going to get in touch with me." I would like to get in touch with my sister.

This split between the notions of good and bad represents an early bifurcation in Eliza that left an indelible imprint on her psyche. The perpetual danger of her early environment when the boundaries between self and other would have been most permeable created confusion as to the source of her felt threat. Was the danger inside of her, or did it emanate from outside? Lacking essential childhood nutriments such as attunement, soothing, and containment, Eliza was prone to see herself as the seat of destruction.

Eliza's story illustrates the circumstances through which psychosis can emerge as a life solution. While her earliest voices helped to fulfill a need to escape the terror pervading her home environment, over time they came to assume a maniacal and contemptuous tone, mirroring her struggle to integrate negative emotions. Eliza's narrative, both in its form and content, exhibits a kind of surrender to psychic distress made unavoidable by the amalgam of early deprivation, abuse, and loss. Her psychotic flight became a kind of solution to the pain of material reality. Communication with the television and with her natural surroundings fulfilled intimacy needs without the risks associated with human closeness. Voices served as the repositories for unwanted, intolerable emotions. Disorganized thinking protected Eliza from that which was too painful to know. Unfortunately these unconscious strategies are double-edged: Eliza found herself very much alone. The tremendous losses that gave rise to her psychic struggles became a self-perpetuating system, confining her to a position of loss, both in terms of realizing life purpose and love. Despite this, her sustained desire for connection, evident in her manner during the interviews as well as in an expressed yearning, spoke to a capacity to love and be loved that transcends the scars left by a lifetime of suffering.

Chapter Eleven

Sarah

Who Am I?

Marilyn Charles, Michael O'Loughlin,
and Secil Arac-Orhun

Sarah, a Caucasian woman in her late forties or early fifties, reported having been coming to Fountain House for about a year and a half. In her description of what led her there, Sarah reported having had "a nervous breakdown," two years before. She had been living on [street] with a friend but couldn't pay the rent and so became homeless. "I wasn't really homeless," she clarified, "I was outside." Sarah described a striking discontinuity between her experience prior and subsequent to the breakdown. In response to Secil's questions, she related in a somewhat disjointed way her experience two years before of her brother finding her and having her committed.

> S: I didn't remember him, I said I didn't, you know, I said that "you're not my brother" and it didn't look like my brother, you know, because maybe 'cause he gained weight, so he called the cops on me, and had me put in [Hospital] for a month and I was taking medication and they gave me a bed and everything and what happen was he visit me but I still didn't remember him, so they said that I had a nervous, I was running away from him and he was saying "get that girl, get that girl," and they handcuffed me and they put me in the ambulance.

In spite of the confusion and distress that led to her hospitalization, Sarah described the hospital stay itself as "nice . . . they fed us three meals a day and I shared it with another girl and they diagnosed me as bipolar disorder." When asked what was nice about it, she replied, "They had people talk to you." In contrast, she depicted her experience of her brother during that time as alien and frightening.

> S: when I first got there, I was scared because I, I tried to tell them that it wasn't my brother, and they didn't believe me and they, I told them that I was an orphan . . . He didn't look like, you know, my brother. My brother was skinny and the other guy was heavy and his face was different, so I got sort of like scared, you know? And he came, he came with his wife, his ex-wife. He's married, he's divorced.

Sarah reported not even knowing her name when first taken to the hospital. "I had a lot of drugs in me, heroin and all kinds of drugs, they cleaned me out." She said that she had been depressed because her mother had died.

Although she gave somewhat conflicting reports of her living situation prior to being hospitalized, in her initial interview, Sarah said she had been living with a friend. This friend moved to Florida, leaving Sarah without a home. Sarah reflected back on the moment of being taken into custody, saying she "had nowhere to go, but I had bags and he said I was homeless, but I wasn't really homeless. I was gonna go home, you know?" It was not clear, however, where home might have been.

At the hospital, after the initial fear and strain, Sarah felt that she was treated kindly. She had been running away from her brother. "He got the cops after me. They put me in the ambulance and they put me in the hospital for a month." Sarah seemed to have been very confused by the information she received from her brother and his wife. For example, her sister-in-law told Sarah that she had a son.

> S: I was surprised.
>
> I: Surprised?
>
> S: Yeah, because at that time, I didn't know, I didn't know. I didn't know because I was confused. I got scared and I thought they were coming to get me and everything.
>
> I: Sarah, can you . . .
>
> S: I thought they were the mafia.
>
> I: Who was the mafia?
>
> S: (laughs) My brother, my brother and his ex-wife.
>
> I: Ok, like what made you think that they were the mafia?

S: The way they were dressed. She had the short haircut.

I: Ah.

S: And maybe her face made me think that.

In spite of her fear and confusion, Sarah said that she feels badly about not remembering her brother. He would come every three weeks and bring her something to eat, she recalled, but then they would also offer information that was difficult to assimilate. "They would just tell me that I had a son and everything . . . I heard he is in jail." She reports feeling like she should go visit her son "and see who he is, right, it's the right thing to do, right? . . . Maybe he'll bring my memory back." Sarah did seem confident that she had never been married, that her son's father had been someone with whom she took drugs. "It was a one-night stand," she said.

Sarah's experience of the hospital seems similar to previous experiences in which her basic needs had been attended to but in which she had been given names or labels for reasons she could not discern and did not seem to question. At the hospital, "they diagnosed me as bipolar disorder . . . schizophrenia," she said, without much sense of investment in these labels one way or another. Most prevalent in her discourse regarding this initial hospital stay is a sense of confusion. She said that she hadn't seen her brother for a number of years, "He said I was missing for like, many years." At the time her brother approached her on the streets, he had a picture of a missing girl, someone who Sarah thought did not look like her, who had a different name. The friend she had been living with called her Kim, and this man called her Sarah. "He showed me a picture of a missing girl, and I thought it was just a missing girl, and he said that was me and 'you were missing' and I said I didn't know what. So I got scared and ran away from him. I was running in the streets . . . I thought he was going to hurt me." She continued,

S: I had something like amnesia, like I didn't know who I was and I was . . .

I: So, you didn't know who you were, you were, and I guess I remember you mentioning that the doctor told you your name.

S: Yeah, the doctor.

I: But, not Sarah, something else. I totally forgot that.

S: Yeah, it was Kim.

I: Ha, Kim, Kim. For example, what impact did it have on you to hear that you were Kim, for example, but then it turns out actually that you are Sarah?

S: I was surprised because, because Kim had . . . had no family and Kim was an orphan and I thought I was Kim.

I: Now that, so, but in our previous interview, you had quite a lot of memories about your parents.

S: Yeah.

I: So, I wonder what made you think that you were an orphan?

S: Well, I didn't, I didn't have any family at that time. I don't know, and my friend Diane thought I was Kim and she called me Kim.

I: She called you Kim. So you met with Diane in the bar?

S: Right.

I: Right? And so you started living with her.

S: Right.

I: So in the bar did you introduce yourself as Kim to her?

S: She asked me if my name was Kim and I said "yeah."

I: Okay, so for years you were Kim?

S: Yeah.

According to Sarah, "Kim had a different life" than Sarah had. "She was different . . . she didn't have any parents." As Kim, Sarah reported working as a waitress and enjoying a close relationship with Diane, playing board games in their free time. But then, her narrative became disorganized. She shifted from her discussion of her life with Diane and being a waitress to what seemed to be a reference to the period of time after Diane had left and before her brother approached her, describing being alone in the city, overwhelmed, "trying to get some money."

I: So, your, like your main source of support was Diane?

S: Yeah, and then when my, when, then when she left, I was walking and then the guy came and showed me a picture of me and said I was missing and it didn't look like me. It didn't look like me and then, and then he wanted to talk to me and I didn't want to talk and then, then I went to the hospital.

I: Do you remember the first day of your hospitalization?

S: They put me in an ambulance, and they took me to the, I asked them, I was in a bed and I asked them, "When am I going home?" and they said, "Soon, soon." And they kept me in a room and this lady came in and she said, "What did you do for a living?" and she said that I was panhandling. I was panhandling. So I said I wasn't and they said I was.

I: What was panhandling?

S: You know, asking for money in the street and she said, "Is that how you supported yourself?" And I said, "No, I worked." And she said, "That's what I think you did." And I was there like about eight hours. I was, they gave me medication and I was sleeping, and so after like eight hours, they told me that. I said, "Am I going home?" and, "Can I leave?" and she said "No," so then um, they took . . .

I: Who was this, by the way, "she?"

S: Doctors there.

I: Mm-hm. Okay.

S: Yeah. So, um they took me to, they brought me to a psychiatric ward and they put me there and the next thing I knew it, I stayed there for three months, and they told me I was going to leave the same day.

I: What did you make of it? Like, why do you think they made you stay there three months?

S: Because, I don't know. They were trying to find out who I was. They didn't . . . they were trying to, you know, find out who I was, if I was Kim or Sarah.

As Sarah described having wanted to leave the hospital, she mentioned grief and crying, but then withdrew her statement. "I wanted to leave and, um, I wasn't really crying." When asked where she would have gone, she spoke of going to see her friend, but then did not seem entirely clear whether

her friend had been in Florida or New York at that point. She then shifted abruptly to thoughts of her brother.

> S: But I, I have no memories of my brother, I don't know why, there's no pictures, you know, photographs, maybe if there was a photograph, maybe I could remember him, 'cause he was running after me, I got scared, I thought it was, I really didn't, I thought something was going to happen.
>
> I: What, what were you afraid would happen?
>
> S: I don't know. I thought he was going to kidnap me or something, yeah.
>
> I: Yeah.
>
> S: Could that happen, Secil? Somebody could say . . .
>
> I: Sorry?
>
> S: Somebody could say that they, they're related to you, right? And then (laughs), and then you don't remember and then you run away from them, they're running after you, wouldn't that be frightening to you, Secil?
>
> I: It would be frightening, I, I, it is frightening, Sarah.
>
> S: I was having nightmares, though. I was having nightmares.

We can wonder, at that point, to what extent her discourse seemed incoherent because she was not sure of the context in which she is speaking. Is crying linked to the need to remain in the hospital? If so, was it important to not be crying? If her actual feelings were less important than whatever meanings were being made of them by others, then how does that affect her speech?

Safety seemed to rest in having shelter and food to eat, the basic accoutrements of "home." After the hospital, "they put me in [residence], and I was living there, it was a shelter, and I stayed there for like three months, and then I moved from there and I went to next door, [another residence], and they put me on [public benefits] . . . and they took most of my check and they gave me three meals a day and I've been living there." Sarah reported unhappiness with her living situation, wanting to move somewhere, anywhere else. "They take a lot of your money," she said. "I don't get much money, they only give me thirty dollars a month, a week."

Sarah still had mixed feelings about her brother. "He released me," she said, recalling that he had brought her clothes and had taken her to [first residence]. And yet, "he's not as warm and loving as I thought he, a brother would be, you know?" When asked what loving understanding would look like, Sarah responded, "You know, a sense of touch, uh you know, if you're crying, he would hold you and you know, support. He didn't do that."

Although Sarah saw her brother regularly she still did not recognize him. "I still don't think it's my brother. . . . He tries to bring back memories and talk to me, but I still don't remember." "Sometimes, I cry because I don't know if that's my brother or not." She did not have much sense that he understood her and she also wished that he would help her more financially, though she did appreciate his help in getting her to a safe living environment. Although she remembered him as warmer and more loving when she was younger, she also recalled that those were times when he had been drinking and using drugs. "My mother was never home," Sarah said. In the absence of a parent to turn to, Sarah seemed to orient towards her brother, going to the park where her brother would hang out with his friends and "then he would walk me home."

This gap, where parental care and comfort should have been, seems linked to what Sarah described as a great deal of conflict in her family as she was growing up. That conflict seems to have escalated after her parents separated. She described heated fights in which her parents "used to throw things":

> S: They used to fight a lot, they used to fight a lot. They didn't get along, mostly about money. They used to fight about money. Even she wouldn't give us enough money to eat and he used to like, when all these, like, poison our minds against our mother and my mother didn't want us to go, we used to have visitation rights on the weekends to see him and, um, he used to, um, talk bad about her, and my, and the, and my brother used to tell my mother, he didn't want to, she didn't want us to go there.

Money seems to have been at the root of a great deal of the conflict in the household:

> S: Yeah, she, yeah it was because like a lot of times he didn't want to pay at, you know support for the kids and he, like I told you what happened he, um, he used to, um, you know poison the minds against my mother and I told you about my brother, right?
>
> I: Mm-hm.
>
> S: Yeah.
>
> I: Uh I remember you once said like he didn't pay so you were, were hungry for a few days.
>
> S: Mm-hm.

I: Yeah. Sarah, I remember last time uh . . . you were mentioning that your fath . . . like your mom had your father put in jail.

S: Yeah, she wanted to put him in jail.

I: Did he go to jail?

S: Did he go to jail? Maybe for a day, maybe.

I: For a day? Do you remember what it was like? Did you know about it?

S: Um . . . when I was coming home, I saw the cop cars and they put him, put him in jail.

I: Do you, can you tell me what happened? What precipitated it?

S: Hm?

I: What, what were the events that led to him going to jail?

S: Because he starved us and he used to hit, sometimes he, my mother used to hit him so . . .

I: Your mother used to hit him?

S: Well, he, when they used to fight about money, yeah.

I: So your mom used to hit him but he went to jail?

S: Yeah (laughs).

I: Okay so he used to stalk you, you said?

S: Stalk?

I: What, I couldn't understand what you said. You said he used to do something.

S: Well, he used to look around for us. He used to look for, he used to come in the neighborhood.

Sarah reported being depressed during this time when her father was relatively absent.

S: Well the way they, the way my mother treated him and um he went to jail and I felt bad and um I wanted to try to help them, you know, get

> together but it didn't work. So he came out but he still used to come around. They told him not to come around. He used to look for me and my brother and um take them to, to his apartment so the cop, the uh judge told him not to, to come around because he, my mother didn't want him around, around the apartment.

Sarah did not recall when her father moved out, but suggested that some of the parental conflict seemed to be in relation to her mother's desire for distance from the father, whereas her father had not wanted the separation. "Maybe because the kids, like, me and my brother, you know. He didn't want to, you know, come, get a, you know, he wanted the kids, to see us, actually he felt that, he was, she, she was taking them away from her, from him. And, um, that's, you know, he was worried, worried about us." In the meantime, her mother resisted his intrusion, in part because the father was "saying bad things about her." The conflict seemed to have been extremely difficult for both children. Sarah described her brother resisting going to their father's house. "Yeah, she, yeah it was because like a lot of times he didn't want to pay at, you know support for the kids and he, like I told you what happened, he, um, he used to, um, you know poison the minds against my mother and I told you about my brother."

Her brother had resisted spending time with their father but Sarah had felt more important to her father than her mother. "He wanted the kids more than her," said Sarah. "He wanted her back but she didn't want to see the same things about her." The fighting seemed to escalate after her parents separated. When her father "used to come home on the weekends to visit us," she said, "He used to follow her around." This conflict was extremely difficult for Sarah, who described her father at one point as "poisoning" her. "It made me feel, I used to cry, feel bad . . . 'Cause he, he should have been more nicer to her . . . He should have gave her a chance." She went on to explain, "Well, he be more sympathetic towards her because she, he, they both used to drink, and, umm, he, shouldn't be, well, he used to drink, and they didn't get along. I think they went to a marriage counselor. . . . It didn't help."

Although her brother avoided their father because of the ways he talked about their mother, Sarah was able to be close to her father and to receive some welcome nurturance. "He used to spoil me, buy me clothes. He used to, I don't know, spoil me. . . . He used to drink a lot, though." During her visits, she reported, he would drink from the time he woke up in the morning. "He used to sleep a lot, lay in bed." When asked what impact her father's drinking had on her, Sarah replied, "I was at that time, I was, I had a baby." Secil asked how old she was at that time. "Seventeen, yeah. My son is in jail now." In this last statement, we see how the elements of her story are linked associatively, without a clear narrative thread through which to order or make sense of her experience.

Although she described her father as drinking daily and being pushed out of the household, Sarah reported her mother as the more disturbed of the two parents. Once again, we see the longing for comfort and care, in her description of a "nice relationship" with her father, explaining, "He used to give me a lot of money. And he used to take me on a ride to [amusement park]. What else, umm. He was there for me." When asked in what ways her father was there for her, she responded, "Well, he was like very, umm, sympathetic towards me and when I had a problem, I used to tell, he used to help me out with the problem. Yeah." In contrast to this idealization of her father, Sarah recalled her mother working as a waitress and being around less. And yet, there were some good times. "We used to play cards, things like that, yeah." In this memory we see a link between the mother with whom she played cards and Diane, with whom she also played games.

In spite of the gaps in her memory, there were some events that Sarah did recall. For example, she recalled coming home as a child and seeing her mother naked and very drunk and her father calling an ambulance to take her to the hospital. It was in this context of chaos and disruption that her brother "used to take care of me, he was older than me," said Sarah. "When I was younger, we had a lot of friends, and my family, my mother was, she used to drink a lot and, this is vaguely what I remember but, and one time, I came home and she was, she has her clothes off, and she was in the staircase and I was coming home from school, and I was looking for my mother, my brother, and I couldn't find him. My, my father called the ambulance and they took her to the hospital, because she was drunk, she was drinking a lot." When asked if she remembered the impact this incident had on her at the time, Sarah responded, "She was in the street with no clothes on, so, I was very young, I was very young. I don't remember. I remember, like, I just have little bits and pieces of the memory, of that." At another point in the interviews, Sarah said, "I was very young . . . I was scared, I was very scared. They put her in a mental hospital." Sarah recalled her mother being oriented, not towards her, but rather towards her various boyfriends. "This is the memories I have, she was never home. She was always out drinking and going out with the men . . . She lost her boyfriend . . . she used to cry, and everything, and I didn't understand. I was 'why, Mommy?' you know, and it was all because of her boyfriend, yeah."

A repeated theme is the extent of conflict in the family, both between her parents and also between her father and brother. In many ways, she felt very alone. She said that her father "starved us and he used to hit, sometimes he, my mother used to hit him so. . . ." She recalled the period when her father was in jail because of the marital conflict as a particularly difficult time for her, "I felt bad, I was depressed." It was in that context that Sarah turned to her brother, who would drink and who also smoked marijuana.

Grief and loss are also recurrent themes in Sarah's narrative. "I don't really have a lot of memories of my family, 'cause I don't have photographs of them, pictures of who they were and things like that." She stopped going to school in the sixth grade. "We used to move a lot," she said, and then when she was seventeen she had her baby. She said that her mother would move to get away from her father, but that he would find them because he wanted to see his children. "I had a sister," she recalled. "She passed away, too . . . ten years ago."

Although Sarah's sister had been dead for ten years, her father for twenty, at the time of the interview, she spoke of these deaths as though they were still fresh, at times describing her father's death as having occurred, not twenty years before but rather "a couple years ago . . . I think about him all the time."

As Sarah talked about her various losses, time, place and person seemed to lose their distinctions. What was left was the thread of grief, isolation, and displacement that ran through her narrative. Sarah described sharing her sadness at the loss of her mother with her brother but then the narrative once again became incoherent as she tried to locate herself.

S: Where was I staying? I was staying at a shelter. I think it was a shelter.

I: When your mom passed away?

S: I think so, yeah.

I: A shelter? How did you go to a shelter?

S: I was on the street and they put me in a shelter.

I: When did you get into the street?

S: When was I in the street? Um, after my friend Diane passed away, not passed away, she left, she went to Florida, um, Diane, I, I was crying and um somebody asked me if I was all right and they put me in a place where, where I, you know, could keep warm, it was cold out.

The interviewer tried to find anchors:

I: So you were in a shelter since your teenage years?

S: Yeah.

I: And then your friend Diane took you?

S: Yeah.

I: She was a close friend of yours?

S: A friend, acquaintance, I met her in a bar, a bar, yeah, a bar.

I: You met at a bar?

S: Yeah.

I: And, like, how did you end up living with her?

S: Well, I told her I didn't have a place to go and she said it was all right that I stayed with her.

I: How long did you stay with her?

S: I stayed with her, not long, maybe about since I was seventeen.

I: Seventeen?

S: Yeah.

I: Until when?

S:'Till now, 'til nineteen, 'til uh, let's see, 1970, to 2009.

I: 2009?

S: Yeah, yeah . . .

I: Mm, so it should have been difficult that she moved?

S: Yeah.

It is difficult to tell from this narrative whether Sarah had spent those twenty years in a shelter or with Diane. Rather, there seem to be important moments that punctuate the dialogue without necessarily providing anchors in space or time. Loss is one such moment; her mother, sister, father, and Diane have all been lost, albeit in different ways at different times. Also lost has been a sense of continuity in relationship; her brother is not the same brother she has known, nor is it clear precisely who Sarah is. Is she Sarah, or is she Kim, and what would it mean to be one or the other? We can wonder to what extent the alcohol and other substances have been used to moderate or even erase the pain of what it has meant to be herself.

Although in one place in the narrative, Sarah said that Diane had named her Kim, in another place in the interview she reports arriving at the hospital and saying to the doctor that she "didn't have a family. I told him I was an orphan."

S: I didn't know who I was.

I: Oh, like, you had no memories?

S: No, I didn't have any . . .

I: Did you even remember your name?

S: I remembered my, a little bit, a little bit.

I: A little bit.

S: Yeah.

I: What would you remember while you were in the hospital?

S: I thought I was, I thought I was Kim W.

I: Kim W?

S: Yes.

I: Who's Kim W.?

S: I don't know, uh, that's what I thought my name was.

I: But, what, how, where that name came from?

S: Somebody said I was Kim W., I asked, some psychiatrist said it.

I: That you are Kim W.?

S: Yeah.

I: How did he know?

S: I don't know (laughs). He said I wasn't Sarah. So that's when I thought I was Kim W.

I: And then how did you realize that you are Sarah?

S: They kept telling me, they kept telling me, "Oh, your name is not Kim, it's not Kim." My friend Steve, he told me my name is Sarah. He used to call me at the hospital. Steve, my friend, and I still keep in contact. I know him thirty years, about thirty years.

The conversation then breaks down even further:

I: So, in the hospital, first the psychiatrist that said you are Kim, but then . . .

S: No, not that hospital, another hospital . . .

I: Which hospital?

S: I think it was _____ hospital.

I: _____ hospital? So, they said that you are Kim?

S: Yeah.

I: And then they said that you are Sarah?

S: Mmhm.

I: And not Kim?

S: Yeah.

I: So, so it would have been very confusing, I guess?

S: Yeah, it was confusing.

I: What impact did it have on you that you didn't even have your . . .

S: I don't know. I didn't have any identification.

When Sarah talked about her current experience of her brother, we could hear threads of her longing for the type of closeness she felt with her father, which had centered around feeling special to him and him taking care of her by "spoiling" her and buying her things. She struggled to make sense of the disparity between her current brother, feeling "sort of sad at seeing him. It, it, we'd go to dinner. He doesn't talk to me as much and his, and his personality is different than, than I thought, you know?" Previously, he had been "a bit more warm and loving" but now he was "distant." She was grateful that he had "released" her and helped her get to her first residence but she also longed for more emotional support.

S: You know, a, a sense of um touch uh you know if you're crying, he would hold you and you know support. He didn't do that.

I: Do you cry . . . near your brother?

S: Does my brother cry?

I: No, you.

S: Sometimes I, I um I cry because I don't know if that's my brother or not.

She continued,

S: He doesn't understand like um . . . my feelings, you know, my feelings.

I: What would you like him to understand?

S: Like maybe you know like um . . . he'll be more open to me uh . . .

I: Like in what ways?

S: My problems, things like he could like help me with. Things like that. I know he's not a doctor but you know . . .

Sarah also wished that her brother would help her more financially, in some ways longing for the type of comfort she received from her father. "Now that I'm working," she said, "he thinks I have a lot of money but I don't, you know?" When asked what her brother had been like when she was younger, Sarah replied that he had been "very loving. You know, he would hug me, things like that. Yeah. He was drunk though, yeah."

We see Sarah lost, not only in relation to her previous life but also in relation to her current life. When she discussed her diagnosis, for example, her ideas about it seemed unclear and remote.

I: Um . . . before being hospitalized, did you ever think that you have some kind of mental condition or, um, like bipolar? Were you aware of that?

S: No, I didn't know. The doctor told me.

I: The doctor told you. So do you remember what it felt like when you first heard that you have something?

S: I was surprised. I didn't, I didn't know.

I: So, can you tell me what that surprise was about?

S: I was sort of like um . . . uh shocked, you know, because I didn't think that um I had a mental disorder and when they told me I, I sort of maybe, maybe I realized it because maybe I did change my clothes a lot and maybe that's part of the bipolar.

I: What do you mean by changing your clothes?

S: Well, maybe I change in different ways, different clothes. Maybe the clothes make me look dis, you know, different. Maybe that's part they think of the bipolar.

I: Can you tell me a little bit about the clothes? What do you mean by you changed them?

S: Um maybe I changed them like um . . . I, I switched my clothes maybe. Maybe-maybe different clothing maybe, I don't know how they thought I was bipolar. I don't know.

I: So, did they tell you what the symptoms of bipolar are like?

S: No, they didn't tell me.

I: In the first interview you say that, that it caused ups and lows.

S: Oh, yeah. Ups and downs. I do get, yeah.

I: So, so like, for example, um, how is uh how does it feel like or what's the experience of feeling high and low? What is that like?

S: I don't know. They said uh sometimes I'm high. Maybe I'm happy and the next minute, I'm depressed.

I: What does happy Sarah feel like?

S: Um . . . happy. Things go my way, I'm happy. I don't know. Getting paid from my job (inaudible) um . . . seeing a friend I didn't see in a long time, good memories. Depression, uh, I want to be by myself, I feel depressed, I think about my family, I wish they would, they were alive, you know? Things like that . . .

I: Is there anyone in your family that has a mental illness?

S: My brother, no, not my brother. No. My mother, no, I don't know. My mother had a drinking problem. Maybe she had bipolar disorder, my mother. She could have had it. Drinking, could be that be bipolar disorder?

Sarah reported a great deal of confusion regarding her bipolar diagnosis. When asked if people treat her differently because of the diagnosis, she replied, "Well, some people ask me if I, if they ask me . . . One of the patients asked me and I told her." Although on the one hand Sarah described her diagnosis as just something "I have to deal with," she also expressed concerns about being "different." But then, she said, "other people had the same, people that I live, I live with have the same bipolar disorder and, um, I usually am around those type of people, but outside I'm not really around the people that don't have the diagnosis. Some people have it, some people don't." She expressed some concern as to how she might be judged by "regular people," fearing "they would judge me":

S: Well, they would, they would, well, it's not good. My, my case manager told them I don't have to tell them and she told me not to, you know, if they ask me to tell them.

I: Do you know why she said not to tell anyone?

S: She didn't say tell anyone. She said . . .

I: Not, I mean to most people.

S: Yeah. I don't know if my brother knows. My family might know. Do, do they know?

I: I mean your brother took you from the hospital so I guess he knows.

S: Yeah.

I: But I'm not sure. You don't think he knows?

S: I don't know.

I: Do you think he would be reacting differently to you if he knows or not knows like would there be a difference in the way . . .

S: I don't think he . . .

I: He treats you?

S: I don't think he would treat me different. Do you think he would?

I: I'm. I don't think so but it's like your interaction but I don't think, I think, yeah, um . . . so because he took you to the hospital . . .

S: Yeah, he took me to the hospital.

I: He took you out of the hospital and you were in the hospital for a reason so um . . .

S: To cure my bipolar disorder.

I: Yeah, so . . .

S: Can I ask you a question?

I: Yeah, sure.

S: Would that, is there a cure for that, bipolar disorder?

I: I mean with medication like a lot of the symptoms can be managed and if you talk to your therapist about it or to your case manager . . .

S: They said if I didn't take the medication, I would, I, I would say that wasn't my brother. I would leave.

We can see ways in which Sarah felt lost within a system that offered her assistance, but on its own terms. She asked for reassurance but also seemed tentative about the response:

S: If I didn't take it maybe I would, I would leave and not know my brother and I would walk away like I did when I seen him in the street. So my medication makes me, makes me calmer?

I: I'm not sure. What do you think the medication does for you?

S: I guess it's a stabilizer like you said.

I: But what does it for, do for you?

S: I guess, like you said, it keeps me stable and um . . .

I: But what, in what way it makes you stable?

S: To, uh, to see if that's, that's my brother or not, you know, and see if that's um . . . my friend Steve, my friend Steve I see. See, see if that's Steve and things like that.

Sarah seemed caught between her dependence on others and her desires for greater independence, to be able to make her own rules and have her own timetable. In her current residence, "you have to leave the place. You have to leave, you have to leave. You can't stay in the room." Fountain House, which she had been attending for a year and a half, had given her "something to do." She had been working in the horticulture department but wanted to move to clerical. "I like to try different things," she said. She liked "being around people . . . talking to people." They also "have events, things like that. They have parties."

We see Sarah longing for home, for a space of her own, where her basic needs are being taken care of and where she can make her own choices about how to spend her money or her time. In her narrative, we see ways in which home has been something to both yearn for and survive in. Paternal care is spoken of in relation to basic needs for sustenance, whereas the moments marked with her mother are those in which they might quietly play some game together and pass the time. In a family in which adults turned to substances to soothe their distress rather than working problems through with one another, Sarah, too, turned to drugs and alcohol. Decades later, we find her still relatively unformed and unformulated, carrying the pieces of her life without being able to organize them into a coherent narrative.

Attuned and attentive parenting is essential for the development of coherence in identity and self-narrative (Main & Hesse, 1990). Meaning itself is built within the context of relationships, through which the child begins to identify self, other, and world. Moments of shared engagement help to build the capacities for understanding and sharing mental states (Lyons-Ruth, 2008) so essential to emotional understanding and self-regulation (Malatesta & Haviland, 1985). When these fundamental attachment processes have been disrupted, it is difficult to construct a coherent sense of self (Liotti, 1999). Such disruptions not only affect self-development but also the ability to adaptively engage with, empathically connect with and, in that sense, know another person's mind. Such engagement forms the crucial underpinnings of *reflective* or *metacognitive* functions, the capacity to recognize and differentiate one's own thoughts and feelings, and also infer the thoughts and feelings of others as subjects in their own right (Lysaker, Gumley, & Dimaggio, 2011). From her descriptions, we can conjecture that Sarah's parents were not sufficiently attuned to her needs and feelings to help her to develop these crucial capacities or to consolidate a secure or stable self-structure. Her story, then, is one in which being known in any real sense was sacrificed to the more pressing demands of survival. The question of "who am I?" remains conditional, in relation to what price or promise might be attached to the answer to that question.

Chapter Twelve

Daniel

Haunted by His Past

Michael O'Loughlin, Marilyn Charles, and Secil Arac-Orhun

Daniel, a man of Latino origin in his early forties, approached the interview with great earnestness. He worked hard to be understood, and he explained his life in great detail. Daniel has had a difficult life and has suffered many comorbid difficulties. Daniel's life did not get off to a good start, and he still experiences pain due to the consequences of the poverty, poor boundaries, abandonment, and exposure to harsh street life he experienced early on. Psychoanalyst Wilfred Bion (1984) noted that we learn from experience. Those unfortunate enough to get off to a poor start in life may not acquire the adaptive skills to allow them to weather later adversity effectively. Because of the multiple risk factors involved in comorbid disorders in cases like Daniel's, it is impossible to pinpoint a single factor as causative of his struggles with psychosis. Daniel has great regret and guilt about his earlier life, and the way earlier events led to an unfolding tragedy in his late teenage years. Daniel is still struggling with the significant aftereffects of the traumas he has suffered and the extreme psychic experiences they have produced. With the help of the Fountain House community, he is striving to build a support network and beginning to explore his artistic talents as he seeks to create the elements of a new life narrative for himself going forward.

EARLY LIFE

The second interview focused primarily on early family history and key life events, and Daniel opened up this interview with a graphic description of the lacunae in his early life. He described a childhood, replete with experiences of deprivation, abandonment, poor boundaries, hard knocks, and inevitably, shame and abjection:

> All right, I grew up in the streets of ________, and um, my mother was, was, we were poor people, poor family. My dad, my pa deserted us and he went somewhere with another female and had more kids with the other female. He deserted us.
>
> Deserted us, okay. So, we were a really poor family you know, and my, my, on my, on my mother's side, you know and, I used to have some uncles on my father's, on my father's side, and my family, you know, my family's a working family and, my mother was poor and she, but she, she raised us up, and then, you know, I grew up and I dropped out of school 'cause I lose my front teeth.

What should have been a rather mundane childhood accident became a source of great shame to Daniel. In two incidents in his family, his younger siblings accidentally knocked out some of his front teeth, and for reasons that are suggestive of a failure of parental care, Daniel abandoned whatever prosthetic device had been installed. To this day his speech articulation is noticeably impaired due to a failure to receive the necessary orthodontic care. Daniel suffered deep shame and humiliation because of this perceived defect and because of teasing from peers. The situation was compounded in that he blamed himself for not having the discipline to follow through with the orthodontic regimen prescribed for him. Nowhere in his narrative is there a realization that his parents may have failed in their duty of care to this eleven-year-old boy. You will notice repeated clarifications in Secil's interview as Daniel struggles to make himself understood despite his articulation difficulties:

> D: You know it's a shame, because um, my two little sisters, one by one hit me with a toy truck.
>
> I: Toy truck? Yeah?
>
> D: Yeah and, and they cut in half.
>
> I: Yeah.
>
> D: Then they, then they, one sister after her, that my mother used to babysit, they hit me again, on the other one, so, and then, we went to the dentist and they did work in there, they, they drilled two holes in my front two teeth and they put some kind of cotton, but then, you know, I start playing with it so, with a needle, I start playing with it and I pulled, and I pulled the cotton out of my teeth.

I: They put cotton on your teeth?

D: They, they were doing that, my sister hit me, right?

I: Yes.

D: With a toy truck, and they drilled two holes in my teeth.

I: Yes.

D: And then they put some type of cotton.

And, somehow, I um, took out the cotton out with a needle and it became rotten,

I: Mhm.

D: And then, we decided to um, take them off.

I: Mhm.

D: So we went to a dentist and they, they took them out my, took them out, everything.

I: How old were you?

D: I was about eleven.

I: You were about eleven?

D: Yeah, that's bad luck, you know what I mean?

I: Sorry?

D: It's bad luck to lose your teeth like that. It's, it's no good, at that age, you know.

I: It got rotten?

D: Right.

I: And you said you felt ashamed?

D: Yeah, to go to school, I was ashamed.

Daniel went on to explain how the shame and exclusion he experienced because of the mouth injury caused him to eventually drop out of school and begin to sell drugs on the street. While Daniel indulged in some self-blame for the failure to have the necessary orthodontic work done, feeling that this caused his life to enter a downward spiral, he also offered some musings that even back then he was beginning to hear voices that attributed misfortunes to forces outside himself. These voices gained in prominence, as we shall see, when he encountered more striking difficulties and setbacks later in his life.

D: You know, let them, when, when they took them out, I was supposed to let it, let heal.

I: Yes.

D: And I didn't do that, they, they, they pulled apart right next to it.

I: Mhm.

D: But after taking my teeth, that's what happened, if I had let them get healed, the gums, get healed, I would have, everything would have been different, it's my fault, you know . . . It's my fault because . . .

I: That's your fault?

D: It's my fault, it's not my mother's fault, it's my fault about my teeth, because remember I told you earlier I start playing with it until it fell out, and also they told me, "You have to wait a while and then we'll put in, and then we'll give you dentures," but I said, "No I can't. Put them in right away." So after they took them off, they, they give me dentures right there, right there and then, they made sure it worked and everything, he said it was going to be all right, but then after the gums healed, they were, they um, the dentures fit me too big, something like that, it's shameful, you know, but it happens with the chosen people, you know, with the chosen people from God, that's why, the devil, you know, they were all around the world, you know.

I: The devil that caused it, you think?

D: Yeah, yeah.

I: In what way?

D: Because he knew that I came, that I was going to work something like that, let me say it clear, he knew that I came from heaven and he knew my mission, you know, so that's why they say that it was his, you know, the devil's work, but you know. They say that it was the, the devil that took all my teeth, his work.

Discussing his father's role in his life, Daniel offered a poignant memory of some of the things he learned from his father, things which are as much a reminder of the lack he experienced after his father abandoned the family, as they are poignant totems of potential father-son bonding:

I: You said your father, father abandoned you?

D: Yeah, yeah.

I: Can you say a little bit about that?

D: Yeah, of course, no problem, um, my father . . . my father wasn't there, you know . . . I mean, there are two things, you know. Let me see if I can put this together. Let me tell you, one time, my father, he used to hustle a lot, you know, he used to do a lot of hustling, selling, selling fruit, he used to have horses, he used to live in the mountains, and he took me there. He, he, he gave me his breed, you know. He taught me how to fish, we went fishing, how to, how to, how to fish crabs from the sea, how to fish, how to fish, how to get crabs from the earth, you know the dirt, earth, in the mountain, there's, there's a crab that comes from the, you know what I'm talking about, so he taught me that, you know, he gave me a really cool breeding, you know.

LACK OF BOUNDARIES

Unfortunately, Daniel's abiding memories of his father revolved around recollections of his father's alcoholism, his reputation for domestic violence, his incarcerations, and his embarrassing public lewdness:

D: So you know my father, I mean, we was embarrassed of him, so sometimes we got embarrassed of him, you know.

I: About what?

D: Because he used to like, uh, he used to get drunk and he used to you know, do, do, do shameful things like . . .

I: Like what?

D: He pulled his, his thing out, you know, in front of everybody, this and that, you know, that's what my sister told me, too, you know. We were ashamed, sometimes, by the way he was hustling. He was like, I don't know, you know, he was like, he was good people though, you know, he had good kids, and . . .

I: When, he would drink, what are your memories of him drinking?

D: We were very good, so we used to sit down in parking [lot], and my father used to do, you know, crazy things when he got drunk.

I: What would he do?

D: He, he, he take his, he take his penis out, show it to people, you know, like drunk, you know.

I: How old were you then?

D: I was young, I was ashamed, that, that part I was . . .

I: You were ashamed?

D: That I was ashamed, I felt ashamed, I was, I felt ashamed, and my sister . . . He was, he was Caucasian, you know.

I: Caucasian?

D: He was Caucasian, my father was Caucasian, he had hazel eyes.

I: Hazel eyes?

D: Yeah, he had, he was light skin, Caucasian, yeah, so he knew things and would buy us stuff, you know, but he, he was trying to do good, he used to do knockoffs, too, you know.

I: Mhm.

I: But then I think something changed . . .

D: Something changed, because?

I: Do you remember what changed?

D: I think he went to jail . . .

I: When did he go to, for, for what did he go to jail?

D: He, he talked to his daughter in the wrong way, I believe that's the truth.

I: Sorry?

D: He talked to his daughter in the wrong way, but he also said that he was innocent, because his wife, the other wife that he had, he used to poison, she used to poison him.

I: Poison him?

D: And, and, and his girl, my father's wife, family was against my father, so, so they got together and plot against him.

Asked for his reaction to these events, and to his father's incarceration, Daniel expressed stoicism:

I: That was . . . what impact did it have on you that he went to jail?

D: I fought, I fought, I hold back my tears, I held them back, I was brave, you know, I was brave.

I: You held, you held your tears back?

D: Because when he, when I saw him in the newspaper, by this time I was in, fresh in [new city to which Daniel had relocated] . . .

I: Oh you were in ________ by then?

D: But it was fresh, because we had moved recently, so my, my aunt said, "Daniel, look," and showed me newspaper and it was my father (inaudible), you know, I felt, I felt, you know, I'm saying your father's going to love you, you know, what I'm saying?

I: So you saw him in the newspaper?

D: I felt horrible. Yeah my aunt showed me, this is _______, your father, so I held back strong, you know, I wanted to cry, but I held back strong 'cause you know, I was seventeen or sixteen, I think I was sixteen.

Daniel had a mother who, by all accounts, was desperately poor and who not only exerted minimal supervision over Daniel, but who, due to their reduced circumstances, welcomed the income that his drug dealing produced:

I: Back in [birthplace], how was your relationship with your mom and your sister?

D: It was very liberal.

I: It was, what did you say?

D: It was very, like, like, free, you know, like, she never said, "Daniel, come home now, now." She let me, she let me out there, she came to live with the way I talked to her, I said "Look, mom, I got this, I'm going out there, you understand?" You know, she let me roll yayos, she let me buy, you know, pounds of weed.

I: She let you do what?

D: She let me roll yayos in my room with my friend.

I: Oh, she used to let you roll?

D: She let me, in her apartment.

I: What impact did it have on you? How did it affect you that she was so free?

D: It's like a liberal thing, you know, like a street thing, you know, it's like liberal, she let me roll yayos, you know, my, my, my friend.

I: She let you?

D: She let me, she let me let my friend in my room and bag the nickel bags, you know, he was, she saw him, he used to buy, he used to buy nickel bags and roll yayos.

I: Yeah, how did it affect you?

D: It's like a lifestyle, you know, it's like.

I: Sorry?

D: It's like a, you know, like a street style.

I: So what do you mean by street style, like is it, like, how was it for you?

D: She was like, she, she let me go out there and do what I got to do, you know? She, she, she was my mother, but she was also my friend.

I: Was it good for you or like, would you rather have her only as friend, or only as mother?

D: Only as mother but, you know, that's how I grew up, you know, I needed the money, I mean, so I start selling, you know.

I: Would you rather that she had a little less free style and that she didn't allow you to roll in your room, maybe, like, uh, do you understand what I mean?

D: Yeah, yeah, yeah, but you know, she, I don't know what to say, you know. She, she trusted in me, that's what I'm saying.

I: Mhm.

D: That's what, she trusted in me, and you know, we used to be poor, but you know, that's how it is you know, in the ghettos, you know, you sell drugs you have money.

While many factors undoubtedly contributed to Daniel's difficulties, he repeatedly turned to the disfigurement caused by the injury to his mouth as a turning point:

D: If I had let it heal, if I had do the right thing, 'cause if I had do the right thing with my teeth, everything would have turned out different.

I: Uh, so, what, what would it be different, what would be different? What do you think?

D: I, I, I would stay back, you know.

I: You would?

D: I, I would have never dropped out of school. I would have stayed back in [birthplace].

I: Mhm.

D: You know, I would have gone to school, I would have married a female if she liked me, like that you know. Things, you know, like that. I would have married a female.

I: Do, do you . . .

D: I would have, you know how, I would have continued school, I, I dropped out of school because of my dentures, I would have continued school.

I: Yeah.

D: So, you know, that's what happened in my life, you know.

LIFE CRISIS

At seventeen years of age, Daniel migrated a considerable distance from the place of his birth to a large city where some cousins resided, and where, after having been fired from his factory position for chronic lateness, he resumed life as a drug dealer. A major trauma in Daniel's life was triggered eighteen months later when he was sexually molested in public while attempting to deliver drugs. His chronology of this event was confusing, but he returned to this event repeatedly and there was consistency across the various narratives. The bare facts appeared to be that he was sexually molested; that he heard voices ordering him to kill the perpetrator; that he did indeed fatally wound the perpetrator with a gun a few days later; that he served a lengthy prison sentence; and that he made a suicide attempt and has had experiences of psychosis since that time. For example, in the third interview, he described the sexual molestation this way:

D: I, I didn't remember the molestation, I didn't remember exactly how it happened, I only remember certain parts, certain parts, certain flashes, about the incident. So, I looked all right but they told me, "Yeah, he did, he, he molested, he did that to you, get him, get him, get him," and I finally was, I finally, you know, got him, you know, I shot that man, you know, and it's true you know.

I: What did you remember?

D: I remember that he took my hand, put it on his testicles, to scratch it, 'cause I was scratching my beard. I also remember that I was nodding, you know (shakes head "no"), my, my, my internal being was saying, "No, I don't want."

I: You were seventeen?

D: I was seventeen, yeah, it's pretty old to me, it's old, it's old.

I: Yes, yes.

D: You, you know better, but I couldn't help it, you know what I mean? So.

I: You were nodding, you said?

D: I was, I was, I was, I was um, um, I was a drug dealer, so um, um, so after that, um, I was nodding he said, he had like, his hand down my pants and I was nodding and he took my pants off nodding. Then, I asked a lot of people, you know, um, I was naked in the playground, naked, and this happened [year], December 11, and then, that happened 11 December, then on the 14th, I got the weapon and then I got him, after that, I became evil, you know, I became, yeah, I became evil, you know, and, and . . .

I: What do you mean?

D: I, I, I was going to finish suicide, you know, when that happened, after that, you know.

I: What made you think of suicide?

D: 'Cause of the molestation, when I say it's my fault.

I: You were . . .

D: I was saying that it was my fault that it happened.

I: How come it was your fault?

D: Because, because, I mean, it's like um . . . I did a whole bunch of drugs, something like that, you know, I, I, I came out of my house and then, I started out doing um, I started doing glue and then I started like, buy some heroin, and then, and then I, I lost it, I lost my mind, you know, I lost it.

His first impulse, Daniel noted, was to commit suicide, but then, he said, "I had a thought. I said, 'Look, how about him? If you die, what's going to happen to him that diss you?' So I got him, you know. I, I, I, they gave me a weapon and I bought the bullets at the corner store . . . and everybody wanted me to get his car, but I end up getting him. I shot him. After that I became mentally ill." Elsewhere, Daniel framed the impulse to retaliate—an impulse he claims was fanned by the perpetrator bragging that Daniel was a coward and would not fight back—in terms of a voice that he heard commanding him to take revenge:

I: Could you perhaps start by telling me when you were hospitalized or treated for psychiatric issues?

D: The first time?

I: Yes.

D: Um, um, my lying, I mean, I started taking medication in [year] 'cause, I mean, my whole mental disruption came about when I was in [city to which he had moved], and I got sexual molested by rude people in public. After that I became suicidal, after that, 'cause they molested me in the streets, when I was delivering uh, delivering some drugs. Um, they molested me, and they, they gave me a heavily beat down you know, so, I was going to you know, I was, I was going to suicide, so I bought the weapon and I bought the, the bullets and everything, and then a voice say, "What about him? If you use that [weapon] (starts laughing) What about him?" Seriously, so I investigated, right, every detail because I didn't remember quite what, everything that happened.

Just as he had done with the oral injury trauma, Daniel identified this sexual molestation and its attendant trauma as a marker event that forever changed his life's trajectory: "I got the weapon and then I got him, after that, I became evil, you know, I became, yeah, I became evil, you know." Readers familiar with the work of Richard Gartner (2001, 2017) on the consequences of sexual abuse of boys, will have no difficulty in understanding why a sexual assault—occurring, in Daniel's case, in an environment in which psychosocial support was entirely absent—could leave Daniel with memory difficulties, dissociative experiences, paranoia, and the kinds of intrusive and persecutory thoughts he went on to describe. He put it succinctly in the first interview, stating that " . . . emotionally, when I got sexually molested, that took a toll, toll, it changed my mind, it changed everything, you know." Daniel acknowledged that he set out in life with high aspirations, including wanting to finish his GED [high school equivalency diploma] and wanting to purchase a home and have "a whole family, wife and kids." He noted that when he first moved to [city in which he was incarcerated] he had gained steady employment in a factory. However, after he was fired, he fell back into his old habit of drug dealing, and this led to his downward spiral.

DEMONS AND VOICES

When Daniel arrived at prison he was advised that relatives of the man he had shot were there, and he said this is when the voices in his head grew more intense. His chronology is hard to follow, but he seems to suggest that he was having some extreme psychic experiences prior to the sexual molestation, but these were greatly aggravated after that incident. For instance, in the first interview, when Secil inquired about voice-hearing experiences, he offered this explanation:

I: Do you remember when you first used to hear voices?

D; Um, it happened after the case of the molestation.

I: After the molestation . . .

D: Demons, demons, they were demons. They were demons, demons, demons.

I: Did you used to hear voices before?

D: No.

I: No?

D: Oh yeah, yes, in the car, yeah.

I: Where?

D: At my friends when I was hanging out, he was saying "yo," they are hearing my voices . . .

I: So, before the molestation you started hearing voices, right?

D: I started hearing demon's voices, demons.

I: Do you remember what was going on in your life at the time?

D: It was like I was, um, being rejected you know.

I: Rejected by whom?

D: By the people in general . . . because they could see my thoughts, you know, truly, truly, you know. They, they saw the flash one night, right, I was in my room in ______. I was praying on my knees. I prayed the whole night. I was being religious, you know.

I: Mhm.

D: So I prayed the whole night on my knees, and the day after they stayed there, the daylight, daylight spirit came into my room. Yes, and it was a big flash and people saw it.

I: What did they see?

D: They saw, they saw a big flash in my room.

Daniel spent most of the third interview attempting to explicate the extreme psychic events he had experienced and attempting to show how they arose from the trauma of the molestation, the shooting, and his subsequent lengthy imprisonment. Attempting to explicate his religiosity and the way in which the Holy Spirit turned on him and caused him to kill his attacker, he stated:

D: Yes, I was feeling bad, bad, it's bad, but that was because of the demons and this and that, you know, 'cause of my faith in God, my, my faith in God, that's what happened, you know, 'cause I was, I was reading the bible, all of a sudden I started hearing voices. The home people, the, my home friends, they um, they say, "Daniel, we can't hear these voices," you know, and after that I went to jail. After jail, I was reading the bible, fasting, and everything, I was going to go to heaven, that's the truth, Secil, I mean, um, the Holy Spirit made me kill that man, you know, and that's the truth, you know, because she say, that's the only way I can let go of the world, not love the world, and let go, so she could take me, that's what happened.

I: When was the first time you heard, uh, the Holy Spirit? Do you remember the first time she talked to you?

D: Um, the first time she talked to me, when I was in [city where he lived at time of incarceration]. She didn't talk to me. I only listen to the [genes?] voices.

I: Sorry?

D: I, the Holy Spirit didn't talk to me when I was in [city where he lived at time of incarceration] in the street, I was only hearing the uh, um, oh, you know what, oh, you know what, you know what?

I: Genes voices? After, after the, after the molestation, then, that was on a Friday, right?

I: Yes.

D: And then the next Saturday, in the morning, I was hearing her.

I: What did she say?

D: Get him, get him, get him.

I: Get in?

D: Get him, you know get the guy that, that, that . . .

I: Ah, get him.

D: Right, right.

I: Get him.

D: Right.

I: So.

D: I mean, after the molestation, I was hearing her voice, and then, you know, um, like that, but, um, yeah, that's, that's what happened, you know, but then, you know, I used to work in the factories, and this and that, you know. In [birthplace], you know, I suffered a lot of scorn 'cause of the bible faith, you know, when I was in [birthplace]. You know, I suffered a lot of, uh, the rejection, you know, scorn.

Daniel went on to suggest that when he returned to his birthplace the family of the man he had killed was determined to do him harm. Recognizing that he had allied himself with the Holy Spirit, they, in turn, allied themselves with the devil so they could hurt him. He believed they could read his mind, and had imputed to him a homosexual motive and a nefarious alliance with God and the Holy Spirit. Notice here also some conflict over skin color that may reflect some ambivalence in Daniel's identification with his light-skinned father:

D: What I'm saying, they knew, it was God's mission and my people were saying that to them. They were saying that they could read my thoughts, because I needed to be, to, to do, to do homosexual acts, gay acts, homosexual acts, to have them shut my mind. So, so that my, my mind, the mental thing that was in my life, 'cause they were saying this and that, it was that, it was the spirit of God, or the Holy Spirit, the spirit or the Holy Spirit in me, that's why they could have seen my thoughts in my molestation and that, that led me to do those other drugs. So, so I think it was proven and then, then, then, Jesus Christ pulled in, in the voice of the cricket in the back of the balcony saying, "Daniel [last name]."

I: Wait, wait, wait, Jesus Christ.

D: Jesus.

I: Pulled in the voice of what?

D: Like a cricket, like a . . .

I: Cricket? Yeah? And what did he say?

D: He said "Daniel, it's my sister's fault."

I: "It's your sister's fault." What did your sister . . .

D: *His* sister.

I: What did his sister do?

D: His sister is the Holy Spirit.

I: Yes.

D: The sister of Jesus Christ, is the Holy . . . the Holy Spirit is a female.

I: Yes, and what did she do?

D: She . . . he, he said it was her fault because I didn't like her, her complexion.

I: You didn't like her complexion?

D: Right, something like that.

I: I wonder what about her . . .

D: I mean I didn't not . . . I'm saying, you know?

I: What about her complexion didn't you like?

D: She was too, she was snow white, you know?

I: Snow white?

D: Not yellow, not pinkish, she was snow white. And her hair was too soft (laughs). That's why.

I: What makes you laugh?

D: 'Cause of the way I am, the way I am, I'm talking, something like that. Listen, but, that's what happened, you know? She was, she was, she wasn't pinkish or yellowish or beige, she was too white for me, you understand?

In addition to suggestions of racial unease in the excerpt just presented, Daniel also seemed to struggle with the imputation of homosexuality implied in his experience of having been sexually desired and molested by a man. In seeking to not have to claim agency for these conflicts—and indeed for the shooting—Daniel continued to invoke an intrusive and domineering Holy Spirit:

I: What about the cousin of the guy you killed?

D: The Holy Spirit wanted me to have sex with him so she could say that it was my fault and not her fault. You, you see what I'm saying, right?

I: Mhm.

D: That's the truth. She, she wanted, she wanted to show the world that it was my fault and not her.

Daniel expressed a sense of a foreclosed future, indicating that because of his misfortune he will not enter heaven:

D: You know, I want, now, now when I die I'm not going to go to Heaven.

I: You are not?

D: No. (Shakes head)

I: Why not?

D: They don't want me there, you know.

I: They don't, they don't want, how do you know they don't want you?

D: Because they're responsible for everything bad that happens to me.

I: So you don't want to go there?

D: I can't go there.

I: You can't go there, you don't feel safe there?

D: It's like, you know, they, they don't want me, so you know, I can't go there.

D: You know, God don't want me, and his daughter don't want me.

I: God and his daughter?

D: Yeah, that's true. You know. (Laughs) Truth, it could be, you know, but I'm saying, he wanted me, you know, God wanted me, even though, after, after we switched souls, you know, he wanted me yet, you know. But, you know, it's not my fault, you know.

In prison, Daniel claimed that he discovered the Koran, and his embrace of the Muslim faith allowed him to take some refuge in a sense of omnipotence:

D: I'm a, I'm a, truly a prophet, I prophesize.

I: Sorry?

D: I'm a teacher. I'm, I'm a prophet, I got power.

I: You're a, uh-huh.

D: I got power, yes it is. It's serious, it is.

I: You're a prophet of which religion?

D: Um, Muslim.

"SCHIZOPHRENIA"

Asked to speak about his understanding of his diagnosis and treatment, Daniel again took refuge in his belief in the influence of outside agencies, in this case the Holy Spirit and Voodoo, as shifting responsibility for his violent act—an act that he viewed as precipitated by the sexual assault that was first visited on him:

D: Hold on, like, like (puts his head down and then mumbles to himself). I'm trying to remember, but it was like, um, schizophrenia, I believe.

I: Schizophrenia?

D: Yeah. Schizophrenia.

I: Schizophrenia, how did it affect you to learn that?

D: Because (pauses). Two things, I'm going to tell you the truth, two things. The Holy Spirit and Voodoo.

I: Voodoo? Uh-huh.

D: And the Holy Spirit. Voodoo was spying and the Holy Spirit.

I: Sorry?

D: The Holy Spirit and Voodoo, that's why.

I: That's why . . .

D: And they shot, basically they shot my mind, my problem. I am shot because of three things, the Holy Spirit, Voodoo, witchcraft, and the shock of the case.

In perhaps the most emotionally open moment of the interviews, Daniel revealed how, when placed on the witness stand, he broke down as he sought to claim innocence due to fact that the trauma precipitated his violent response:

D: Yeah, Secil. I was gonna suicide, you know. I took the jury stand, um, Secil. They put me in the jury stand, with a whole bunch of jury, the case was holy, Secil. They put me in, they put me in the, in the, in the jury stand, and they were seeing me, they, they wanted to hear me, why I killed that man, you know.

I: They put you on the stand?

D: Yeah.

I: How did you, how did it make you feel?

D: I was, I had to tell them why I, why I killed that man. I had to tell them. You know, that's why everything happens in my life, this is back in [year], you know. It, it's like, you know . . . The lawyer asked me, "What happened after that, after, after that case? What happened after the molestation, what did you do?" I, I started sobbing, crying.

I: Sobbing, crying

D: I was crying.

I: Why were you crying, Daniel?

D: Because I was going, I felt self-pity because I was going suicidal. But, but after that I kept on, you know, you know. That's what happened, you know what I mean, Secil? Back in the day, I'm not the only one who cried in a case, right Secil?

I: Sorry?

D: I'm not the only one who cried in a case, this happened back in the day, you know. So that . . .

I: Do you, do you feel . . .

D: . . . that, that, I'm saying because, they know, they know, Secil, they know, my kinds of people know that I'm innocent. Therefore they protect my life. Because if they touch me, they're going to get hurt bad.

I: I guess . . .

D: But people have to believe me, because I proved my point innocent, Secil.

When asked about his use of medication, Daniel's answer was unequivocal: medications help him maintain a level of emotional regulation that has improved his capacity to be in the world. His response, again, is tinged with some perhaps necessary grandiosity, but ultimately he understands that he is still vulnerable to emotional dysregulation and the risk of being flooded by traumatic memories:

D: They work. They, they, they are, they are normal without medication. I, we cannot do that.

I: And.

D: For real, Secil, I can't do that. I laugh, I cry. The way I feel, you know, depression. For real, man. They, they, they, they think, sometimes they jealous because haters [say], "No you don't need medication," but it's not that, I do need medication. See, when I was in the church there, I wasn't getting medication and the way I felt, you know, it's just awful, you know?

I: You felt . . .

D: I felt like, you know, the sunshine, you know. I couldn't take it.

I: Couldn't take it, it was too much.

D: Yeah, I had, I need, I do need medication because I'm hard true world, even though I'm high functioning, that's why. They say that because I'm high functioning, you know. You know, so, I mean I got powers, I got powers. Yeah, I think, I, they, they like my powers, I make [birthplace] very powerful. I gave power to [birthplace]. I feel it, you know. I gave power to [birthplace] and they say they could fly without wings.

I: Without wings?

D: Right, they say they could fly without wings.

I: What, what, what did they mean by that?

D: They mean that, the power I gave them, I gave, gave, you know, uh, uh, excellent power, excellent power.

I: Excellent power.

D: I gave them excellent power, yes, Secil. I gave them letters, grammar and forming letters, right, I gave them two hours.

I: Mhm.

D: And it's not, it's, it's not sealed, nothing, nobody's power. It's proven, Secil, that my power, don't drive and not very effective. No see, body power, it says give power. So that's what they said, I give them power.

Daniel continued, suggesting that medication was vital to his emotional regulation:

I: But uh, you said that like, you can't do without medications.

D: Right.

I: So do you find medication helpful?

D: Yes, I do, Secil.

I: In what ways is it helpful for you?

D: Way you, way, way your, presentation, way you act, you know, way you feel. I mean I know, I know, I could become, sarcastic mean like, you like, what's sarcastic mean?

I: Sarcastic?

D: (Nods)

I: Sarcastic is when like, you make jokes, but like. Mmm, I mean, I know what it means but . . .

D: I know because, I know, I know, I know without that medication, it's worse now, before it was, because, uh, like I said, I laugh a lot, I cry, I mean, it's . . .

I: A lot of feelings.

D: Right, you talk, the way you talk, you know, it's just. You have to be careful, you know. The medication help you, you know. In, in doing the day, you know? Wake up in the morning and go about your day, that's why it's helpful.

CONCLUSION

During the interviews, Daniel came across as sincere, and he struggled mightily to make his life narrative relatable. He endured layers of trauma and adversity in his early years that left Daniel poorly equipped to handle the much more traumatic events of his early adult life. The complexity of Daniel's case resists articulation of simple causal explanations for his current psychiatric struggles, but it is inescapable that psychosocial factors loom large as risk factors. In Daniel's case, psychosocial factors include risk factors such as poverty, adverse childhood events, inadequate boundaries, sexual molestation, and so forth, as well as the evident lack of living and containing structures in Daniel's childhood that might have better equipped him to manage later adversities. Daniel has received psychiatric care, and his medication regimen may, as he claims, be facilitative of his current positive level of functioning. However, as in so many cases in this book, there is no evidence that Daniel has received opportunities for sustained psychosocial or therapeutic support prior to his arrival at Fountain House, two years prior to these interviews. With the rise of incarceration as a mechanism of containment for persons with psychiatric struggles, we are increasingly worried that persons such as Daniel run the risk of becoming rudderless and disconnected as they are pushed toward experiencing their own experience only as decontextualized—or perhaps unmetabolized—fragments of trauma. We, psychoanalysts, often speak of metabolization, containment, holding, and other such terms that imply that persons suffering psychic distress need to be in the presence of persons who bear witness to their experiences, and who create receptive spaces that allow them to begin to re-narrate their own histories in ways that diminish fragmentation and intrusion, and increase capacity for re-storying experience. It is not yet too late for Daniel to benefit from such possibilities. The tragedy for Daniel is that he had harbored aspirations for a good life, and now he is reaching for an explanation for his disappointment:

> D: But listen, that can't happen, if that molestation didn't happen, I wouldn't be here today. I would have been in [city where he was incarcerated] working, and married with kids. She didn't take me, if the Holy Spirit didn't take me to [birthplace], that's on her. Ain't nothing I can do about that. That's all I'll say, you know. No rush.

However, now he appears to have tempered his expectations. Apart from his artistic endeavors, he merely wishes for a life free of intrusions and complexity:

> I: How do you find Fountain House? What's your experience like here?
>
> D: I just, I just, you know, been given another chance even though, I'm a client. Even though I take medication they, they, they find, uh, um. They give me a chance.
>
> I : Even . . .
>
> D: In the, in the neat way, you know . . . I been here and they give me an opportunity. You know, to do something positive with my time.
>
> I : You said.
>
> D: Some people say, "Oh, you work too hard," this and that. But, but, I like to work you know? It's my business, it's what I do with my time, you know. Some people not high functioning and they get jealous, you know. But, you know, this place gave me another opportunity. It gives me, a good, a good, a good opportunity, I'm grateful, you know. Even though everything . . . even though I'm not going to go to the glory of God, forever. I, I mean I found um, I saw a new day, you know.

And, unfortunately, his aspirations now are somewhat foreclosed:

D: I don't want no kids or married, whatever. I just want to be left alone, do what I gotta do, and enjoy my life, you know.

Chapter Thirteen

Jamie

Seeking Comfort

Michael O'Loughlin, Marilyn Charles, and Montana Queler

Jamie, a Caucasian woman in her late forties, approached her meetings with Montana with a very pleasant, if obviously anxious, disposition. Jamie's life story in some respects follows a typical path for persons with psychic distress in our society. She experienced what she described as a "mental breakdown" shortly before her sixteenth birthday. Her struggles with psychic intrusions have dominated her entire adult life and have caused her considerable suffering, including difficulties in earning a living and in establishing sustained, intimate relationships. As Freud astutely noted, opportunities for success in love and work contribute greatly to satisfaction in life, and disappointment in those areas can create conditions for shame and stigma. Another feature of Jamie's struggle—and one that is not atypical, as many of the life stories in this collection indicate, also borne out by the struggles Lucy Newlyn (2018) reveals—is that the capacity for recovery is often compromised by the debilitating and aberrant nature of the experiences. Perhaps most destructive are the adverse reactions of others, which risk stigmatizing, shaming, and further alienating the person already suffering psychic distress.

The big unanswered question that Jamie's story raises is why she was never invited into a sustained talk therapy experience that might have allowed her greater insight into her struggles. That opportunity might have allowed her to find more success and satisfaction in the life tasks of love and work. That the interview was punctuated with anxiety is hardly surprising, as Jamie was put under the stress of facing and examining both her life difficulties and the internal psychic experiences that she constructs to make daily living more bearable. Inevitably, of course, hidden within Jamie's struggles there is also a story of resilience, courage, and humanity as Jamie continues to live her life with persistence, dignity, humor, and grace.

Jamie began recounting her story by noting that while she had earned a college degree, she was unable to land a professional position. As she so poignantly put it, "Nobody wanted to hire me for a job." Jamie often used the term "sick" to describe her mental condition, and such a reference led her to reflect back upon her first crisis, which occurred just before her sixteenth birthday. She reported being hospitalized for two months. It is notable that while Jamie sometimes used the terms "sickness" and "mental illness" to describe herself, she seemed acutely conscious of the stigma associated with these terms. She was careful to point out repeatedly that, although she accessed vocational services at Fountain House, she was not "mentally ill" like her peers, and she avoided participating in other activities with fellow members. The net effect of this self-isolation was to deprive Jamie of the solidarity and fellowship that is one of the core healing mechanisms of the Fountain House community.

Jamie's description of her initial crisis reflects the complexities of her thinking about the psychic difficulties she has experienced:

> J: After two months from September to Christmas, and they said you know I was diagnosed, you know when I first got sick I wasn't diagnosed with a mental illness. I was diagnosed as a severe nervous breakdown.
>
> I: Uh huh.
>
> J: There was no mental illness issues when I started getting, when I was in [Hospital].

It took well into the interview sequence before Jamie was able to venture close to the difficulties in family dynamics that may have precipitated her initial breakdown. Right at the beginning, however, she revealed the social estrangement and rejection that she experienced in high school—a set of symptoms that suggest how deeply rooted her difficulties were:

> J: Yes, I told my mother, my friends were being very mean to me at that time and another boy was being very, I like, I was really obsessed with this boy in high school.
>
> I: Mhm.
>
> J: He used to come pick us up from [Place] and I really liked him a lot, he didn't treat me good at all and my friends didn't treat me good, as far as I understood that I would give my life for them and they weren't, as far as

the feedback to me from them, from my family they weren't good friends to me. They were very jealous 'cause I was very pretty I had a beautiful shape, and I had, I was an A+ student and they were just very jealous, and the whole thing is I got sick.

She also revealed how understandably bewildering the whole experience was for her:

J: And then my family had no choice, they didn't even know what was going on 'cause they didn't, we didn't know what mental illness was. We didn't know mental illness existed, so that, they, the doctor that they talked to you know, said you know I think we're going to have to take her to the hospital and I didn't know about this. They took me in the car to [Hospital]. I didn't know I was being, going to the hospital and I ran away, and they you know, they took me in the hospital, they put me in the seclusion room and they gave me an injection, and as far as that I've never, I've been seeing a doctor ever since then.

I: Do you remember what you were feeling at the time?

J: I tried to go back to school in junior year at [School], and they, you know, were like giving me the work and I couldn't do it.

I: How come . . .

J: Then I got one hundred percent better, and I don't want my record to say in it I went back to [School] and they wouldn't take me there.

I: How come you were having trouble doing your work, what was it that was happening?

J: I wasn't focused, I just wasn't feeling good.

I: What were you feeling?

J: Like, like anxious and nervous.

I: Mhm, how did you deal with that anxiety at the time, what did you, what kinds of things did you do?

J: I didn't know what to do.

I: Did you have certain things that you would do to try to manage it?

J: No I had no idea about mental illness, I didn't know it existed.

What is most striking is Jamie's difficulty, even in retrospect, in understanding precisely the source of her distress. Her recollection was punctuated with uncertainty, captured in statements such as "I wasn't focused, I wasn't feeling good." And "I was anxious and nervous." This distress apparently culminated in a diagnosis of schizophrenia at age sixteen:

> I: And how did you understand at the time why you were in the hospital?
>
> J: How I understood?
>
> I: Yeah, how did you understand it at sixteen years old?
>
> J: I didn't understand nothing.
>
> I: What did you think was happening?
>
> J: I didn't know I was mentally ill, I didn't think I ever was.
>
> I: Yeah?
>
> J: Then they diagnosed me when I got out, they diagnosed me as schizophrenic.

Six years later, suffering severe symptoms, Jamie was back in the hospital, again feeling unsure as to why she was there:

> J: So. Uh, they put me in a seclusion room for ten days. I don't know why, I wasn't even doing nothing wrong, and they wanted me, they wouldn't make me, I had to go to the bathroom on the floor, I had no clothes, just a thing, yup that was left by my brother.
>
> I: So they left you, they neglected you, is that what you're saying?
>
> J: My brother, [Name], this is, this is the story. They tried, they would call the hospital, and they would say, "Don't call this hospital, your daughter's very sick and she's not doing good." And they would hang up the phone on my mother. So after they found out what was going on, I mean there was no police to help me, nobody to help me, you know, nobody helped me. My brother got me out of there, and we found out about [Hospital] from a friend, that it was a really good hospital. And ever since then it's been history.

Montana's attempts to probe Jamie's understanding further revealed the difficulty she still has, thirty years later, in understanding the extreme experiences she endured:

I: So when you were sixteen and you were eventually diagnosed with schizophrenia, did you understand why you were given that diagnosis?

J: Nope, I didn't understand, I just agreed with it.

I: Did you have symptoms that . . .

J: 'Cause I started hearing voices or something.

I: Do you remember hearing voices?

J: (Shakes head no)

I: You don't remember?

J: No.

I: So you don't, you've never heard voices even like in your adult life?

J: Yeah I've heard, that's the diagnosis they give me 'cause I'm hearing voices.

Jamie assumed that her experiences of voice hearing earned her the diagnosis of schizophrenia, but she claimed no concrete recollection of the experience. She did, however, report salient memories of social rejection and abandonment that may well have been attributable to the discomfort her friends had with the symptoms of anxiety and distress she was manifesting:

I: And your friends, they were not very nice to you either?

J: No.

I: Did they tease you?

J: Uh, they wouldn't call me no more. I used to call them up, and they said, "Oh my daughter's busy, don't call back," yeah.

I: Was that before you went to the hospital, or was that afterwards?

J: No, before.

I: It was before?

J: Yeah.

I: Did you have some kind of falling out with your friends?

J: Nothing.

I: So for no apparent reason they just stopped . . .

J: Yup.

I: . . . wanting to hang out?

J: Yup.

I: And what'd you think about that, how did you feel about that?

J: I didn't care.

I: You didn't care?

J: I cared, when I went in the hospital the first time I wanted them to come see me, they wouldn't come, then my, then I said, "Ma, you better bring my friends here right away." Then they came once, they didn't even talk to me, they didn't even talk.

Later in the first interview, Jamie offered some insight into the relationship between perceived social rejection and the voices she reluctantly acknowledged still hearing:

I: What does your illness feel like to you now?

J: I don't feel mentally ill at all. I feel calm, relaxed, peace of mind, I feel fine.

I: Once in a while you have this ex-boyfriend's voice pop into your head?

J: Yeah, I don't know why.

I: And what does it say to you?

J: Oh, "Get out of my neighborhood, I don't want to see you, move far away." Uh, then I hear this voice saying, "Oh yeah that's right, we're not your family."

While acknowledging lifelong difficulties that have prevented her from holding jobs for more than brief periods of time over the past thirty years—even after receiving specific job training and psychosocial support at Fountain House—Jamie at times denied the attribution of "mental illness." At other times, however, she used the term freely to describe herself. This seeming contradiction is not as inconsistent as it might appear. Jamie appeared to be making a distinction that persons with psychiatric distress often make, between the relative mildness of their own symptoms and the symptoms of others with more evidently severe psychiatric impairments that they might view as constituting "mental illness." Referring to a cousin, for example, Jamie noted:

J: . . . they have a problem with their daughter too, she's very sick.

I: With mental illness?

J: Yeah she's really sick. I have, uh, my doctor said I have nothing to do with her. He's right, exactly.

I: What does that mean, what do you mean you have nothing to do with her?

J: (laughs) She has different issues from me.

I: Oh, your issues are different.

J: Just like here, that's what I meant when I told you I have different issues from people here.

I: Yeah.

J: Exactly.

I: So how are your issues different from the issues that you see in the other people at Fountain House?

J: 'Cause I'm not severely mentally ill.

I: Mhm, do you think that you have ever been?

J: No, never.

Later in the interview, speaking of her current medication regimen, Jamie noted: "I'm not sick, though. I'm not sick, I just need the medicine to stay well and that's the end of it," she stressed, and then laughed. Acknowledging that she heard voices and experienced other atypical psychic phenomena, Jamie sought to normalize her experiences in a way that would not be out of place, for example, at a Hearing Voices Network meeting:

J: I'm a separate individual, and I have a separate mind, and I have a separate issue from everybody else here.

I: What, what, how would you describe your issue?

J: Well, my issue? (laughs)

I: Yeah, if everybody else has a different issue than you, then how would you describe your issue?

J: I have a different issue too.

I: What's your different issue?

J: A lot to do with uh, you know, like the thoughts I get.

I: Yeah.

J: That they're not real, that's the main issue. I'm you know, I'm like contemplating in my mind but I know that you know that so.

I: Is it constant . . .

J: 'Cause I never looked sick when I was young.

I: Mhm.

J: I never looked sick, I never felt sick, even when I was seeing all these doctors I never felt sick you know.

I: Yeah.

J: They just don't want to take me off the medication because they think I'm going to get sick.

I: Yeah.

J: But I don't feel sick I don't have no symp . . . well little symptoms, not a lot like anybody else 'cause people are getting disturbing thoughts and they're not sick and it's, and they have to distinguish if they're real or if they're not real.

I: Yeah.

J: You know but don't, my mother says you're not getting off the medication 'cause we're afraid you're going to get sick again.

We wonder what might have happened if Jamie had been afforded either peer support or therapeutic opportunities to embrace her psychic experience rather than being left to feel a need to disown her own thoughts.

JAMIE'S "FIXATIONS"

Jamie described two lines of thought that she experienced regularly. The first of these concerned a series of religious apparitions, and the second revolved around an identification with Elvis Presley. Jamie revealed a clear awareness that these experiences were not part of the consensual reality of her family and peers, yet they were expressions of her vulnerability and she held onto them tenaciously.

> J: . . . You know what, they, I know God is with me and I've seen the true face, this is another thing, I've seen the true face of God, nobody's, I saw him, I don't care, I wasn't hallucinating.
>
> I: Can you tell me about that experience?
>
> J: Yes, I, it was the best experience of my whole life, and he came to me, he goes, "I want to put my fist through the wall, now you know why."
>
> I: That's what God said to you?
>
> J: He was mad and it was him, and I'll tell you I saw the afterlife and the Virgin Mary and Joseph and the Holy Spirit and the Virgin Mary too, and I was more beautiful than her, and I saw her, and you know what God said? You're more beautiful than her.
>
> I: How did that make you feel?
>
> J: Very good, and I'll tell you Montana, this world did not come from God.
>
> I: What did this world come from?
>
> J: I don't know 'cause God has no part of this world, but I know there's a Holy . . . I know there's a Holy Spirit.
>
> I: How do you know that?
>
> J: Because I see him all the time.
>
> I: You do.

In the third interview, Jamie returned to these mystical visions, particularly in relation to the Italian Capuchin monk Padre Pio:

> I: You mentioned before we started talking on the record, that um you've been seeing the signs?
>
> J: Yup.
>
> I: Is that part of what you see as your illness or is that something separate?
>
> J: It's not the illness. I disagree totally.
>
> I: So what are the signs?
>
> J: I disagree totally.
>
> I: Okay.
>
> J: With the, with the nun here and my doctor. I disagree. They said it's uh the illness, I don't agree with that.
>
> I: What are the signs?
>
> J: I really believe that I'm seeing all those visions.
>
> I: Can you tell me what those visions are?
>
> J: I don't care what he said. I know, I don't know if you ever heard of Padre Pio?
>
> I: I don't know about him, no.
>
> J: He had the stigmata of Jesus, his hands would bleed.
>
> I: Mhm.
>
> J: And his feet would bleed.
>
> I: Mhm.
>
> J: And when Jesus, when they, when they uh striked the sword in his, in his chest, Jesus when he was crucified, all water came out, and Padre Pio used to get blood coming out of his chest from the stigmata.
>
> I: Mhm.

J: And it used to be soaking wet, at the end of the day they had to take the, the shirt off him and yeah. And his feet would bleed like Jesus when Jesus was crucified and the hands would bleed too. And he created many miracles.

I: Padre Pio.

J: Yeah. And I see him and I know what I see.

Jamie was clear as to the function of these visions:

I: What do you think the purpose is of these visions?

J: For me to be well. One hundred percent. And listen to what they're telling me.

I: What do they tell you?

J: They say everything in your head doesn't exist and that Elvis [inaudible] (laughs).

I: That includes the Elvis story?

J: Yeah Elvis is done. I tell you I saw, can I skip the subject to Marilyn Monroe now?

In the cases of both excerpts above, Jamie immediately segued into what she described as her "fixation" with Elvis Presley:

J: I have an uh, I have an uh, uh, uh, a fixation about Elvis too.

I: What's that?

J: That I think my brother's doing these things because of Elvis (laughs).

I: Why?

J: 'Cause he's like, I'm hearing his voice like I'm not your brother, I'm like, oh my God, I went to Tennessee, I had no symptoms about Elvis or nothing, I was perfect, no illness, I swear, this is what I don't understand.

I: Yeah.

J: I had no illness, I had no nothing. I was there, I was fine. I have a fixation with Elvis, for many, many years I thought he was my father, sometimes I think I look like him too (laughs). Well I don't think I do and Marilyn Monroe.

I: What about Marilyn Monroe?

J: I think she was my mother (laughs).

I: You do? You laugh about that though, do you, do you actually think that?

J: I don't know what to think.

Jamie was clear that while she experienced pushback for her beliefs, she held firm:

J: My faith? They say I'm seeing nobody.

I: But what do you believe?

J: I believe I'm seeing him, even the nun told me here, she said, "You're not seeing this." So, believe what you want, but I know what I see and what I feel (crosses arms).

I: Mhm, and what do you feel?

J: That I'm really seeing him, Padre Pio.

I: And when you said that you saw the afterlife, can you tell me more about that experience?

J: It was, it was not from this world.

I: What did it look like?

J: It was, all I know was it was a while ago, I don't remember a lot, but it wasn't from this world and there is a world after this, they say there's no proof of it but there is.

I: Were you awake or were you sleeping?

J: No, I wasn't sleeping, I was awake.

I: You were awake, and what were you doing at the time . . .

J: There is a life after this, I know, we're all going to go when we die but I know where I'm going (laughs) but it's like a thing like what about other people, you came to me, where are all the other people in this world going to go?

I: Maybe they go to the same place but they just don't get to see it like you . . .

J: I hope to God, I hope to God, I love everybody in the world.

I: Did it look like a nice place?

J: Beautiful.

I: It looked beautiful.

J: It's like you know when you see the moon at night?

I: Yeah.

J: It's like behind the moon.

I: It's like behind the moon?

J: Yeah.

I: It's like a place behind the moon?

J: Yeah and I'll tell you . . .

I: And is it light, is it bright?

J: But God created this world, he told me I, I created this world and they say I'm just seeing, I'm glad I'm saying this because.

I: It feels good to talk about it?

J: Yes, and I've saw, you know like the burning bush?

I: Mhm.

J: You know the burning bush with Moses?

I: Mhm.

J: I closed my eyes and I saw it, and I saw God, and he said, "Jamie, I created this world for a reason, and I put you in this world, I did this to you, I put you in this world for a reason," but he wouldn't say why. Can we talk about something else now? (laughs).

FAMILY DYNAMICS

In the second interview, Jamie explored her early family life and, in explicating the relationship with her father, she returned in due course to elaborate more on the function of the Elvis fantasy in her thinking. The closest Jamie actually came to articulating family stressors as a precipitant for her own struggles was when she described her father's penchant for violence toward both her and her mother. With respect to herself, Jamie noted:

J: One time my father hit me. I was all dressed up.

I: Uh huh.

J: You know, no illness, no nothing. I was one hundred percent and he hit me. I don't know why. [inaudible] wasn't because you were one hundred percent. It was for something else. He, he maybe he thought you were going out with boys because he was very jealous if a boy would come near me, yeah.

I: How old were you at the time?

J: My father?

I: Were you?

J: My first boyfriend was him, Tony.

I: So you were like fifteen?

J: Fifteen, my first boyfriend.

I: So you were fifteen years old when your father hit you?

J: No, this was years ago. I used to go to country clubs and meet the boy and my friends and we used to hang out at the corner, and my father used to come get me every night, and he would start hitting me. He goes, "You're not hanging out at the corner."

I: How old were you then?

J: My mother goes, "She's not doing nothing wrong, leave her alone." But he was like, he didn't like the idea. That was sitting at the corner, we didn't do nothing wrong.

I: Had your father ever hit you before that?

J: Never.

I: And how old were you then?

J: Fifteen, fourteen, fifteen.

I: When he started hitting you . . .

J: I had the best life in the world.

I: How did it make you feel when he did that to you?

J: I didn't care. I used to still go out (laughs).

I: Were you angry though with him that he would do that to you?

J: No, I wasn't angry with him. No, I just went out again (laughs).

I: Yeah?

J: Yeah.

I: Did you have a close relationship with your father?

J: Yeah, he was good to me.

I: In what ways?

J: He paid for my college. I have no, I have no outstanding debt.

Jamie emphasized that until she became symptomatic, her relationship with her parents was untroubled. However, once she began talking, she revealed a troubling pattern of domestic abuse by her father against her mother. In describing her child self, she seems to describe herself as viewed by her parents, and she explained how this led her to offer a rationale for invoking Elvis as her idealized father:

I: Do you remember what your relationship was like with your parents when you were little?

J: Very good, excellent. I was a good kid. I never got mad, I never gave them a problem for fifteen years, until the day I started getting symptoms.

I: And up until then, what, what were they like with you?

J: Fine, my mother loved me, my mother was good to me. My father loved me. He didn't like when I'd go out with boys, that was the whole thing.

I: What was their marriage like?

J: It wasn't good.

I: How do you mean?

J: My father used to hit her, a lot, from his jealousy.

I: What do you mean?

J: When my mother was pregnant of me, they lived in [Avenue] in [City].

I: Mhm.

J: And one night, she was talking with the neighbor and they, they were just talking, "How you doing . . ."

I: Mhm.

J: And that night he, she went to bed, he was, he started, she was pregnant of me, and he beat her up really bad. And she almost had a miscarriage.

I: Your mom later told you?

J: When she was pregnant of me. She almost had a miscarriage.

I: Wow.

J: But I was born, and I'm here.

I: Did she later tell you that?

J: Yeah, she told me, when I was in, when I got older she told me.

I: How old is older?

J: She said I don't, don't talk to me about it, I don't want to think about it.

I: Why do you think she told you about it?

J: I don't know. Well she knew, my father was hitting her when we were young, my brothers were upstairs and he would start beating her up and we used to hear her screaming.

I: And would you and your brothers like hide out together . . .

J: We used to say, my brother went down there and goes, "Stop hitting her." When my brothers got older, my father, my brother grabbed my father and goes, "You hit my mother one more time and I'm going to kill you," and he stopped doing it. He got scared. Yeah.

I: How did it make you feel . . .

J: One time he beat up my mother and she banged her head against the, the piece of wood in the living room, and ever since then she suffered from severe headaches because of that.

I: Hm.

J: Yeah. I get along with everybody. I have nothing against . . .

I: What did you think about what was going on between your mom and your dad?

J: My father was good to me but if you have a different relationship with your father than your mother, but I didn't like what he did to my mother, that he had to beat her up from jealousy. I think [older brother] has got the jealousy from my father, in a different way, that's what I'm thinking.

I: Were you afraid of your dad?

J: Yes, I was.

I: What were you afraid of?

J: That he was like mean.

I: Were you afraid that he would . . .

J: He never hit me.

I: . . . do something worse to your mother like he could put her in the hospital or something?

J: What do you mean physically?

I: Yeah.

J: No, he wouldn't do that to her.

I: And were you afraid that maybe he would turn on you . . .

J: My mother doesn't like that I talk about these things. My mother, she doesn't like that I talk about these things.

I: Because?

J: It's upsetting to talk about it.

I: Do you feel like you want to talk about it sometimes?

J: Yeah, sometimes.

Continuing, Jamie revealed how the anger she could not express as a child led to her adoption of Elvis as a benevolent father figure:

J: That's why I started thoughts about Elvis. Because he was being bad to me. Then Elvis Presley was on TV and I said, "That's my father," from anger.

I: You said that to your dad?

J: To my mother, my mother heard. She came in the room, she smacked me, she goes don't ever think that again (laughs). And ever since then it's been history with Elvis (laughs).

Jamie then went on to elaborate how an idealized Elvis could be a substitution for the idealized father she lacked so intensely:

I: Would you rather Elvis be your father?

J: Yes.

I: How come?

J: He's like my idol, I love. But I'll tell you when I was young, all these people loved Elvis.

I: Yeah.

J: I didn't even like him.

I: Yeah.

J: I didn't even know who he was until I saw him on . . .

I: When did you start liking him?

J: High school. Isn't that weird? He was dead when I was in high school.

I: What do you think he would've been like as a father?

J: Very good father.

I: In what ways?

J: Loving, compassionate, make you feel wanted and special. And there's that song, I don't know if you ever heard of it, Father Figure.

I: I don't know it, I don't think.

J: (Sings) "I will be your father figure. That's all he wanted, someone special, someone sacred in your life" (laughs).

I: It sounds like a sweet song.

J: Yeah, then he sang another song (sings), "We're trapped in a world that's trouble with pain" (laughs).

I: Yeah.

J: It's like I think I have connections with this man. Then when I was with, then when I was in [College], there was this limousine that used to be outside. Listen to this, the license plate said PA, PA. Not Pennsylvania, PA. And when I was in school, listen to this, listen to this, when I was in [College], I used to write all over my books, PA, PA, PA, PA. Then I go outside and I see this limousine all the time PA. And it was a, it was a Rolls Royce limousine and in the back they put a red sheet so nobody could see who was in it. What am I supposed to think? (laughs)

I: What did you think?

J: I got very, very curious.

I: Yeah?

J: Yeah. Like they're hiding that from me. About the mafia too, that the mafia's after me. (laughs)

I: Why would the mafia be after you . . .

J: Because Elvis is my father.

I: And why would they be after you because of that?

J: Because he's my father. That's, I think sometimes that's why these people took me.

I: What do you mean?

J: From my family, Elvis.

I: Yeah?

J: Isn't that weird? But they say it's the illness doing that.

I: Doing what? Making you think what?

J: About Elvis, and everything associated with it.

Addressing a later conflict, in which Jamie's family rejected the new wife of one of her brothers, Jamie astutely explained how the latent stressors converged to make her symptomatic, and how reliance on God gives her peace of mind:

J: Yeah, I just want peace in my life, Montana (blesses herself).

I: Yeah.

J: I ask God, let me find peace of mind.

I: Yeah, sounds like there wasn't a lot of peace in your household though when you were growing up?

J: Yes, that's why I got sick.

I: Sometimes we internalize that environment.

J: That's why I got sick, Montana. It was a breakdown.

I: Yeah, so . . .

J: No if's and's or but's about it.

I: Tell me what happened. Your brother, you said, moved in because he was having difficulties.

J: He was getting sick. From his wife, she was, I don't want to curse.

I: This is, your older brother, this is one of your older brothers?

J: The oldest.

I: The oldest.

J: This is how mental illness started in my house. From him, from his wife, from his wife mistreating him.

I: How did she mistreat him?

J: Uh, I don't know, just weren't getting along, and my father said, "You're not going to marry her." She was pregnant of a boy.

I: Mhm.

J: And uh, and uh, my father goes, "You're not marrying my son, my son has to finish college and get a good job." He didn't listen, he snuck and married her. Biggest mistake of his life. Biggest mistake of his life to marry that . . .

I: So none of your family was present for the wedding? It was like a secret wedding?

J: No it wasn't a wedding, city hall. They snuck and got married.

I: Mhm.

J: Biggest mistake of his life, biggest mistake. Biggest mistake.

I: How come?

J: She was another jealous one, she used to look at me and make these faces and make me sick. Dr. [Psychiatrist] said she couldn't make you sick but I thought she was making me sick. Where was Dr. [Psychiatrist] when I was fifteen? (laughs). He goes, "She couldn't make you sick," but I thought she was. She was a B-I-T-C-H. Jealous, we didn't get along.

Returning to Elvis later in the interview, Jamie shared how she had become coy about her relationship with Elvis because she received so much pushback from both her psychiatrist and her family. Regarding her psychiatrist, she noted:

> J: Yeah. I don't know, Elvis isn't Elvis (laughs). Is Elvis behind it? Nah. I mean Dr. [Psychiatrist] said Jamie, that's your birth certificate. I even gave it to Cheryl, (laughs) on Wednesday.
>
> I: But you feel like Elvis would've been a nice dad?
>
> J: (Nods yes) I just don't want to think it no more because it, it caused too many problems for me.

Jamie noted that her mother "doesn't like when I get thoughts, she wants me to be perfect all the time." As for her brother, he said, "Jamie, if you think Elvis is your father one more time I'm going to hit you." As Jamie succinctly noted, "He doesn't want me thinking about Elvis." In the final interview she related:

> J: Well Clozapine, you have to get blood work done once a month for that, I don't know if you know that? Yeah you know that, of course you know that. And there's uh, my nurse practitioner, [Name], she sees me at [Hospital] once a month too.
>
> I: Okay.
>
> J: To give me my medication, check your blood pressure, things. And she asks you about your symptoms.
>
> I: So they ask you about these visions that you're seeing?
>
> J: Yeah.
>
> I: And what's that conversation like with them?
>
> J: No, I don't disagree with them or nothing, I just you know, that's what they have to say.
>
> I: What's what they have to say? What do you mean? What kind of things do they say to you?
>
> J: They say it's the illness, I'm hallucinating from the illness.
>
> I: But you, inside, disagree.

J: Inside I really believe that I'm seeing, I hope I'm seeing them, because it's beautiful.

LONELINESS AND ISOLATION

Perhaps one of the gravest consequences of the psychic struggles that people such as Jamie suffer is the risk of social isolation. If a person grows up with parents who fail to contain and nurture a child's psyche—becoming in effect what Wilfred Bion (1984) called *wilfully misunderstanding objects*—that child will grow up with a hunger for the acceptance and embrace of loving adults in their later lives. Ellyn Saks (2008) and Lucy Newlyn (2018) clearly benefited from partners and mentors with such healing qualities, and Joanne Greenberg (1986) and Catherine Penney (see Dorman, 2003) found healing, containment, and love from their respective therapists, Frieda Fromm-Reichmann and Daniel Dorman. Jamie was not so fortunate, and she explained poignantly that sexual and emotional intimacy have eluded her, as has the opportunity to have children of her own. She desperately seeks intimacy, but as the dialog reveals, she also wards off intimacy, denying its importance because of the lack such an admission would entail. Sadly, she expressed that meeting "somebody without a problem" is difficult "because they don't want to be with somebody with a problem," nor, as she later remarked, does she want to be with someone who she perceives as having problems:

I: Are you in a relationship with anybody?

J: No, I haven't been in a relationship for a long time.

I: How long is long?

J: Long, maybe, oh my God, twenty years. Nobody.

I: How come?

J: I don't know, I never met nobody no more. I don't know how they're going to feel seeing that I'm coming here to Fountain House, but it's hard to find somebody who is going to understand me.

I: Yeah.

J: You know, somebody without a problem because they don't want to be with somebody with a problem. Because it would be very difficult, if he has a problem, I have a problem. I need to be understood.

I: Yeah.

J: You know.

I: Yeah, are there people in your life now that you feel do understand you?

J: My mother understands me. She said, "Jamie, you do have an illness." I know, you know, as of now I guess I do.

I: Mhm, how does it make you feel to say that?

J: It doesn't bother me.

I: Yeah?

J: But I feel like I could help myself one hundred percent.

I: You feel like you have the ability to help yourself?

J: Yes, oh yeah, all the time.

I: It sounds like you feel empowered.

J: Yeah, it's good, right?

I: Yeah.

J: Everybody's good to me here, I have nothing against nobody.

I: Was there a time that you were hoping that you would be in a relationship with somebody?

J: (nods yes) I blew it.

I: How so?

J: With [Name].

I: Was that the last relationship?

J: '88?

I: That was the last one?

J: Before [second hospital].

I: And how did you feel . . .

J: Because ever since [second hospital], it changed my life [second hospital]. It gave me life again.

I: Yeah.

J: And Dr. [Psychiatrist] says you're not like these people, you're just like when you go to [second hospital]. You see people sick, you know very sick some people doing well, just like [second hospital], he said. You know?

I: When you say you blew it in that relationship . . .

J: With [Name].

I: What do you mean?

J: Uh, you know, he liked me a lot but he owned a body place. Handsome.

I: Yeah?

J: Very handsome guy.

I: Yeah?

J: Everybody in my family liked him.

I: Yeah?

J: And sometimes I did things that I shouldn't have did.

I: Like what?

J: He gave me his picture and I ripped it up.

I: Why did you do that?

J: I don't know, I was just mad at him for something, I don't know why.

I: Did you feel like he understood you?

J: Uh, a little bit. He was nice to me but not nice to me all the time.

I: Do you remember how he wasn't nice to you?

J: He used to make fun at me sometimes. Yeah.

I: What kinds of things, do you know?

J: We went out to dinner and I said, I said, "What is swordfish, like steak?" He goes "How could swordfish be like steak?" I'm like, "Okay I guess it can't be like steak" (laughs).

I: Yeah. So you were asking him kind of genuine questions and he would kind of throw them back in your face?

J: Yeah, and then he goes, "You want to dance a little bit in the living room?" He goes, "Oh I thought you knew how to dance" (covers face).

I: So he embarrassed you too.

J: Yeah, yeah. Maybe it wouldn't have worked out. Maybe my father was right.

I: What, about what?

J: Not to be with a man.

I: Your father told you not . . .

J: He liked some of the boys I went out with but . . .

I: Did your father not ever want you to get married?

J: Yes, bottom line.

I: He didn't want you to.

J: My mother said she curses him because, "If it wasn't for him you would've been married with children, had a whole different life."

I: Do you agree with her?

J: Yes. But I'm saying you know what, sometimes I think if I would've gotten married, what happens if it wouldn't have worked out, what if I had children and that would be really stressful.

STRUGGLES WITH WORK

Jamie related having made strenuous efforts to enter and remain in the workforce, but vocational stability has eluded her, as "something always gets in the way."

I: Yeah, you're starting a new job pretty soon. What kind of work will you be doing?

J: It's a [inaudible] position, nothing, nothing educational, but it's a job, I don't care.

I: Nothing that you can use prior education . . .

J: I care about it, but it's not my education, not what I hoped for in my education.

I: What do you hope for, or what did you hope for?

J: I tried to get a really good job, but it's always something.

I: What do you mean?

J: It's always like something in my way, you know, it's the story of my life, always something in my way.

I: What is that something?

J: It's probably the illness, standing in my way.

Jamie was unclear as to the reasons for her many terminations, even from vocationally sheltered positions:

J: I went to [Company] for nine months. And that was it. I got another training experience after that on Wall Street and they fired me, I don't even know why.

I: No?

J: No, I was doing a good job.

I: Did you get feedback?

J: They told me to come in and they said they fired me. I don't know why.

I: And they never gave you any feedback (interrupted)

J: I did a good job. They didn't tell me why either. They said that I wasn't meeting up to their uh expectations or something because my father just died in September and it started I think in October, so I was upset about my father dying and I used to cry sometimes. Then they said you can't sit down on the bench while you're waiting for work. And sometimes I used to sit down, but I did the work okay.

I: It sounds like it was a hard time for you.

CONCLUSION

Despite the disappointments and struggles in her life, Jamie has preserved a sunny, if anxious, disposition and she has shown remarkable perseverance in seeking to enter the workforce, despite many setbacks and disappointments. She has repeatedly used the services of Fountain House to receive training and supervised placements in order to gain a toehold in the world of work, though as yet she has not succeeded in holding down a job for the long-term. Fountain House, of course, offers considerable psychosocial support to members, and, by arrangement with a local hospital, therapeutic services are also available. Jamie has chosen not to take advantage of these opportunities. This decision could be because of her sense of being stigmatized as what she calls "mentally ill," though it is possible, too, that the only kind of therapeutic encounters she has experienced have been with intrusive mental health professionals who try to debunk her beliefs. Through invalidating the fantasies in her psychic structure rather than in seeking to gain understanding of these experiences in Jamie's internal life, psychiatric care might have inadvertently strengthened her adherence to these ideas. We wonder how different Jamie's life trajectory might be if she were to receive sustained, affirming support—what psychoanalysts refers to as containment and holding—that could allow her to develop a sustaining and regenerative narrative for her life story.

Chapter Fourteen

Jesse

Mr. Misunderstood

Secil Arac-Orhun and Michael O'Loughlin

Jesse, an African-American man in his forties, was born and raised in the United States. At the time of this study, Jesse did not hold a high school diploma because he has had a history of psychiatric and behavioral difficulties beginning in early childhood. Jesse has spent time in residential treatment centers, in psychiatric hospitals, and in prison. At the time of the interviews, Jesse was living in a supportive housing program and working in a creative field.

Jesse's history was filled with trauma. Several important figures had failed to keep him safe, and he spent many years in various institutions. At the beginning of the interview, as Jesse was signing his name on the consent form, Secil noticed that he added "A.K.A. Mr. Misunderstood." At the end of the interviews, he explained that this signified how deeply misunderstood he felt by many of the people around him. Jesse's life story revealed the complexities of a person struggling with significant persistent psychiatric difficulties.

EARLY YEARS

Jesse was born into chaos and trauma. He said both his parents had struggled with alcoholism. In addition, his father grappled with mental health issues. Jesse explained his parents' difficulties:

> My mother and father met in . . . there's a psychiatric institution in [State]. . . . My mother and my father met there. I don't know exactly, I

> don't really know my mom, so I don't know exactly what happened. That's where they met . . . I . . . I know my father was paranoid schizophrenic, and I also know, and found that later, my father was a rapist.

Jesse's parents were unable to take care of their children. The children were found malnourished, they had been sexually and physically abused, and they were in crisis when Jesse's grandmother adopted them. Jesse explained why his grandmother took custody of him and his sister:

> My grandmother got custody of us when I was eighteen months old . . . I'm glad she got custody. I'd probably be dead. My mother was trying to kill us. She was starving us. She wasn't feeding us at all. We were malnourished. We were bruised. When they got custody of me, they said I had a broken thermometer in my rectum that they had to remove. Eighteen months old.

Jesse remembered having psychological difficulties as long as he could remember. He reported being a hyperactive child and having behavioral problems:

> I had such an intense mania as a kid. Like today you see this stuff on television and the news and stuff, a lot of kids—attention deficit disorder—kids that run around and all this energy and whatever, they can't focus on anything . . . they thought that I was . . . because my mother, when she was pregnant with us, was using all kinds of drugs. So I had this extreme mania to the point where my thoughts were moving so fast that I couldn't speak . . . because I was hyperactive, it was impossible to teach me anything . . . they suggested that because my situation was so extreme that I needed to be put on medication.

Jesse was put on Thorazine before he was ten years old. He reported, that by the time he became a teenager, the dosages of medications were so high that he was unable to think clearly:

> I started taking it [medication] at such a young age that my tolerance was up, but it got to the point when I was in . . . that I couldn't, um, especially with Thorazine, where I could not read, I couldn't learn in school, because I read, I read one line, and by the time I started the next line, I forgot the one that I just read.

The trauma did not stop after Jesse and his sister moved in with their grandmother. Although he viewed his grandmother as a savior, she had significant limitations as a caregiver. Jesse explained that she used Jesse and his sister to elicit praise from others for the good she was doing:

> My grandmother constantly, all through her life, sought the attention and the praise of a mother who was unable to give that to her, for whatever reason . . . I think part of the reason why my grandmother went out of her way to get custody of me and my sister, my grandmother . . . look, I'm not demonizing my grandmother, nobody's perfect, I love my grandmother. But I think a part of her motivation for getting custody of us wasn't just the fact that we were her grandchildren, but also because, "Look at me, world! I'm saving two babies, I'm going out of my way to do something noble. Notice me. Give me attention. I've done something good!"

Reflecting on how his grandmother's need for attention negatively impacted her caregiving, Jesse noted:

> My grandmother tried to make me the focus for herself. In other words, I wore glasses that I don't . . . I never needed . . . I wore shoes . . . orthopedic shoes that I don't believe I ever needed. For years, my grandmother told me that doctors told her that I had something called excessive hip rotation. If you mention that term to a doctor, they will tell you that's not even a medical term. So my grandmother was making me sick, even though I wasn't sick, so that she could receive attention from people.

The profound limitations of Jesse's early caregivers, and particularly their failure to contain him or keep him in mind and safe, set the stage for deep psychic and emotional struggles in adulthood.

SEEDS OF MISTRUST

Jesse's early environment lacked important figures that he could rely on for safety, trust, and stability. This contributed to problematic attachment and a tendency to distrust authority figures. Jesse explained that his development of mistrust and defiance began when he found out about his father being murdered. He related that he reached a turning point in his mistrust of the world around him when he was ten years old and he was expected to identify his father's dead body:

> Somebody called our house . . . and told my aunt, "Your brother is dead on the next block." So when I heard my aunt starting yelling and run out of the house, I followed my aunt out of the house, and we ran to the next block. There was a big crowd of people, and as we approached it, I guess the police stopped my aunt when you get up to the tape, but I was smaller and everything, so I ran under the tape and I got past the cops, and as I got up to the front, and I'll never forget. . . . This big black cop gets in the way, and he's got this big smile on his face and he's laughing about

> something, and he stopped me and he says, "Hey where are you going?" and I say, "That's my daddy." He said, "Well, you think you can identify the body?" I say yeah. So he said, "Okay, you want to see it? Fine," and he let me through. And um . . . that had a traumatic, traumatic effect on me. I mean, I remember at first . . . at first I couldn't . . . I couldn't . . . there was so much blood on his face that I couldn't really tell it was him. Except my father had a silver tooth in the front of his mouth, and his mouth was open. Both of his eyes were open. When I saw the tooth, then I recognized him.
>
> [My uncle] got past the police line, and when he got up there, he started arguing with the cop for letting me through, and then when he turned to his brother, my father, he closed both of my father's eyes, and his, my father's left eye popped back open. And in my mind as a child, to me, I felt as though my father was getting his last look at me.

Jesse stated that he wished he had been stopped from seeing his father's body. He longed for an adult figure that would provide the protection he needed as a child. He elaborated on the way he viewed his father's death and the way the authority figures handled it:

> Like it was a game. And to me . . . um, I think even at that young an age, to me, unconsciously of course—unconsciously, because my brain was overloaded because of everything that was in front of me, unconsciously, not subconsciously, unconsciously, I was developing a hatred of authority figures. Because even as young as I was, they stopped my aunt, the adult, but I got past. And then I run into the person who's supposed to stop me. And he still allowed me, while laughing. Like, like . . . this is just an everyday thing. Just another dead n___. And the thing that gets me about it is, this is, this was a black cop. And . . . unconsciously, I believe that I was beginning to develop a hatred for authority figures. Right then, it started right there.

He reported that he began to challenge the authority figures in his life:

> That had a traumatic . . . it messed up my school. Um, authority figures couldn't tell me what to do. I would tell teachers, "You're not my father, you never raised a black boy," and then that turned into, that turned into violence, and I started fighting.

While Jesse and his sister were living with their grandmother, their step-grandfather sexually abused Jesse's sister. Jesse's account of the abuse reflected a seeming ambivalence around viewing his sister as a victim. At moments his comments conveyed a belief in her complicity and even culpability for what she endured:

> She was extremely, extremely promiscuous. To the point where the school would tell my grandmother to make sure that my sister wore shorts and stuff, because she would like, tempt the teachers . . . just extremely, extremely . . . promiscuous at a very young age. So, um . . . one particular night, I saw them in the living room—in the dining room, whispering. I wanted to know what they were whispering about and when I walked into the room, they both jumped up and acted like they weren't whispering, whatever. I wondered what was going on. But I remember the next night, my grandmother was in the basement, and I was going into the bedroom. I had my own bedroom. My sister had her bedroom, and when I was going into the bedroom, when I opened the door, my sister was laying in bed with her legs spread and my grandfather was [slang word for sexual molestation] her. He had his finger in between her legs. And when I saw it, my grandfather turned around, and he was—he said . . . "Sh, sh, sh."

When Jesse's grandmother, armed with a gun, finally confronted her husband about the abuse of his sister, Jesse found himself in the role of mediator:

> I tried to get in between them to break them up because I was thinking . . . I was thinking that if grandma goes to jail, what's going to happen to me and my sister? . . . so I'm trying to tell my grandma, "Grandma, if you go to jail, what's going to happen to us? Who's going to take us? Where are we going to go? . . . I don't want you to go to jail, Grandma." So he's just stupid . . . when she pulls the gun out, she flips the couch over, and she raised the gun at the door. He's on the other side of the door in the hallway, banging on the door: "Baby, let me in, let me talk to you." So I get in between the door and her, and I say, "Granddaddy. Get out of the house. Go for a walk and come back later. Get out of the house. She has a gun. She has a gun. Get out of the house." "She's not gonna shoot me, she won't shoot me." I said, "Granddaddy, get out of the house. Please." So then I turned to my grandmother and said, "Grandma, Grandma, if you shoot him, you're gonna spend the rest of your life in jail. You're gonna go to jail if you do this, I don't want you to go to jail." And she threatened to kill me. She said, "If you don't move, I'm gonna shoot you." So I moved out of her way. I moved out of the way, and I was yelling to my grandfather to get out of the house. Some kind of way, a ten-year-old was able to plead with a grown fucking man, talk some sense into him to get him to leave the house. To come back when she's not angry. So I actually talked him into leaving the house.

> You know what, you know what the strange thing about this is? Even to this day? I wasn't too young to process what I was doing. That particular night, I was saying to myself, this is some bullshit, I'm a kid. I was saying it to myself, I'm a fucking kid, and here I am with adults. And then I started getting angry with myself. I never should have told her, I should have kept my mouth shut.

Jesse found himself in a parentified position, serving as a caretaker to his parents, a role he too often had to take up as a child without trustworthy caregivers.

ANGER AND EXTERNALIZATION OF FEELINGS

Jesse told his grandmother about a time when his step-grandfather had hit him. Although he had asked Jesse to keep this a secret, Jesse felt compelled to tell because he feared what his step-grandfather might do:

> I started wondering, if, if he could do this to my sister, maybe he would try it with me. And I was already scared of him after, you know, I felt how strong he was when he hit me, and then I said, well, I gotta take care of myself too, I can't have him coming into my room. So I decided to tell her.

After he hit Jesse again, the neighbors called the police, and Jesse was taken to the hospital. In the hospital, he reported that his step-grandfather was molesting his sister, which led to his sister being taken away from his grandmother and placed in a group home.

After these events, Jesse talked about his growing rage toward his step-grandfather. When I asked Jesse how he felt about his sister leaving, he related:

> I wanted to kill my grandfather. He is too big and too strong, and I didn't know how I was going to go about doing it, but there were a few nights . . . 'cause he used to snore, and it was easy, and a few nights, a few nights, like maybe three or four times, for a half hour, I stood over him in bed with the knife in my hand. My grandmother next to him, both of them snoring, where I contemplated cutting his throat. For years . . . one particular night, we got into an argument, and my grandmother got in between us to protect me because he would have destroyed me. Got between us to protect me, and when she got between us, over her shoulder, I said . . . I told him, "You know what I'd do, mother fucker? You know what I'd do? You know how many times, I mean nights, I stood over you while you

slept and wrestled with killing you? Do you know how many times? I'm gonna cut your fucking throat when you go to sleep."

REJECTION

The chaos, conflict, and violence at his grandmother's house, along with his "hyper behaviors" led to significant difficulties at home, and Jesse reported that a short time after the incident with his step-grandfather, he began to live and move from one residential treatment center to another. As a teenager, his grandmother did not want him in her house, so, Jesse found himself without a home. According to Jesse, the admission of his desire to kill his step-grandfather was the reason he ended up in group homes and eventually homeless. When his step-grandfather heard Jesse's threats, he told Jesse's grandmother that Jesse needed to leave. Jesse explained his thoughts with regard to his grandmother's decision:

> J: That's the only thing he ever stood up to her on . . . I think he could look in my eyes and see the fear and the hatred; he had no idea that I stood over him three or four times, I'm not sure exactly, three or four times in the middle of the night for like a half hour, saying to myself I should just stab this mother fucker in the throat for what he did to my sister. You're a grown man, and you would molest a child, and my grandmother is still with you over some material shit. I, I, I, I hated him . . .
>
> I: How did you feel about your grandmother staying with him?
>
> J: I understood it. My grandmother never worked one day in her life. She dated judges, policemen; she always had men to take care of her. She was married five times. The other marriages didn't work because no man in his right mind would put up with her shit. No man. But she found the one man out of seven million that was dumb enough to put up with her shit. And she wasn't letting him go. 'Cause she knew she was impossible. She knew she wasn't gonna find a man with a three-story house, with money in the bank, with a pension, and two cars . . . she didn't give a shit about my sister anyway! Now, had it happened to me . . . had he molested me, it may have been different, but it was my sister. She didn't love my sister. Parents are full of shit.

Jesse's reaction points to a repeated message he received in various contexts: that he did not truly matter. This generated feelings of melancholia and depression. Jesse went from one institution to another and became so dysregulated and aggressive that he was deemed "incorrigible." He explained:

> What happened was that I was in so many juvenile placements in [State], getting kicked out of them for basically fighting, assault, and disruptive behavior that . . . the division of youth and family services in the state labeled me incorrigible, or something like that. And no juvenile institute in the state would take me. So then, uh . . . I got sent to [another state] because nowhere in [State of origin] would take me.

After Jesse had to move out of his grandmother's house, he could not find a safe space or institution to serve his need for containment. The institutions in place to help traumatized teens had rejected him. His life story during his youth was filled with dislocations, fights, aggression, and further trauma:

> It was very hard to stay in line . . . at that particular time, it was very difficult to tell me what to do . . . I used to have to get restrained all the time, and I would attack staff, and I would attack teachers, and, and I would throw, like, pool balls and stuff like that . . . when I first went there, like I said, when I was young at that age, and I was scared of everything, and what happened was every morning for at least a month, the first time that I went there, every morning they did this to me as the only kid in the cottage with funny-looking shoes and funny glasses. So they used to pick on me, and I was the smallest and the youngest kid in the cottage, so every morning we'd have to get up, make our beds, you know, straighten our lockers out, go downstairs into the TV room until the staff member would come down, make us line up, and we'd go to the cafeteria. Every morning when I'd go downstairs, it was every day, everybody would get down there before me on purpose, and as soon as I walk into the TV room, they would push the couch in front of the door and they would jump me. The whole cottage . . . for fun. And I would get down on the ground and ball up in a circle, like this, so, to try to keep them from, you know, hitting me, and then they'd start hitting me in the head, and they'd kick me and beat me up for sport.

Jesse's story fits the trauma model that explains how boys respond to trauma with aggression, identifying with the aggressor, and at the same time reenacting the trauma they experienced. According to this model, the child takes defensive measures for survival that are usually maladaptive. Secure attachment, self-esteem, and trust suffer, and problems such as aggression, hyperactivity, irritability, and learning disorders arise (Krugman, 1987). Jesse recalled a counselor from one of the many residential facilities, who was empathic toward him, and in some ways served as a temporary good object:

> And then one particular day, the staff member there, named, um, Mr. Y. Mr. Y., I'll never forget him. He used to give me drawing lessons, he used

> to spend a lot of attention to me. As a matter of fact, I think part of the reason why I went, why I acted out at the other school and made sure I got myself sent back to [the same residential facility] a second time, was 'cause I wanted to be with Mr. Y. He was like a father figure. He was so cool. But anyway, he pulled me to the side one day. He said, "Look man, I could lose my job for saying this, but I'm gonna tell you this anyway, man." He said, look, he said, "You've gotta defend yourself, you cannot just let them beat you up. You have to fight back" . . . He's the one that t-told me how artwork can be a self-defense mechanism . . . And that's what I started doing.

However, for Jesse, fighting did not stop there; as he found an outlet to express his anger and was able to defend himself, he discovered a pleasure in physical combat:

> I would attack a staff member, or grown man, before one of the kids. Because the kids would fight back, and it would be like, well, a lot of these guys are scared to lose their jobs . . . and then it got to a point where even when I lost the fight, I loved it. I started to love it. The adrenaline, your heart beating fast, the—the feeling of power that you get from hurting somebody. The, um, even, even like, you know, getting punched in the eye, the pain of seeing, uh, the flash of light, and all this stuff. It started to get to the point where I was like, alright, so what if I get my ass kicked and I got a fat eye or cut or bruise, or whatever, or whatever. I actually like looking at bruises on my face and shit, you know. It reminds me of my life . . . And then, then my assaults became much more, much more aggressive, and much more, much more violent.

The pleasure Jesse derived from being beaten up can be seen as a reenactment of his childhood abuse.

WITHOUT A HOME

Jesse's difficulties, including not having the safe haven he so much needed, continued beyond his teenage years and eventually he found himself on the streets, homeless. The lack of safety and exposure to trauma continued, and sadly, Jesse's traumatic encounters continued:

> Every day, you know, people do fucked-up things to, to the homeless. People do fucked-up things. I'll give you an example. These couples approach me, I'm out there panhandling, right. These couples approach me, they say, "Yo man, are you hungry or whatever?" . . . So they come back and they got this bag, and they give me the bag and everything, and

> they . . . and I know this, that they keep kinda giggling amongst themselves, so I'm wondering, are they stoned or what's going on, whatever . . . So I go, I go to bite into this sandwich, and something said to me "Look at the sandwich first." I'm thinking maybe they spit in it or something. I open it. They took razor blades . . . and had inserted razor blades at all different angles in the meat in the sandwich.

Jesse did not have the adequate safe environment growing up, and as he continued to be traumatized on the streets, he developed increasing paranoia:

> I got so paranoid in the street that I couldn't even listen to my Walkman. And I would do—you know what I would do? I would take a ladies' compact . . . I'd find a ladies compact in the trash, you know, with a mirror on it. Then I'd take a rubber band and then put it on my Walkman, and I'd take a rubber band and wrap it so that when I walked down the street, I could look into the mirror and see who's behind me, because I was that paranoid from my drinking that I didn't know if somebody was gonna roll up on me and shoot me. That's no way to live. And you have no privacy when you're in the street, you have no privacy.

Compounding his difficulties, Jesse also developed a substance abuse problem. Having been failed by his family and society, Jesse reported that he gave up on life and lost hope. His resentment manifested in a flagrant disregard for the rules of society:

> And then my paranoia was growing from the drugs and, and mental illness, and I was . . . I, you know, I used to think everybody else was fucked up, and that I was the sane one, and now that I'm older and I look back on it, I was really fucked up mentally. And I would do things that would scare people. What, what I realized was that it was menacing behavior. I didn't realize . . . I honestly didn't believe that the thing—I had an excuse for everything. I honestly didn't believe that doing this or doing that was unacceptable behavior in the eyes of society . . . I'll give you an example. I used to masturbate in the park. But I used to do it in a way that . . . I felt like, okay, I'm in my world, I'm not bothering anybody else. I would go to a bench with a table like this, or whatever. I would go to the one in the corner of the park when the park was empty when nobody else was in there. I'd wear baggy pants, whatever, cut a hole in the pocket, and I would go, look around, make sure nobody's watching, and do my thing. But I didn't realize that that's unacceptable. The way I was rationalizing is, I'm homeless, where am I going to go?

NO HOME, NO HOPE, NO FUTURE

Jesse explained that he had been incarcerated several times. In his mid-twenties, after the longest period of incarceration in his life as a result of being both high on drugs and breaking into people's homes for robbery, Jesse tried to reconnect with his mother and sister in an attempt at repairing their relationship. However, his sister rejected him. After recounting this rejection, Jesse began to describe again how he became homeless and self-destructive. He spoke to his feelings of worthlessness during this time:

> There are different kinds of homeless people . . . you have homeless people, and then you have bums. They're not the same thing. They're not the same thing. There is a difference. The difference is: A bum is a person—and I was a bum for a while—a bum is a person who has given up on life . . . a bum is a person who has absolutely no love for himself, they don't care about themselves, they've given, they've reached a point where they just don't care anymore. They're ready to die. Many of them are conscious of it. A homeless person usually . . . well, they all start out homeless, and you eventually become a bum. But a homeless person is a person who just doesn't have a place to go, who's—who hasn't been on the streets long enough to have completely lost himself and still has a glimmer of hope or expectation still within them. . . . So in the beginning, I was just homeless. . . . And then when the drug addiction, addiction took over, I completely lost myself, and all I cared about was using the drugs. I prostituted myself, I robbed people, I broke into people's cars. I just, I didn't care about . . . and remember, my grandmother was always telling me this was just . . . everything that she would tell me, you're just like your father, you're gonna be homeless, you're gonna do this and this . . . this was just reaffirming everything that had already been planted in me. Once you become a bum, it is very difficult to just go back to being a homeless person. Something profound usually has to happen. I cannot tell you those twelve years how many people I've seen get killed, overdose, get locked up, um . . . kill themselves, and that's how the vast majority of the people that you see out here are . . . they're walking dead. They're gonna die soon.

Many circumstances led Jesse to disregard his own life, including the way he grew up with his grandmother and the role his father had played in his life. He explained:

> Something that my grandmother used to do intentionally . . . Now that I'm older, I realize that it was intentional. My grandmother used to call me [Bruce] all the time. [Bruce] was my father's name. My father was

> home—he was drug-addicted, paranoid schizophrenic, homeless out there on the streets, completely dysfunctional, out-of-his-fucking-mind crazy. And my grandmother used to say, "[Bruce], go get me . . ." or "[Bruce], go do" anything—act like it was an accident: "Oh Lord, why did I call you [Bruce]? Jesse, go do this, go do that," whatever, because she was programmi . . . she used to tell me over and over and over again, for years and years, you're going to be just like your father, you're going to be just like your father. You're going to be homeless, you're going to be a drug addict, you're going to be dead before you're twenty-eight, over and over and over again, to the point where . . . when I got to my twenty-eighth birthday, I actually prayed that night, I couldn't believe that I made twenty-eight, because I had it in my mind that I was never going to see twenty-eight years old. I actually believed that I would be dead before then.

Through all the hardship and trauma, Jesse has several strengths and talents, one of which was his artistic talent. When Jesse was accepted to college based on his artistic talents, despite lacking a high school diploma, his compulsion to enact his father's fate stood in the way of his success. Jesse recounted:

> J: So by the time, by the time I got to college, by the time I got to [School], especially after [residential center], after the, the abuse that I suffered, I was getting into fights on campus. Worse, actually worse, now that I think about it, because there was nobody to stop me, and then looking at these little, these rich white kids, and I'm saying to myself, "You mother fuckers don't know nothing about, about hardship and pain and suffering. I mean, you, you know, you don't, you don't, you can't possibly understand who I am, what I been through, and where I come from."
>
> I: So a sense of not fitting in?
>
> J: Yep, exactly. But then there's also that self-destructive side of me, the side of me that says you're not gonna live to be twenty-eight years old. You're gonna ruin it. You can't graduate from school. Your father didn't graduate from school. You have to fuck this up.

Despite his talent and potential, Jesse did not graduate. He engaged in significant self-sabotage and used drugs and alcohol to regulate his emotions. However, this attempt to self-medicate was not up to the task of containing Jesse's rage. His outbursts led to both psychiatric hospitalization for bipolar disorder and incarceration for robbery and violence. He compared these experiences:

> A lot of people [in prison] are sick mentally and don't even know it, and can't keep a job, or they don't want a job, or they're just lazy. It's so much easier to be in jail. You don't have to pay bills, you don't have to be responsible for your kids, you don't have to be responsible for anything. Yeah, somebody telling you what to do, but we can deal with that because we learned how to . . . we learned how to survive . . . I don't care what anybody says—of course, I haven't been to all of them—people don't get better in psychiatric hospitals. I would rather be in jail and prison than be locked up on a locked psychiatric unit because it's just like—you know how they say that laughter is infectious? Now you take somebody that's already mentally fucked up and then you put them in an area with a whole bunch of people, other people that are fucked up, mentally fucked up, and then you create a system of control by which people look bored and don't have anything to do and they can't express themselves the way that they normally would . . . medication deals with the symptoms of the illness. Nobody in medical science either, nobody is dealing with the underlying causes that create the conditions in the first place. Everybody wants to deal with the symptoms, but nobody is really dealing with the reasons why we is sick in the first place.

For Jesse, psychiatry's approach to treating his difficulties was not ultimately effective. He has acute awareness of how the medical model failed him and he recognized that a system focused only on suppressing his acting out and violent behavior was insufficient to help him change the self-destructive trajectory of his life.

"A.K.A. MR. MISUNDERSTOOD"

Early attachment figures did not provide adequate trust or healthy attachment models for Jesse, and even at the time of the interview, relationships were difficult for him to navigate. As noted previously, when signing the consent form, he signed his name as "Jesse, A.K.A. Mr. Misunderstood." Jesse's explanation for calling himself Mr. Misunderstood revealed a longing for connection with someone who might see his most authentic self as well as a political critique of a society built around inequalities:

> I'm Mister Misunderstood . . . For a lot of reasons that I haven't even touched base on right now. But I am, look, whether we want to realize it or not . . . we have two justice systems in this country. And I've seen it a million times. We have two justice systems. We have a system for the rich, and we have a system for the poor. And, anybody who can't see that is either in denial or dumb . . . For that reason, I'm not—I'm not a patriot. Me being a black male in this country, when people first meet me, be-

> fore . . . before they, before I even open my mouth—and this is other black people, too. Even my own people, when . . . as a particularly black man, whenever you first meet somebody, before you even open your mouth, they're already started formulated an opinion about you. And if you are a police officer in this country, and 80 percent of the people you're arresting are black and Latino, and you been doing the job for five years, whether it's conscious or not, in the back of your mind, at some point you're going to associate, this is how these people are. If you're black, Latino male, this is how you are. Even consciously, you know, you say, well, they're not all the same, but in the back of your mind, and that's gonna affect your, your attitude when you're dealing with them. And so, there's nothing that can be done about that.

Jesse observed the way society's judgments about his race and social class have impacted him. When his father was killed, Jesse believed the black police officer thought, "Like . . . this is just an everyday thing. Just another dead n____," leaving Jesse feeling vulnerable and hopeless in a situation he could not control. Reflecting on how he has dealt with these feelings, Jesse related:

> There is duality in me. There's part of me that don't give a fuck. There's part of me that says you think whatever you want, I don't really care how you feel . . . the masochist in me, the dysfunctional side of me, will put myself in positions to give people the wrong impression of me. And then, I do it unconsciously sometimes, and then when I realize I, I'm, I shouldn't have did that, I did this, and then I try to change, then people look at me like this guy's a Dr. Jekyll, Mr. Hyde, they don't know which one, which person is there.

As Jesse explained, a part of him had given up and consequently felt indifferent to the unfair situation he had experienced. As multiple levels of trauma drive the individual to the edge, a sense of indifference forms, perhaps as a defensive stance against intolerable trauma and rejection (Hammersley et al., 2004).

RECONNECTING THROUGH HIS TALENT AND STRENGTH

Jesse is a very resilient, smart man, and his ability to survive through so much trauma and his verbal ability to tell his story in such a detailed, visually evocative, cohesive narrative speaks to his inner resources and capability. At the time of the interview, Jesse was trying to turn his life around. He began to build a life for himself, was staying sober and creating art. His artistic talent was a major asset, serving as an outlet for him to symbolize his feelings.

Jesse has also been in therapy for a decade with the same therapist, and utilized the therapy to make sense of his life story and to utilize his artistic talent to produce art. Furthermore, Jesse was very reflective, speaking about his own defenses. He took responsibility for his therapist not understanding who he truly was, as he recognized that he had defensively presented her with a façade out of self-protection. He was able to focus on bodybuilding and creative expression in an attempt to work on healthier aspects of himself and to find ways to more easily coexist with people:

> I just lost 70 pounds. I was 285 pounds, and, and really muscular. I, I what I did was, is, I took the negative addiction of drugs and, and alcohol and everything, and I replaced it with bodybuilding, and bodybuilding helped me for a lot of reasons, because it helped me sleep at night, it helped me feel better about myself and more confident, it gave me a chance to release pent-up hostility and frustration in the gym, and all of those—all of those things, you know, were good for me . . . when you're, when you're big and muscular like that, when people approach you, they're already intimidated, already just by your physical presence alone. So I'd go out of my way sometimes to try and make people, to make people feel comfortable with me.

Jesse also used his artistic talent to connect with others:

> One of the things that I did at the gallery was, when I first started volunteering at the gallery, I noticed that music is one of the great dividers, and one of the great connectors. So . . . when I first started helping them out there and everything, we were remodeling it, so I would bring my radio with me, and I'd bring all the CDs that had, "White music," on them . . . which is silly—white, black—because music is music. . . . So what I did was let them see, and then, while the music is playing, I'd sing along to the music, so that they'd say, "oh, he even knows the words." You know what I'm saying? It's not like an Uncle Tom thing where I'm trying to act like a, act like a white person, but the reason that I did it was to say, "Hey, you don't have to be intimidated by me" "I'm a person just like you, I even listen to some of the same music that you listen to; you don't have to be afraid of me." And even when you do that—it's not even a racist thing . . . even when you do that, people are still, like, I bet he has something to hide. And they're right. Because there is a monster in me too. There, there is the side of me that, that's potentially violent, can fucking hurt you, and so . . . but I do my best in life to keep that under wraps and under control.

Several factors played a role in his resilience, desire, and ability to change his life. He saw several of his friends die on the streets, scaring him into seeking treatment for his drug and alcohol addictions. His intellect was also a significant asset, allowing him to begin the work of processing and symbolizing his life experiences, giving him the ability to narrate his life story in such a detailed way speaks to his capacity. His long-term relationship with his psychologist proved instrumental in this regard, as he spoke repeatedly of his high regard for her. He relayed that his therapist saved his life, and he gave her the credit for turning his life around. His commitment to therapy and to his therapist speaks to his capacity for making and keeping meaningful relationships. Through all the trauma, hardship, and betrayal he survived in his early life, the glimmer of hope and trust he has in relationships speaks to his resilience, inner strength, and capacity for human connection.

A growing spiritual sensibility also supported Jesse in his path toward recovery. He had several experiences that he felt were spiritual moments, where God was influencing his decisions and helping him make good choices. In many ways, spirituality allowed Jesse to find a good object that prevented what he called his internal "monster" from becoming destructive. Jesse explained:

> There's too many coincidences . . . I'll give you an example. There have been times where, I have a Bible, and I'd say to myself, I'd say to myself: "Lord, if you're real, if this is true, if this is really real, this is my problem, this is what I'm going through now. If you—if you want me to—to yield and do the things that you tell me to do, I'm going to just blindly open this book, and—and if you're really real, if you really exist, speak to me directly." Not maybe, not kind of directly. And over and over again, out of all of those pages, the one passage I went to completely and, and honestly fit exactly the situation and the answer that I was looking for. Now, people can say whatever; I know that you have a lot of religious nuts out there and people that—you can look and say, oh, this guy is mentally ill, you know, maybe he's delusional, whatever. I'm not delusional.

In addition, throughout the interview, Jesse described his psychotherapist as a valuable source of support in his recovery. Jesse's trust in her gave him hope that his capacity for interpersonal relationships was not totally destroyed by years of cumulative relational trauma, and that he could still form important, fulfilling, meaningful relationships.

His primary caregivers, social support system—including those that were responsible for his protection—mistreated and failed him. A potentially positive space could have been the psychiatric facilities that were tasked with helping Jesse in his psychic struggles. Yet, he felt rejected and failed by the psychiatric system as a developing boy and as an adult as well. His early experience with psychiatric medications also proved unfruitful, as he was so highly medicated that he was unable to think for himself. Jesse's willingness to create a new life points to his resilience in the face of trauma and discrimination. He has significant inner resources including his intellect, artistic talent, faith, and drive, all of which have been assets through the hardship. Furthermore, he was able to utilize psychotherapy, which increased his ability to understand himself and his willingness to seek and create a new life path for himself and transcend the abject horror of his early life. Therapy helped Jesse utilize his inner resources and intellect and afforded him the opportunity to make meaningful changes in his life's trajectory, to overcome self-destructive impulses, and to begin to re-story his experience in fruitful and generative ways.

Chapter Fifteen

Roundtable Meeting of Team Members to Discuss the Book Draft

Elliott Madison, Andrew Schonebaum, and Mario Pinot in Conversation with Michael O'Loughlin and Montana Queler

Note: This is a lightly edited transcript of a roundtable meeting that took place in November 2018 at Fountain House. Participants had read all of the book draft with the exception of the afterword. Andrew, Elliott, and Mario have been affiliated with Fountain House for many years.

Andrew: So some of the general impressions that I got when reading was that in many, if not also in all of the videos, is there seemed to be a different tone in reading it. The videos seemed to be more hopeful than the reading. It didn't come across in the specific excerpts and also in terms of the commentary on it. To give you an example so one of the people, I don't remember her stage name . . . I won't use her real name, but she is the person who is with the hearing loss.

Michael: We called her Faith.

Andrew: Yes, Faith. So . . . talking to her in real life, seeing the video, and also last night we had a fundraiser and she was highlighted in a video there . . . talking about how wonderful her life is now. Even though she didn't fulfill the dreams she had when she was younger, she's very . . . she talked about being very fulfilled now with her life and how meaningful her life is and that did not come across to me in reading the chapter.

Michael: Interesting, okay.

Andrew: And that seemed to be a common theme. You talk about resiliency in it but it is almost as someone who was a survivor, not in the way that of someone who thrived after that. One person, is a male, and it talked about you know what he could achieve . . . he didn't achieve his dreams and I'm thinking to myself *well he might've not achieved the dreams he had when he was younger*. I sure as hell didn't. I wanted to be a doctor growing up and then I didn't do well enough my first couple years of undergraduate. Then, I wanted to get my PhD and I ended up having to leave graduate school early and so I didn't achieve that dream. And so then I came here and now I am happier than I could ever imagine with something that is not any of the dreams I had when I was younger. And so to have a statement there saying you know what he could have achieved, what he did . . . well maybe he is . . . maybe he does have a meaningful life and that didn't come across that way in that chapter.

Michael: Yes, okay. That's a good point. Do you think it would be feasible and worthwhile for us to sit down and have a few minutes with at least some people and catch them up on their lives and put a postscript at the end rather than leaving it the way it is?

Andrew: I think that would. You know, "What is going on in your life today?" Maybe some people.

Elliot: Well some of the people, you're not going to be able to get a hold of.

Michael: No, I understand that. But, for somebody like the one you just mentioned, it could provide a corrective.

Andrew: Yeah she's there. Assuming that the video last night was an accurate representation of how she was feeling, she wasn't just putting on a show.

Michael: That's a reasonable assumption, of course, yeah.

Andrew: She seems to be in a good place.

Michael: In a good place, yeah.

Andrew: And it's nice to see that. Whether or not it had something to do with that much, and it would be great if it had something to do with Fountain House, but even if it didn't . . . so that was the general impression. The other thing that also struck me is that while it's very clear that the person's trauma plays a very significant role in how their mental health issues. But, there are several times where, it was not insinuated, it was really said explicitly that the trauma was the cause of psychosis. And it wasn't anything that was in the transcript, it wasn't the person saying "Oh well you know childhood trauma made me hear voices." It may have caused those voices to be what they were, but not necessarily what changed the brain chemistry to make the person hear voices in the first place.

Michael: Absolutely, and that is part of our bias as we approach the work. We have been pushing back against the more chemical hypothesis, that it's something that you're born with, but it is a huge inference, I mean and undoubtably it is complex. It's never a simple factor. What our goal was to try and complexify the story so that it would not be over-simplified, but we might have over corrected in doing so. It's a good critique.

Andrew: And then the third thing is that it might be biased coming from your backgrounds, but it seemed like there was a heavier emphasis on, much heavier emphasis, on psychotherapy versus a community support. There was some talk about Fountain House, and it didn't necessarily have to be Fountain House, but just talking about people's social networks and other support systems they had and may have played a large role in their resiliency then was evident from reading the chapters.

Michael: That's very helpful too.

Mario: I thought, in talking about psychotherapy, and the narrative that community was given kind of an emphasis that you need a community somewhere. I almost vaguely remember something about the community of the hospital. Someone there to talk with and to kind of express yourself and something about how general practitioners being more sympathetic at times than "trained therapists." More casual, more whatever you want to call it. I found that kind of interesting. Sort of a community and kind of a relaxed atmosphere where you can actually think about "Well my father was an alcoholic, my mother was a drug addict, my brother went to jail because he killed someone," and all those traumas that . . . who wants to think about that? You know? You don't think about that always, but when you think about them, you "process them," and then you kind of unexplode them. They detonate, even though that's a hard word.

Montana: Defusing.

Michael: Detonate or defuse, right?

Marco: Defuse (chuckling), that's what I mean. Very big difference.

Michael: Very big difference. Well, Lucy Newlyn, that English poet whose poem opens the introduction, she had a breakdown in her forties, and she said that the person who helped her most was her family doctor because he was a human and he listened. He didn't see her as a category, he just was there for her, to listen to her. That I think is . . .

Elliot: That I think comes across in some of the stories. I think, I think we might have a bias also.

Andrew: Oh yes, we definitely have biases.

Elliot: Because we . . . it's voluntary when people come in here and we get a chance, which is kind of unique probably in mental health, to get to see people at their best for the most part. It's unusual to see people at their worst here. It sometimes happens, but for the most part by and large, the 280 people that will be coming in today . . . they're having a good day. And not only that, they're coming into a place that is engineered to maximize that, to extend that. Focusing on their strengths and creating a mood of positivity and hope. So, I was a little less struck by the, I don't want to say pessimism, but the kind of more dreary tone because I think that occurs once they leave this place. This place is not their home, this place is not their life. That, you know the person we were talking about, Faith. I know her very well. I was her worker for many years and would regularly go out and see her. I, I don't think her story is an unmitigated positive. I think a lot of her . . . she is . . . she deals a lot with depression, just not here. So, I think the role when members talk about Fountain House it's sort of like children talking about recess when they're talking about school. Sure you have some children that get bullied and recess sucks but for the most part recess is set up to appeal to what children want to do. Fountain House is set up to appeal to how and moving people's lives forward, but I think it would be an unbalance, and we tend to have an unbalanced view because the rest of their life is set up against them.

Andrew: That's true, that's true and I understand. I would say that we're more than just the recess. We're not just a respite, a short respite. I think it's a little more life changing. Before I came to Fountain House I worked at a residential program and so half the people in that residential program were members at Fountain House. So, I got to see people in two different environments and so I saw people beaten down at this residential program come to Fountain House and be leaders knowing that they'd be going back down to be beaten down again. But this was still a full part of their life and part of the reason they got beaten down at the residence is because they were so hopeful . . . they saw something that was different and was better. And so coming back to the residence they were, one person I can remember in particular, was quite rebellious against all of the rules and the structure. And I think that was something that he learned being at Fountain House and realizing that there was hope and there was something better.

Elliot: I'm not saying recess in a frivolous way. I'm not saying what we're doing isn't life changing. What I'm saying is that in the end it's only part of the experience. What we often forget is that a lot of our members are treated outside of here . . . Where they are treated with respect and they have potential and they have opportunities that a lot . . . and I think you hear it in the stories, they feel a lot of those don't exist outside of here. They feel penned in, they feel poor because they are poor. They feel they don't get a choice in their housing and who their roommates are. This is all true. It's not true here. They have choice and they have respect and they have potential. So, I guess, I think, in some type of ending highlighting that might be useful. That this resiliency, and some of them mention it in their stories, that there's this problem of how do you . . . like in the story you were talking about . . . you go back to the residence and they don't care that you had choice for eight hours during the day. You're still just a resident here. You're going to do what they want you to do, and in some ways that creates even a greater difficulty, right? If you believe "All right I do need people to take care of me," and it's kind of like this split of where here (Fountain House) I am an adult and I'm making choices, meaningful choices and there I'm being . . .

Michael: Infantilized, yeah.

Elliot: I could see why many members struggle with that. In some ways it's even harder just accepting the fact.

Andrew: Yeah because you can see what you're not . . . you can see more clearly what you're not having because you have the hope. There was one particular person, what he did, because there were staff-only rooms, he stole his own copy of the staff key. So, he could go into the staff office and use the water cooler when he wanted, you know. When he's outsmarting everybody there . . . he took advantage of that.

Elliot: I mean for us, I think it is a more depressing reading because, again we don't always get to see . . . we certainly don't get to experience many members most depressing stuff before they came to Fountain House because they don't necessarily feel like they want to share that. They're here to focus on something positive.

Michael: And you're not doing therapy so you're not asking them necessarily to share that.

Elliot: Right, and that's kind of like here is a place where I'm respected for my skills and my contributions. I don't know if I want to muck that around by saying I was "Oh yeah I was also an addict and abused." I could see where that's a rational, reasonable choice. Like, "Hey, I want to focus on the positive stuff here."

Michael: Well, it's a chance to build a new identity. One that's not filled with that baggage.

Andrew: No, but I think it's a positive that could come off a little bit stronger.

Michael: Okay, good.

Mario: That's kind of interesting because I remember I wanted to start therapy several years ago, start therapy up again. The place that I went to was kind of run down and looked shabby and there were signs all over, I think I counted six or seven signs, that said "Do not eat in the waiting area." And I'm like, "Gee, seven signs of that? What's going on here?" And I remember that the therapist was somewhat late, of course they never apologize because they're late. And, and I just I'm thinking about that when you come to Fountain House maybe I was spoiled to expect . . .

Elliot: Human decency?

Mario: And if I didn't find it, I would just, I left the therapy. I think she called me on the phone and I think I said to her, "Well I've been spoiled by Fountain House," you know? And I think I missed out on therapeutic interaction, processing things, and diffusing them because of this attitude that I had that wasn't always, that isn't always a constructive attitude. I mean I have to be flexible to say that this is not Fountain House, this is an emergency room in a Hosptial and I have to wait for them to take care of me. And complaining about the fact that I'm depersonalized and objectified and moved around isn't really going to be very helpful to me. Quite the contrary.

Andrew: Wait a minute . . . unintended negative consequence. But on the other hand, you . . . you realized that you deserve better than that.

Mario: Yeah, you realize you deserve better but you're not going to get better. What you're going to get is nothing.

Andrew: But the next step is learning how to deal with that, but knowing that you're better than that and not accepting it because you're not worthy.

Elliot: Exactly, exactly, good point.

Andrew: But understanding that there are some things you just can't change, but you are better than that.

Mario: Right, right.

Elliot: I thought the language in the narratives was very true. Having spent now eighteen and a half years here. Forty hours a week plus with folks in conversation I didn't find that, which I think is really difficult even with video tape because I have an anthropology background so I've done plenty of transcribing, I thought that was very, I felt the language felt true. That these conversations, they're, they're not really conversations, they're more of edited monologues which I think is difficult to make sound true because it's not how many . . . 99 percent of our members don't speak in monologue. There are some members that only speak monologues. But, I think most speak in . . . so I thought that was really well done.

Michael: And part of that we owe to you because when we had the first meeting you said, "Well you can't do this work unless you're here and people know you and you know them." And that was, that's how this, came to be, and the authenticity came from that suggestion.

Elliot: I thought that what was interesting is that it's almost hidden and I wonder why that was done. Because I would walk by while you guys were on the fourth floor doing your interviews and I would see you laughing and I would see you talking, and all of that is kind of . . . and we watched the videos and you guys are engaging and I mean that's an important part of Fountain House is this idea of engagement. And it reads, truthfully, but it reads as if, were Mario sitting in a room, putting the camera, and saying "Okay Mario tell us about your life," and those are not the people you were interviewing. The people you were interviewing, you had to engage them. Now you had experience with them months ahead of time so you knew how to best engage.

Montana: Yes.

Elliot: But, some of the people you picked are not that easy to engage. They're not used to doing self-reflection and coherent narration. And, to be honest, I can't believe all of them were quite as coherent in narrative. There had to be jumping around.

Michael: Oh God, yes.

Elliot: And you guys were able to, and that's part of engagement, is being able to understand where people are coming from. I'm just curious why that, I know that because you probably, well I don't know I am just going to leave it at that. I think you should, in your introduction or something, explain the reasoning that, you know, this was not a monologue per se.

Michael: Well, actually, I can raise my hand here because it's really my fault because Montana and Secil had written extensively about their experience, about being in the experience, and I took it out. But, that maybe we should consider having a little bit at the end of each one. A reflection on the experience of *being with* so that you capture the dynamic vibrancy of the experience, don't you think? Because we had that.

Montana: Yes.

Michael: And I said "No, no we don't have room for that," because we were playing with other constraints, but I think it might be worth it.

Elliot: But, I think, like, if you took any of those people especially some of them . . . [Name] . . . I forgot what his name was in there.

Montana: I think we called him Dylan.

Elliot: If you took Dylan and you tried to replicate . . . or I wanna do a follow-up and see where Dylan is now . . . and sat him down and said "Okay Dylan" . . . it wouldn't work. It took a level of engagement, a level of sophistication to be able to kind of cut through the fantasy stuff and the wish to impress and try and get to that, and I think that—I don't know if that's always useful—but it seemed like a big part of this process that's completely not mentioned.

Michael: And he's a particularly nice example because he was intensely engaged with Montana. In fact, I think all of them probably were.

Andrew: There was one chapter where it seemed to come out. The person was talking about their childhood and it was pretty wonderful until the questions got more probing. Then you heard about the drinking and the spousal abuse that was there. But, in the beginning the person was "Oh yeah happy childhood, we went to the beach," or whatever it was and all that. And then it took the deeper probing to get to that.

Elliot: Because part of this, I see for me, as the program director, is that this is a valuable . . . what I'd like to see is that this is a valuable document for people in school, people thinking about working with our folks. And that was the original way you kind of pitched it to us. You know that we think it's too one-sided, it's all about the medical diagnosis and not about the narrative. And so I think the only thing is that without, and I'm not saying it has to be after each one in the introduction, is that it involves an engagement to get to the narration.

Michael: That's a very nice point.

Elliot: And that the narration is not . . . this is not easy. You're not just going to like, what I think many therapists think is that if I just ask the right few questions you're just going to tumble out in this very linear order.

Michael: And give me the story.

Elliot: Yeah and the narrative doesn't happen that way.

Andrew: And that's why it's so important also maybe in the introduction talking about the relationship development. Like you said when you're meeting with your therapist for your fifty minutes and you're asking questions, you don't know that person. And here they develop relationships with all of you and it really changes the dynamic.

Michael: That's a great point. We'll work on that for sure. That's very helpful.

Mario: But there's also a, correct me if I'm wrong, but there's also a . . .

Andrew: I will.

Michael: We will.

Mario: Ah, I just lost my train of thought. There's also something at Fountain House where, it is kind of an informal practice I guess, where if you . . . if the member wants to sit with the staff and have a therapeutic discussion and conversation it is kind of pooh-poohed. You know it's sort of like, "We have this to do and we have that to do and I don't know how to do this and I have to find, could you tell me how to do it?" So there's turning to members for help but there . . .

Elliot: And that's why we don't get the narrative. That's what I'm saying is the language read true, the kind of despair and the deepness of the struggle, it was new to me. I knew some of these people pretty well because we don't do that. And I'm not saying we should, I'm just saying. But, that's a value additive to work like this because we're not going to do that.

Andrew: Generally, I mean it depends on the person. There are plenty of people I have worked with over the years who are open books and they'll talk very freely about the trauma they have had in their lives. We were talking about these particular people who were interviewed.

Mario: And they're not lengthy conversations. They are sort of, you know . . .

Andrew: You get bits and pieces.

Mario: Yeah, yeah, yeah, yeah because I know when there's a staff at the front door, which is just basically sitting there and greeting people as they come in, and members sit there with the staff, it seems to me like an opportunity to process certain things and remember certain things.

Elliot: Yeah but the focus mostly at Fountain House is on the present and the future. Probably a little more on the future than the present. What are we going to do next week? What are we thinking about school? When's the scholarship application? You know? Whereas a therapist traditionally is more focused on the present and the past; they're moving that way. We're moving this way. We have the present that we share, not that the therapist never hears about what the person is planning for the future and we never hear about the past, but we both have different focus.

Michael: Different focus, yeah.

Mario: Right and how do we know that focus is actually correct or is it off?

Elliot: Oh, they're both correct. I think if handled well they both make a lot of sense. It's just what makes us different and it's probably difficult. I mean probably the question of "well why wouldn't you have a system that focuses on the entire thing?" Right? I'm not sure you actually can. I'm not sure that that actually . . . because sometimes folks can be too caught up in the past and just keep repeating it, repeating it, and repeating it. That doesn't mean that they don't need to do so, and the same about the future. People are the same about the future, "Oh it doesn't matter that I have a drug addiction, I'm going to be a doctor, I'm going to do this." I think you need both but they probably do need . . . I don't know if they need to be as siloed as they are but . . .

Michael: But let me ask this question, since I work with teachers who are not psychologists, and they're never going to be psychologists. I work a lot with children's emotions so to sensitize them to the idea of being sensitive even though they won't do it to the level as I would do it in therapy. I wonder if the material in this book would be useful in training to sensitize workers, even though they wouldn't practice it in their daily work. Could it sensitize them to the complexity of the backstories.

Elliot: Definitely and I think we will use, or parts of it, when it comes to . . . when it's available for our training of new staff. I think it does a couple of things very nicely that's useful for our staff. One is that we pride ourselves on taking a holistic approach, but where the holism may fall apart is that sometimes we don't know anything about the past of the person. Not that we need to know the past of each individual, but maybe understanding some of these narratives . . .

Andrew: Usually the only time we learn about the past, about someone we're working with is when we have to. When we start working with someone we don't go to their file. If we have to write a psychosocial for a housing application or something, then we go into the file, we talk to the person about their past, but it's only in that context. Sometimes things will come up in conversation, but nothing to this degree of depth.

Elliot: And I think that even though you're doing great work here, this is part of the subjective experience, part of the subjective world the person lives in. Because sometimes I think it gets frustrating for new staff like "Mario's doing great here, he's very involved and then why did he . . . why wasn't able to go to school or do this or that?" and then he comes back. It's, it's that lack of the holistic experience. Yeah, it's optimistic and positive here, but that doesn't mean that when he leaves here there aren't huge struggles that he has to know that he could toil over. And I think that this does a little bit more of balancing that; of kind of being the subjective . . . that it isn't just linear. You can have in a single day positive stuff and negative stuff, and the negative stuff can really throw you.

Andrew: Something we do to try and reach out beyond our walls . . . The transitional employment program is a way to connecting to the outside world of employment with still a lot of the . . .

Elliot: That's positive.

Andrew: I know that's my point.

Elliot: We do very little to reach out to the negative.

Andrew: I know, I don't disagree with you. What I'm saying is that we . . .

Elliot: And I'm not saying we should.

Andrew: But what I'm saying is that I agree with you that we don't do that. But what we do is try and help ease people into that role and develop the strengths, internal strengths, to be able to cope with those challenges in the world. So, if you just throw someone out . . . one of the reasons we do transitional employment is, instead of getting someone a job, is a lot of other programs get people job right away and they're actually better at job placement than we are. But, those people don't stay on the jobs nearly as long because they don't have those coping mechanisms fully developed. So that what I'm saying is we're not negating what's going on on out there, and we're not always aware of what's going on out there, but to some extent we try and help people develop their strengths to be able to handle what's out there.

Elliot: And I'm just saying that as a new staff it can be confusing where you're getting . . . you know it would be like having a student that's getting A's, at the top of the class and then at some simple standardized testing, you know, scoring really low. And that happens with our members because of outside influence, and I think new staff sometimes are like "Why, why is this happening?" Because they're only seeing the person in a positive environment, talking about the future, and I think that's right. But, I would like them to at least know they're up against something huge that's decades in the making and that there's a lot of negativity poured into them. And I think it makes them feel like "Okay, I need to really roll up my sleeves. I don't need to know Mario's particular story, I need to know what I'm up against." The fact that we give people jobs or people are positive here at all is a huge accomplishment which is too easy to be taken for granted.

Andrew: I don't know if this is along the lines of what you're saying but I remember one person in particular, he could talk to any stranger anywhere, but in a job interview he would sit with his head down and mumble, and no matter what, he couldn't pass that point of being able to communicate in a job interview.

Mario: I've heard that, I've heard that. People are excellent workers, you know, and they're Transitional Employees and then they go for a permanent part-time job and they're at the interview and there's a meltdown. But I like the idea of how we try to treat people in a normal kind of way. That's why no one lives here. People have housing, they have apartments, they live, they get up, they have breakfast, they don't have breakfast, they get on the bus or the train, they go through those everyday experiences which can be positive. They can be part of "Oh the train was late again," and there's just this commiseration out of people saying "Yeah I know."

Michael: Yeah, normal stuff.

Mario: Normal, everyday experiences as opposed to living in a . . .

Michael: Well there's two parts. There's a part of their internal history and then there's a part you mentioned earlier of the way society reacts, and society doesn't provide support structures. So this is an abnormal support structure because it's supportive. Out in the world, often, there isn't a lot of support, and there is often a lot of stigma and lack of support, and that's what makes life hard for a lot of people, I think.

Mario: Yeah and I think that's an interesting point. It's sort of like in a fucked-up society where greed is . . .

Michael: "Greed is good."

Mario: Greed is good and that's the predominant virtue that people are encouraged, there are these movements to ameliorate the situation which are absolutely essential and very important. I mean then you go forward, the funding is cut, and you have to go backwards. It just seems like an uphill climb to try and reform society, which is a good thing. Reforms are really good.

Elliot: What does this have to do with the book?

Mario: I have no idea. I'm shooting it out there, you know? I mean it's a fucked-up society. People are not happy, they're alienated.

Elliot: Yeah I don't think this book will fixed the fucked-up society. That's a criticism I have. You know you made that promise.

Andrew: But Mario had a point, and it's not just about fixing the fucked-up society. You might not have had a point, but if you had a point it might be along this line. It's about it being recognized that there are all these barriers. Even if the trauma is in the past, the barriers still exist today, and still you have to overcome that. Like you said, when you went to that clinic that barrier was still there and that barrier was not caused directly by what happened to you in the past. But, what happened to you in the past got you to the point where you had to go there and deal with that barrier, where someone else might not have to.

Elliot: I'm going to say a controversial statement.

Michael: Go ahead.

Elliot: I think another advantage to this book, and I think this is what you were getting at, but I'm going to come at it from the opposite . . . Fountain House should be agnostic on the causes of psychic distress, the reason people are here, and how they define there. You guys are not agnostic, you're on the other side and your concern is, you were trying to be nice, but you were saying to us, "C'mon there's a biological, medical cause of psychosis you're not addressing in this." If anything, I think Fountain House has moved too much onto accepting the status quo of the diagnosis. We should not be in that discussion at all, we should be completely . . .

Michael: Agnostic, as you said.

Elliot: Yeah because it doesn't . . . we can do our work better if we can accept if it's witchcraft or psychosis or early trauma or anything because it doesn't. What we're saying is it's environmental . . . we're doing this environment where we heal folks through these relationships and we don't have to define it. So, I think again for new staff this might be useful because it goes against probably how they've been trained in school and everything else they're going to read because the medical model is the current model.

Andrew: And so surprising to you, I do actually agree with you, and my point was not to . . . The point I was trying to make was not to promote the biological argument. It was the pushback on a specific different argument talking about what actually caused it. Now the environment, and this is where neither of us is agnostic really, the environment plays a tremendous role in causing the harm and also in creating the health. And whatever the biological influences may be, we have little ability to change those. We have limited ability to change any of the structures out there. But, what we do have the ability to do is create a supportive environment where people can change and grow.

Michael: And funny enough I would actually agree with that as well because as a therapist you have to be somewhat agnostic. Your work is your intuition, it is the here and now with the person. And we can take out positions and debates, but when I'm in the room, if I were in the room with you, or you were in the room with me, I have to receive you and you have to receive me, and that's what you do here. That's appropriate. In practice you have to work with the person who's with you.

Elliot: Which I think is easier said than done. I mean if you come already with a medical mind-set or a trauma-informed mind-set, or both of those actually, I see it play out with new staff, that does effect their efficacy in doing social practice which is the model we have. For example, if I believe it's really medical, I can't help but have a cognitive blinder. Like, "Oh you're not taking your medication." If I have a trauma thing, I can't help but to be like "Oh this is triggering, the environment is triggering."

Andrew: So I came from a third background actually and I see this a lot. Now our society practitioners are only hired with masters degrees and most of them are social workers so they really get inundated with the medical model. I came with a sociology background so for me it was all social structure. When I started here, mental illness was a social construct imposed by society for people who are different. And so I had to partially unlearn that. I still have that part of me, because it's the social justice part of me, but as we were saying earlier we all come with different biases. But, I think nowadays because we have so many people coming from social work that that particular bias is so much more prevalent.

Elliot: I think that we have the clinic . . .

Andrew: We're connected to the clinic. I think there are a lot of reasons why, but I think it might be more prevalent now here, as opposed to when you and I started, because of those changes that we've made.

Elliot: So that's why this is a nice balancing . . . why it would be helpful for new staff. Not even that what you're saying is accurate because I have no idea if what you're saying is accurate . . . you know your conclusions. But, it's just a way to be like, "Okay here's a different way this group of people, and the member themselves, are framing it." That they can frame it in a different way that is actually compelling. It's not crazy, it's not voodoo, it makes sense. And, that's why, you know, those narratives may be difficult to penetrate and confront and you don't need to. I would say our job in social practice is not confrontation and changing those narratives.

Michael: Yes, yes of course.

Elliot: Because I think most people are like, "Well no it's like diabetes." I hear new staff drop a line . . . like, "You need to take your medication" and it's like, well, yes, if you accept the biomedical model. And clearly not all of our membership does accept that, and some do accept it as a biochemical but in a completely different way than you're expecting it.

Andrew: And there are some advantages to accepting it in a biochemical way that are actually more societal and about the individual, and so that it can be helpful in that if you're deaf you can always get back on social security. I have friends that are deaf and they lose their jobs. They go right on to social security because their disability never disappears. But if you have a mental illness and you go to work and you lose your disability payment and come off work, then you have to prove all over again that you're disabled. So there are some societal advantages to that. If you say it's like diabetes, it's a chronic illness that doesn't go away and therefore if we can convince people of that then people would be able to get the support that they need. There are some larger advantages. It's just on the individual and trying to label them as something that they may or may not be.

Michael: Interesting. I was not aware of that. That's very troubling.

Andrew: And it's a big issue for a lot of our members. The top two reasons why people don't go to work are (1) fear of failure and (2) the fear of losing your benefits. And unfortunately, and it's not just an American thing, every Western country that has a full safety network . . . going back to work hurts. So it's a big impediment to people, it's one of the biggest barriers we have.

Mario: And also we talk about recovery and members having recovery so that. And I assume that recovery included medication. Like you would be hearing voices or be depressed and you would take medication and I didn't really get an anti-medication, anti-therapy thing from the chapters.

Andrew: Well definitely pro-therapy.

Mario: But it was more sort of like, the big pharmacies are pushing these medications and their lucrative and all this other stuff. I lost my train of thought here.

Michael: You were saying that you didn't get the sense that the book was anti-medication.

Mario: Right. It was sort of like emphasizing that people who had been in therapy for years, and years, and years, and years, and years and nothing-—they're not really moving anywhere. Even with medication. So, I thought that what had happened several years ago, some time ago, was that, "Hey you know that the medication works, the medication will tone down your voices." The therapy might work, it might not work, it'll take five years, it'll take one year so let's pooh-pooh that. So that whole aspect of the therapy which was talking, exploring, and medicine, together to help the person as kind of . . .

Montana: Turned on its head, it looks like you're saying. Flipped.

Mario: Yeah, yeah. So, one was eliminated altogether. You can still get therapy though. Processing things, thinking things over. And when I was reading, I was asking myself, "Well how many trauma have I had in my life?" Then I thought about when my parents would get drunk on the holidays, just on the holidays, and they would get into fistfights. But that was only once or twice a year. I remember I was run down by a bicycle another time, I was hit by a car another time, I remember my neighbor beating her child for . . . it seemed like a very long time, and there were all of these things. I had a pet cat and the cat attacked me. And I'm like. "Well gee this is fucking shit," you know? Fucking little cat, I raised it, gave it a little bottle of milk, and ten years later. Then I'm all traumatized and I'm hallucinating cats, I'm screaming. My mother doesn't know what to do. So just thinking about those things.

Andrew: See you have another chapter right here.

Mario: Just thinking about those things is different than not thinking about them. Thinking about them is sort of like, I think it's mentioned, you take ownership and you're coping with it. You're sort of like diffusing the thing and so it was sort of like bringing back the talk therapy that has been eliminated and pooh-poohed. Which a lot of people pooh-poohed.

Michael: And the insurance companies don't want to pay for it as well.

Mario: That's it exactly.

Elliot: It is nice to see members own their own stories, too. But, again, I would like to go back to I think the relationship between the interviewer and the . . . as an anthropologist, you know, I think that's a . . . you know you guys were doing participant observation. You were there doing stuff and you had a shared language that you could talk about.

Michael: We're going to put a piece in for definitely, for sure. We, meaning Montana and Secil.

Elliot: My favorite kind of "we."

Michael: But I think it will enhance the book.

Montana: I wonder, Elliot, if you're also suggesting that even the way we have presented the narrative material in the chapters conceals the fact that there's more of an exchange?

Elliot: It totally conceals it the fact that there's . . .

Montana: And if you're suggesting that it would feel more accurate, and therefore better, to actually portray some of what we as the interviewers were saying.

Elliot: I'm not sure if . . . Yes. The answer is yes, but I'm also a person who knows trying to get something published. I think you can get 99 percent of the way there with a brief thing of like deconstructing one bit. Maybe at the beginning or at the end. You take a section and you explain this is how it is written in the book and this is why we made the stylist choice to not have my voice. But, this is how it really went down and what I want to highlight is that there's a relationship. You're not speaking into the darkness. There was a human hearing them. There was a human, who wasn't a therapist, they weren't expecting to get cured by you. They built a relationship. This is how I helped them and this how they helped me understand, and you could do that instead of rewriting all fifteen.

Michael: And, if you read through the chapters you'll notice a change. The first chapters, which are Montana and Secil's dissertation, they're more, "Pull out quotes and talk about what they mean." But, in the later chapters that I did with Marilyn Charles and Veronica using that work, we put in a lot more samples from the dialogue. For instance, Secil is working with the gentleman we called Daniel, and she spoke English less fluently, and he's also not a native English speaker, and they didn't understand each other all of the time, and you can really see them trying to find a meeting point. It's very helpful to see the back and forth, rather than to just see the answer.

Elliot: And they were very close, those two. They had worked very closely together.

Michael: He was not going to let go without her understanding, and she wasn't going to let go without understanding him so it worked out very well. But, you can see the dialogue. We can do a nice note so that it would contrast that so you could see.

Elliot: I don't think you have to redo it. Just kind of highlight the relational . . .

Michael: Nice point.

Elliot: Which also then informs the conclusions you're making throughout is based on more than just a cold reading of said statements, you know what I'm saying. I think people from the same guild, given the same statements, would not have been able to make the exact same conclusions you were because of the relational.

Michael: I think that's 100 percent true.

Montana: Do you think knowing the members who were interviewed, that if they read the chapters about them, they would have a positive reaction to them? I mean I've been sort of curious about this since we met them.

Elliot: That's a good question. I think it depends on . . .

Andrew: It depends on the person, clearly. But also, it depends on how their psychosis manifested. For example, there were a number of times where it was referred to that what the person experiencing was not reality based and that person may think it was reality. So they might think that or have an adverse reaction to this and say, "Hey I told you all of this stuff and you're saying it's not true?"

Michael: There are some very clear examples of that, yeah. In the case of one woman, I forget what we called her, she had the Elvis fantasy and so on.

Montana: We called her Jamie.

Michael: Jaime, yes, and I mean Jaime says that everyone has been persuading her that she is having delusional thought. She sees it as reality. That could really feel like betrayal if she read that.

Elliot: I think that what would be most interesting is, and I wouldn't be surprised, is that if some of the people you interviewed have no interest in reading it. They just don't. I don't think they have . . . I know most of the people because most of them came out of horticulture.

Michael: Yes, they did. All of them, I think.

Elliot: And I think the real reason they were doing it was because you guys asked them to do it. I mean that was clear. I mean you guys that, that wasn't a surprise. It wasn't like burning desire to do this. They had a desire for you to understand. Everyone that I knew that went to the interview, and I'd ask them because I have to especially at the beginning . . . "How was it?" and they'd say, "Oh we had a good time." That was pretty much the standard, "It was a good time." They enjoyed spending time with you and Secil and that made sense because they enjoyed spending their time. I think specifically because they knew you were not staff. You know, "I don't have to tell you . . . we're friends . . . I'm telling you the story and you seemed interested" . . . because you guys were genuinely interested. But what I find with most members is that they don't have that genuine interest in telling the story. Some do, but generally they don't. Like you (pointing to Mario). You're not like "Oh let me tell you about my cat." I think most of them will not pick up the book. I'm going to tell them that it's available, but most of them will never read it.

Mario: I think if I'm talking to someone that I may not see again . . . it's like the stranger that stops you friendly . . . you're walking your dog . . . and sort of like dumps on you.

Andrew: But what I was also going to say is a lot of actors have never seen themselves in movies and TV shows. It's just something they don't want to deal with, you know?

Elliot: I think it's really different. It's like watching a video of your birthday party or your wedding. Most people don't. They don't mind it happening because they realize it's being shared with other people. No one has ever asked me, of these people, "When is the book coming out, how's the book going, why isn't it done?" Not once, this entire time. Sometimes they'll ask me "Hey what happened to Montana, what happened to Secil? . . . as individuals, but never once asked about the book, the work because to them it's not their work. It's not the work that is interesting to them. So, I wouldn't expect a lot of in-depth psychic . . .

Andrew: So we're not going to have a reading is what you're saying?

Montana: And just the concern is that we're telling people's stories, we're re-telling people's stories in a way, and we're interpreting their stories and I think all along we were very mindful of re-telling people's stories in a way that might . . . the danger is it being exploitative.

Andrew: And the thing is, the people who know the people here, you're going to be able to figure out who's who. Even with the changed names, you know?

Michael: Do you see any danger in that? Is there any worry from the things you read?

Andrew: Well, I don't think so. Like you said, most of the people at Fountain House in general are not going to be interested in . . .

Mario: It would be interesting to try to get a dialogue and say, "This is your dialogue that you gave us. What do you think of it?"

Michael: The worry is that it could be triggering.

Mario: Or, "This is somebody else's dialogue. What do you think about that?"

Andrew: So we actually had them, after the earlier stage and everyone did the recordings, there was a group of us and there were a couple of other members on that, we had them watch the recordings and give feedback at that time.

Elliot: You're also assuming from a kind of privileged position, too that most of these members, when you look at their stories . . . yeah, people have interpreted their stories, people have written down their stories. All of us folks know their psychosocial and their psych-evaluations, most of them have seen it at Fountain House. Do they agree with all the stuff in the psychosocial? No! They're often like, "Oh, well that's not my diagnosis." It's just the cost of doing business. People are going to write. I'll see people go "Oh they have addiction on here and I never drank in my life. I don't know why that's there!" Then I say, "Oh maybe we should [change it]," and they just say "Never mind."

Andrew: And it is kind of sad in a way because most people are not used to having their whole lives examined so many different ways. So many people here are used to it. They say, "Oh I have to tell my life story again because I'm seeing another doctor, another therapist, and I have to put all that out all over again."

Michael: But the bigger question, and this gets at Montana's question but widens the lens a bit, is that we want to be sure that there's no risk that does harm to the image of persons with psychic distress. That it's a book that enhances people's understanding rather than increases the stigmatization in any way.

Andrew: Well that, what my initial point was, is while it's touched on in pretty much every chapter, that resiliency . . . I think it can be done in a stronger way and not just as survival. A little bit more emphasis on that strength.

Michael: No that's really important actually. We want to make sure we do that because we don't want to make something that can be misused by any policy maker or politician or anybody else that can enhance ill treatment of persons with psychic stress.

Andrew: Because I don't want the people being interviewed to come across as being broken people. They're strong people who have come through some of the worst things imaginable and are still here.

Michael: Absolutely, you're absolutely right. So we will work on that as well.

Andrew: And even the people who might not feel satisfied with their lives in a lot of ways, they are still important people. They're giving back to people all of the time. So even if they haven't found that place of contentment for themselves, what they're doing for other members of Fountain House or the community at large is often immeasurable. You know, Mario might be having an awful day but if he's helping someone at Fountain House their day might be better because of it, and that's very significant.

Mario: There is also this thing of humility. Where you don't want to acknowledge that you are helping someone. You don't want to develop that pride. You almost want to do it, you almost want to do it anonymously.

Michael: We call that self-effacing. Kind of keeping down your . . .

Mario: Yeah, yeah very humble, very . . . and that can be very therapeutic. But also just say "Hey, you know what I had a hard life but I have helped someone, a couple of people, people have helped me." That realization is not prideful.

Michael: And that's the emphasis on the importance of community.

Andrew: And you're absolutely right. Part of the culture of our community is that you don't hear staff saying, "Oh, well, look at all these people I helped today." You hear staff talk about, "Well this place has helped me grow as a person, being here." Staff will often talk about what they get out of being here and not what they're giving, and I think it's all a part of our culture here. So a member will talk about "Oh well Fountain House is helping me this way and that way," but not talk about all the multitude of people they helped along the away.

Mario: One thing that I heard in all the years . . . I've been here since 1977 . . . I think one or two staff were like, "Well members should give back to the club," and that just really pisses me off. I didn't sign a contract. There isn't a sign that says because Fountain House accepted me as a member, I have the qualifications to be a member here, that I now owe. You know this is kind of out of left field. But I have heard it twice in all those years.

Elliot: I'm sure you've heard crazier stuff in your forty years here. But that just annoyed you, it stuck.

Mario: That just annoyed me, yeah.

Andrew: Well I think some people have interpreted it that way, and I have definitely heard it at other clubhouses, people talking about that and I find that disturbing. On the other hand it's what happens naturally in this type of environment. It is not that you owe anyone anything, but it's about you getting that satisfaction out of doing it because you want to. The core principle of the need to be needed, and so it's not "Oh because we're helping you, you need to do this." It's helping me to help others.

Mario: You don't hear it addressed to staff. You don't hear staff saying, "Well staff have gotten jobs here so they should feel grateful to Fountain House and they should give back and work extra hours for nothing." Somebody might be single and they can spend extra time here. Somebody else might have a husband, a wife, a significant other, children, pets . . .

Elliot: A black and white cat.

Mario: A black and white cat! And so they can't, even though would like to spend extra time, volunteer, give free time. It's just sometimes, it's not a big deal. Just little irritations here and there.

Elliot: I like your irritations.

Michael: So we have about fifteen minutes left at most. Is there anything else you'd like to put out there? Is there anything else you'd like to say?

Elliot: I might ask once it's out, or when it's getting close, have some people from the book come in and speak to the staff about the book and answer questions. It'll be staff and members, that's always how we do everything, but it'll be primarily for new staff you know?

We do these things called Lunch and Learns so we'll have you in the library and you guys can talk about, "Well this is what we made" etc.

Michael: We'd love to come in any time.

Mario: This is a complex book. It's got all kinds of philosophical stuff and you have someone just graduating . . .

Elliot: Right, not an educated elite like yourself.

Mario: No, no I couldn't understand half the stuff. Winnecott and crazy children and the fucking dialogue and shit. Fascinating stuff but I was like, "Oh I can't understand them!"

Andrew: The social workers just read this last year, so they're all familiar with it.

Elliot: Well that's why I think having them come in to just talk about it is better than just "Here's the book, read it, and understand it." Our culture is much more of an oral culture.

Chapter Sixteen

The Idea of Fountain House

A Place for Recovery in the Community

Kenneth Dudek and Alan Doyle

Fountain House is about an idea in psychiatric recovery whose time has come.[1] Most people who know of Fountain House think of it as a place for people with psychiatric illnesses[2] located on West 47th Street in New York City's historic Hell's Kitchen neighborhood. They associate its founding in 1948 with a group of ex-patients and their wealthy sponsors amid high hopes of helping one another to reenter society upon their discharge from a mental hospital. They may even be aware of the formative influence of John Beard, who labored for more than twenty-five years on the early design and development of Fountain House. Most are unaware, however, that Fountain House is more than an operational endeavor that achieves recuperative results with its membership. It is an idea whose expression combines both a compelling ideal of human nature, i.e., *community*, and a treatment methodology, *social practice*, that has inspired its replication in hundreds of places throughout the world.

The recovery paradigm (Anthony, 1993; Hogan, 1994; Whitley & Drake, 2010) holds out the hope of recovery for those who live with an illness that was once considered to be chronic and progressively debilitating. The paradigm affirms that they can live active, productive, and assimilated lives in society and asserts the rights of people with serious mental illness for self-determination and control over the treatment of their illness. Consequently, any topical discussion of broad-scale public policy for improving mental health services must integrate consumers of mental health services as active participants in their own recovery and be able to demonstrate the outcomes of personal empowerment and social inclusion with tangible evidence (hence, the call for evidence-based practice).

In point of fact, Fountain House, as we shall describe here, established all of these ideas and practices as essential to recovery and the social inclusion of people with mental illness decades before their broader public recognition in the 1990s. Long before these ideas became accepted practice in Community Mental Health, Fountain House had charted the basic coordinates of employment and housing for people with mental illness, as well as other current practices in mental health (Sowbel & Starnes, 2006). In Fountain House, we explicate how the values of hope, empowerment, evidence-based outcomes, and social integration are translated into practice and how our idea of a *working community* speaks directly to the needs of today's broken mental health system.

DEINSTITUTIONALIZATION AND RECOVERY

We believe that the present mental health service delivery system in the United States is in need of repair. We see it firsthand every day in the lives of our members, who without adequate community support services are left completely to their own devices. Under such circumstances, many people who suffer from serious mental illness tend to withdraw. Former patients spend inordinate amounts of time at home with their families, live alone in a room, or are trapped in a jail cell. In effect, social isolation has become an all too common experience for people suffering from mental illness. While this group now lives in society and no longer in asylums, they are for the most part not really a vital part of that society.

Nor are we alone in this assessment. The editors of the *Psychiatric Services Journal* devoted the May 2012 issue to a review of social inclusion for people living with mental illness. They concluded that, while gains exist, the high hopes for advancing this issue have been disappointed. It is unimaginable that a society would deny patients upon leaving the hospital the rehabilitation services they need to support their productive reentry into society. And yet that is what occurs every day for people suffering from mental illness. While ample funding exists, principally through Medicaid, to address crisis episodes with hospitalization, most receive no form of ongoing rehabilitation. And people living with mental illness, who remain for the most part divorced from primary health care services, die on average twenty-five years earlier than the general public does (Parks et al., 2006). Suicide annually claims the lives of a significant number of people with serious mental illness. According to an October 9, 2006, World Health Organization news release, 90 percent of all suicides are associated with mental disorders.

LOSS OF PLACE FOR RECOVERY

The idea of having a place for recovery—a niche, so to speak, in society—is not new in mental health practice. It was the original idea behind the asylums of the nineteenth century. Patients were removed from congested urban places, which were thought to precipitate their illnesses, and given refuge in the tranquility of the countryside. These asylums gradually evolved, however, into the state mental hospital system, which by the late 1940s, while providing comprehensive medical and social care to people suffering from severe mental illness, had become overcrowded, underfunded, and hardly reflective of the humane and therapeutic approach of the moral treatment upon which the institutions were originally patterned. With the introduction of psychotropic medications, the passage of the Community Mental Health Centers Act (Pub. L. *88-164*) on October 31, 1963, and the subsequent waves of deinstitutionalization, a new chapter was opened in the care and treatment of people suffering from mental illness. In the United States more than half a million people with severe mental illness moved from life totally spent in institutions back into their communities (Grob, 1994). Mental illnesses were no longer considered chronic, deteriorating diseases, and recovery from mental illness was now seen as a real possibility.

While it was right to do away with these bureaucratic nightmares, it was equally wrong not to replace them with adequate resources to help people with mental illness to live in the community. Deinstitutionalization was implemented without sufficient social supports in place and even less understanding of the impact that co-occurring conditions such as homelessness, unemployment, and drug addiction would have in their lives. Statistics reported by Klein (2006, p. 35) are alarming:

> Approximately 35 percent of homeless people are suffering from mental illness.
>
> The closing of inpatient psychiatric beds has resulted in the transfer of care from the hospital to other institutions that have not been able to adequately deliver effective services.
>
> U.S. jails and prisons currently house people suffering from serious psychiatric disorders in greater numbers than do public institutions.
>
> Discharge planning has not been successful in decreasing re-hospitalization over the long term.

And employment, which is the ultimate measure of success in recovery, remains elusive. Adults with serious mental illness face many challenges in attaining and retaining employment. As summarized by the President's New Freedom Commission's Subcommittee on Employment and Income Supports (2003), people with serious mental illness have the highest level of unemployment of any group with disabilities—fewer than one in five are employed. Unemployment occurs despite surveys showing that the majority of people with serious mental illness want to work and many could be working with assistance. The loss of productivity and human potential is costly to society and tragically unnecessary.

Nor does public funding for mental health services support the goal of recovery in society. Fifty years ago most mental health dollars supported the state mental hospital system. The majority of these hospitals have since been closed. In their place have emerged psychiatric wings in general hospitals, which concentrate on acute care and offer only limited access to community support services upon discharge. The largest share of current mental health dollars in New York State, for example, pays for inpatient beds located in general hospital units reserved for psychiatric and medical services for people with serious mental illness. Only a small portion of the dollars saved from closing the state mental hospitals has been retained to sustain community-based mental health recovery options.

At the same time, the states, as a cost-saving device, have shifted their mental health expenditures to federal reimbursements under Medicaid funding. Clearly, the reason for this shift is that the state then pays only a portion of the cost. (In New York, for example, the state pays 50 percent and the federal government pays 50 percent of costs.) The irony of this transfer is that while costs of Medicaid behavioral health care are still spiraling out of control, federal regulations attached to the funds severely limit the social service options and community support programs that could be made available to help people with serious mental illnesses survive in society. While we consider community support programs involving employment, housing, and education as key to a person's recovery, federal Medicaid laws, even under the rehabilitation option, limit refundable activities regarded as educational or job-related. In sum, current public funding for mental health has created a dysfunctional system in which Medicaid-funded psychiatric services are costing more and more while the community support services, which are necessary to reduce these costs, are being depleted. Whereas government rhetoric says recovery in the community, federal funding is primarily promoting medical services in the hospital and community health centers, ironically reinstituting the medical model as the primary intervention in psychiatric community support programming.

Nor will the new wave of managed care end such disconnects in the funding system. Government-managed care is designed to control Medicaid and Medicare expenses, paying solely for medical services. As long as most of the funding for mental health services is distributed through Medicaid or Medicare, the emphasis will remain on a medical model, and community support and recovery services will continue to disappear. This is occurring despite the promotion of parallel policies that combine psychiatric, medical, and community support recovery services to address the high health costs incurred by people with severe mental illness. Last, as the states and the federal government reduce Medicaid coverage in order to save money, there is no state or federal replacement funding for recovery or community support services emerging on the horizon.

The real tragedy throughout this period, in our opinion, is the abandonment by state governments of their role to provide community support services to help those who are the most seriously ill. States are not reallocating the monies saved from closing state mental institutions and the subsequent transfer of mental health costs to the federal government. In effect, the states have abrogated their responsibility for mental health care and, under pressure to cut costs in public services, continue to reduce the funding that is necessary for the community support and recovery of people suffering with serious mental illnesses.

Thus, even though the idea that people with mental illness are able to live in the community was accepted decades ago, society has failed to provide anywhere near the range and depth of services needed so that those discharged from mental institutions can live in a meaningful and productive manner. Something is clearly wrong with the structure of the current system in addressing the needs of people with serious mental illness.

A PLACE FOR RECOVERY IN THE COMMUNITY

The idea of having a place like the Fountain House *working community* is what is needed and missing in the community mental health system of today. Despite decades since the acceptance of the idea that people with mental illness can live in the community, society has failed to provide anywhere near the range and depth of services needed so that they can live in a meaningful or productive way. As mental health policy makers and practitioners strive to design such a recovery system, a strictly medical approach of hospitalization and symptom reduction no longer offers an adequate path in mental health services. Moreover, while a range of services along different dimensions of recovery are popular and include employment, education, social functioning, and even spirituality (Whitley & Drake, 2010), still a question exists as to how best to deliver these services and achieve the results expected.

The current debate revolves around the best way to promote the social inclusion of people with mental illness within the community. One view advocates that the professional and related services be delivered directly to individuals in the community. This is known as a *natural supports* or "in vivo" approach (Rapp and Goscha, 2006). Within this perspective, social inclusion is a form of normalization where "individuals with disabilities live, work, play, and lead their daily lives without distinction from and with the same opportunities as individuals without disabilities" (p. 28). Consequently, proponents view any arrangement where people with disabilities associate in a place as "segregation" and in violation of the "in vivo" ethic. In effect, promoters of a *natural supports* approach bypass traditional assembly places and community centers. Instead, they intend to exploit the individual's resilience and the natural resources of the environment to support their living within the community independently.

An alternative view, the mutual-aid approach, which arises out of the Fountain House experience and the self-help movement (Chamberlin et al., 1996; Clay, 2005; Mowbray et al., 1988), advocates for the establishment of places in society in which people living with mental illness can meet, organize, and utilize their talents to help each other. Within this perspective Fountain House represents a collaborative recovery center where those with mental illness and those without associate on a daily basis in a productive manner to support the advancement of people living with mental illness in society.[3] We suggest here that having a place like the Fountain House *working community*, which promotes its members potential for psychiatric recovery through the mutual assistance of the staff and members together, is what is needed in the community mental health service system of today.

SUPPORT FOR RECOVERY

Social isolation has become the number one problem that people suffering from mental illness face. Most people who suffer with mental illness tend to withdraw and isolate. The reality for many is a life of quiet desperation. As we have discussed, many former hospitalized patients live in society but are not really a part of it. Families understand this issue better than most professionals because they are often the caregiver of last resort. But even families with great resources are stymied by this problem as they watch their children ending up living at home well into their adult years. We have also seen how people without purpose or meaning in their lives, and who feel helpless, turn to drastic measures to alleviate their pain. Social isolation in the extreme can lead to suicide (Trout, 1980).

The most common form of support in the community for people with serious mental illness up until the last decade was the once a week visit for therapy and a monthly medication check with a psychiatrist. Today, however, this practice of using a therapist as the main support person has been curtailed and patients simply meet with their psychiatrist once a month for medication monitoring and changes in prescription, usually for fifteen minutes a visit (Lehman et al., 2004). In its place some form of case management has become the rule.[4] In addition, access to community-based social and medical services is complicated by their disparate locations within a service delivery area. Clients are required to travel to a variety of locations or agencies in order to get the help they need, in effect compromising the stated objective of continuity of care in a comprehensive system. Since it is often hard for the individual client to navigate this array of services (all too often, the clients get lost in the process), the additional role of the case manager has been introduced[5] to connect clients to a disparate, uncoordinated array of community services. As described by Rose (1992, p. vii), "continued fragmentation within large provider systems and across different service delivery systems characterize the setting for case management practice." Case management promises a continuum of care that provides comprehensive and integrated services for a population whose ability to cope is impaired in the face of such complex structural environments.

The basic formula for the case management model is similar. The nature and extent of its professional responsibilities usually consist of weekly meetings, benefits counseling, and linkage to housing and medical or psychiatric services. In more recent times, job placement assistance has been added to the list of services. Some case managers and their teams are meant to directly assist the client in securing benefits or an apartment, but the majority of case managers are coordinators who are meant to find others to provide this support.

Such a service system is viewed as comprehensive in design because it offers an array of programming options which are made available to the client based on an assessment of their needs. For the most part, these initiatives also follow an individualized service system approach that features focused roles for individual professionals who are expected to provide a service to the client or patient. Such an approach is considered to be characteristically American in design. Time-limited, discreet services reflect the American ideal of rugged individualism (Hofstadter, 1944) as applied in its design and approach to social welfare. As Lamb (1994) has noted in comparing American and British mental health community support systems: "Americans emphasize skills acquisition and the importance of a skills based approach in helping people function as independent as possible with the minimum of support" (p. 1019). Such a system is premised on the belief that once one or more of these interventions are successfully completed, be it therapy or supported employment, the individual is expected to have successfully recovered and will launch into independence in the community. In Great Britain, on the other hand, skills acquisition tends to take second place to helping people to adapt to their circumstances. Our solution, *the working community*, is an empowerment strategy, not just a "fix it" strategy that embraces a way that involves our members in their own recovery.

Many of these programs also advocate an *in vivo* or natural supports arrangement. Their premise is that, once living independently in community, sufficient non–mental health supports can be found which offer a variety of opportunities or "natural supports." With this understanding in mind, case workers are expected to help their client access the resources in the larger community that will support them on their road to recovery. They further assume that the larger community is welcoming to people suffering from mental illness and relatively stigma free.

There is little evidence to suggest, however, that this is what actually occurs for the majority of people living in the community. While the approach appears on its surface to give people a certain level of independence, it can just as often leave people to fend for themselves. Actually there is increasing evidence that the potential for supporting *in vivo* reintegration efforts is disappearing (Putnam, 2000). For the members of Fountain House, as well as people anywhere suffering from mental illness, society can still be a hostile environment. The stigma against people with mental illness is strong and real in many facets of the larger world whether it is on the job, at school, in an apartment, or in a restaurant. An example of the dilemma faced by people living with mental illness is how disquieting the issue of self-disclosure is for students returning to school (Dougherty et al., 1996).[6] Most people choose not to disclose their mental health issues to their employer and many are scared to death to tell their boyfriend or girlfriend about their mental health experiences. Our members live in the real world, not an idealized one. In reality, people with serious mental illness live in a world where they have daily encounters with various forms of stigma that causes them to be viewed with both fear and suspicion. In our future idealized world, we may eliminate stigma. But in today's world, having a safe accepting place to freely be yourself is a crucial part of recovery.

It is equally true that many people with mental illness have behaviors that are often misunderstood by those in the larger community. In the real world, bizarre behavior or emotional rage in public can easily lead to trouble with the police, which is why so many people with mental illness end up in jail. To build an effective support system there has to be a recognition of the realities of these negative behaviors and the resulting trouble people with mental illness find themselves in, within the societies in which they reside. In place of a focus on individual human deficiencies, however, Fountain House approaches the problem more holistically—as the attendant consequences of social isolation and the need for niches of human company for support—and suggests there be a place where people living with mental illness can gather to overcome their sense of isolation and find meaning in their lives and a circle of friends for support.

PEER SUPPORT INITIATIVES

One positive direction in community mental health services that supports this direction has been the development of peer support programs (Clay, 2005; Solomon, 2004). Peer support programs operate community resource centers that sponsor various self-help initiatives, attempting to create supportive social networks among adults with mental illness. These programs view peer-operated resource programs and peer advocacy as the future base of support for ex-patients living in the community. The evidence for these approaches is still limited but it is demonstrating constructive effects in psychiatric recovery, particularly in its use of peers as a strategic resource in a mental health team.[7] In a related vein, Mandiberg (2010, 2012) has advocated a shift in focus from professional services to a community development perspective that offers the potential for social inclusion through businesses owned and operated by people in recovery and their organizations.

Fountain House was an early proponent of mutual aid in supporting member recovery (Anderson, 1998) and the clubhouses which follow its example continue to foster a socially supportive network of professionals and peers (Carolan et al., 2011; Waegemakers Schiff et al., 2008). Consequently, we suggest a different approach, especially considering all the individuals who do not benefit from the dominant individualized service system approach and the number of existing programs that overlook the impact of social isolation upon those living with mental illness in the community. It holds the additional advantage of cost effectiveness as studies have shown that the costs associated with *working communities*, where services are provided by members and staff working side by side, are one-half to one-third of those offered in traditional professionally operated treatment programs (McKay et al., 2006).

COLLABORATIVE RECOVERY CENTER

The Fountain House *working community* (i.e., a collaborative recovery center) clearly comes out of a communitarian tradition in American society (Hofstadter, 1944) where living in a community derives an attendant sense of relatedness and social responsibility. Living in community is more than location. As discussed earlier, community is relational and involves the sense that I as a person am an integral part of a larger event (Sarason, 1974). Truly living in community is to have a "place" in that community where one takes part in its movements and gets recognized as an integral contributor. Place therefore is an important component in the social needs of every human being but most especially among our members, many of whom have lost their place in this world.

Being established in a place does not mean Fountain House projects an institutional approach. It is in the nature of a place, as opposed to a location, to establish a defining presence for patients and clients. In an individualized service system approach, there is no "place" for people to come to. Mancini (2006), for example, reports narratives by people from the consumer movement who speak about an entirely different experience of *place* where they:

> Were isolated in negative environments that reinforced the message that they were sick, fragile, and incompetent. They were bombarded with diagnostic labels that reinforced their identities as "mental patient." This resulted in an overwhelming sense of despair . . . These messages were effectively communicated via professionals and systems that were coercive, paternal, and indifferent. (p. 17)

At Fountain House, in contrast, being a member of a community means members have a place to go where they do not have to be subjected to stigma on a day-to-day basis. Just as with other groups, such as immigrants (Mandiberg, 2010), people with mental illness rely upon social networks to support their successful inclusion into society (Carolan et al., 2011). Or, as Beard (1978) once described it, people need a place where they are:

> Needed, expected. They have to be missed. They have to have people to give news to, good and bad. They have to have people to tell their secrets to. It's a terrible thing to have a secret and no one to tell it to. (p. 18)

In providing a place in community where its members come to regain their personhood, find meaning, and be among a socially supportive group of friends and associates, Fountain House has consistently related a positive narrative concerning the treatment of people with mental illness. Many members, when they first arrive at Fountain House, do not have any clear goals. We understand that the person, at the moment that is right for them, will take the first step to make a contribution and begin their reentry into the community. Sometimes the motivation comes from a big thing like a job or an apartment. But it can just as easily come from going to a baseball game or cleaning a dish. It is never certain which activity or event will trigger the first steps, but it is the sense of being needed which is the key to motivation. Their gradual participation in the community and the momentum of those activities builds motivation to work on individual goals. Also, having fellow travelers, other members as peers to share the experience, is as crucial in recovery as having a caring staff professional.

Practically, having a place of one's own, which is both part of and separate from the larger society, allows our members to come and go with ease on a daily basis playing whatever role they wish in the society at large and returning when necessary for nurturing and reinforcement, only to return again into the larger world. With the *working community* adding backup and support, every member is encouraged to balance their time between our *working community* and the larger community. Walter, a longtime member, came to Fountain House as a young man. He left to go to work for Con Edison for twenty years but kept up his connection and returned upon his retirement. He now gives back to his community of choice, Fountain House. Thus, moving between a world full of stigma and a place that tries to minimize it, we build the personal strength necessary to succeed. In fact, members describe Fountain House as "a place to come, a right to meaningful work, a right to meaningful relationships, a right to a place to return."[8] Thus, it is out of a sense of place and its attendant values for social networking within society that our *working community* approach was born.

We are often asked in creating a meaningful and caring environment whether we are holding people back from moving on with their lives. Annual enrollments indicate that most members, in fact, move on; most only stay one or two years at Fountain House (but they do come back to visit). Irrespective of how long a person stays, they all have the right to long-term support and the ability to access its resources in a variety of ways. We have learned through our practice that having a place to come to and a place to return to is crucial for everyone, but particularly for a group of people that often find themselves socially isolated. Our members have lost these connections, or more likely have some support but not enough to thrive. As Ronald, a member of Fountain House and a staunch Baptist, explained: "The church people try but they just don't understand people with mental illness." Or, as Michael, a member of Fountain House who served as a board member and supported employment placement manager, stated, "I am not hiding from the world at Fountain House; I am helping to make the world a better place."

In a *working community*, the place is constructed to foster the association of people with mental illness and those without in a collaborative manner in support of member recovery. Our sixty years of practice shows that an effective non-exploitive environment can be successfully created. If we cannot create places in the mental health system for this integration, what hope will we have for achieving it in the larger society? Our *working community* operates in the space between the mental health service system and the larger society. Unlike sheltered environments or asylums of old, working communities have open borders; they are porous to the larger world while maintaining a clear skeletal system of support. In this way, our *working community* is an "emergent community" (Lewin, 1992) serving as a portal for our members that encourages movement and growth into the larger community. Having a place to come and return to is crucial to the recovery of our membership. Having these *working communities* throughout a geographic area will provide a different kind of intervention to support people with mental illness and provide them with the services they need, such as employment and housing.

They reflect a self-energizing community that works for the recovery of all its members. Consequently, we have consciously chosen to raise half of our funding from private sources in order to further connect our membership to the larger society.

COMPREHENSIVE COMMUNITY SYSTEM OF CARE

Fountain House has always projected a comprehensive approach for people with serious mental illness in the same vein as a community mental health center. While we have always recognized that the biological issues of mental health and mental illness are real and will not be fixed solely by environmental interventions,[9] we find the opposite view to be equally true that these problems will not be fixed by biological or clinical interventions alone, be they medication, therapy, or some other medical intervention. Denial of the reality of the clinical nature of the problems does not serve our membership well. But it is also true that not being aware and not factoring in a person's day-to-day life is equally shortsighted. Recovery means acknowledging that there is something very real and unique about the mental health issues that people face. Fountain House began at a time before medication existed with a belief in the fundamental resiliency of the human spirit and we continue to operate on that belief to this day. But to achieve this goal, Fountain House has always recognized that partnerships with other agents within society are necessary. Foremost has been its partnerships with employers (i.e., through the transitional employment) and its partnership with community psychiatry.

Over the last fifteen years, Fountain House has been developing a community-based recovery approach that partners its *working community concept* with a health service center (the Sydney Baer Center), including psychiatric services. The Baer Center along with Fountain House is designed to provide a Comprehensive Community System of Care for people with mental illness to live in society (Aquila et al., 1999). Given the high incidence of serious physical health issues afflicting those with mental illness, current research has emphasized combining psychiatry with general health services (Parks et al., 2006). Fountain House has taken this concept one step further adding a *working community*. The resulting amalgam of medical and psychiatric resources in concert with a *working community* creates a team of people focused on the recovery of the patient/member.

Such an alliance addresses the limitations of a strictly therapeutic relationship of brief encounters that focus solely on the symptoms of the illness with only partial information available for diagnostic purposes. In its place, the Community System of Care has come to add significant value to the process of recovery by introducing both the member and his or her staff worker as active agents in the process. Both the medical and psychiatric staff and the social practitioner appreciate the subtlety of the role of choice in the recovery process. At their discretion, members invite their staff worker from the clubhouse or residence to accompany them to the storefront clinic (or any other house member, friend, or family member). The social practitioner and others who have spent a great deal of time with the member is in a position to provide insight to the doctors about the unique reasons why, for example, someone is not taking their medicine or is facing difficulties in handling ordinary functions. Additionally, such an alliance structure broadens the scope of any inquiry so that the whole team sees the goals of employment, health, housing, and education as vital to the long-term well-being of the member. In concert with establishment of the Baer Center, Fountain House has also added a wellness unit (The Lewis Wellness Center) to its basic house operation to emphasize the crucial role that diet and exercise play in the recovery of someone with serious mental illness. Consequently, the alliance has resulted in the timely detection and treatment of major medical conditions, such as diabetes and heart disease, and in a yearly re-hospitalization rate of less than 10 percent.

Fountain House has also found that it is difficult to attract psychiatrists and general practitioners to work in the community with people with major mental illness. The absence of an adequate funding stream limits any ability to effectively practice. Fountain House, on the other hand, is constantly trying to create a satisfying job for the psychiatrist and facilitating long-term relationships between the doctor and the members, especially within a recovery emphasis. Our storefront psychiatrists and general practitioners have in effect a different kind of health care practice where physicians resemble more the old-fashioned general practitioner whose knowledge of their patients' lives informs their treatment, or in our case, their recovery process. Each of our doctors is able to spend more than the standard fifteen-minute routine with their patients and is attuned as well to their patients' recovery goals such as jobs, school, or housing, as well as physical health. The extra time available to the psychiatrist in working with the member and staff person ensures there are no confounding factors to impede progress.

Our hope is that a network of these *working communities* in conjunction with medical and psychiatric recovery clinics spring up to provide the combination of medical and social support necessary for a person with major mental illness to survive and thrive in today's world.

Fountain House began at a time that predated the advent of psychopharmacology and deinstitutionalization. Even so, Fountain House began with a belief in the resiliency of the human spirit and the need for a place in the community where its vision for a better life for those living with mental illness can be realized.

We have argued throughout that the continuity and success of Fountain House is ultimately founded on the social nature of its enterprise. Fountain

House is a community of people who work side by side in support of the psychiatric recovery of its members. As such it incorporates methodologies that have long been the staple of both psychiatry and social work: task group methodologies that offer purposeful opportunities and diverse, meaningful roles; a mutual-aid framework commonly employed by immigrant and afflicted populations; and the public advocacy of the settlement house movement. Our methodology integrates the professional expertise of the *social practitioner* with the ideals of social justice, human respect, and member empowerment, which inspires both professional and volunteer alike. Adapting and integrating these strains of practice, Fountain House has evolved over the years through innovation and reflection a signature approach in psychiatric recovery, the *working community* that is highly transportable, cost effective, and capable of adoption the world over.

Fountain House appreciates the deep sense of isolation suffered by people with mental illness. Our goal is the social inclusion of people who are excluded from the larger society. It is a goal shared by today's mental health establishment. We have, however, resisted the narrow boundaries of their strategies and suggested instead a more expansive approach. Fountain House presents the tradition and benefit of community—largely either ignored or jettisoned by the mental health establishment—that is founded in humanistic and progressive thought as its antidote. Like those in the post-civil-rights era, we understand that the passage of laws or the affirmation of rights, while honorable acts, are insufficient in realizing the dream of participation in society by people living with mental illness. We applaud the consumer movement and demand with them that there be places in society to bridge the chasm between the mental health service system and the larger society. An emergent *working community* is one which functions like a sturdy bridge that spans the chasm between the chaos of the world and the cocoon of the mental health care system and constantly supports the forays of its members into the larger society. *Working communities* in society give members the time and space they need to explore and understand what it means to live a full life and for communities like Fountain House to continue developing innovative techniques that support these efforts. Additionally, its collaborative nature is capable of gathering the diverse interests of various public agents and stakeholders (business and health sectors in particular) with whom it forms pragmatic partnerships to provide as comprehensive a community of care as a society is able to devise. We hope in explicating here the theoretical underpinnings of our unique form of *social practice,* the publication of this book will encourage interest and discussion in the greater application of the *working community* in achieving our common vision that people with serious mental illness can live and thrive in our communities.

NOTES

1. This material has been adapted and extended from material first published in *Fountain House: Creating Community in Mental Health Practice*, (2013), by Alan Doyle, Julius Lanoil and Kenneth Dudek, and adapted here by kind permission of Columbia University Press and the authors.

2. Note, the community mental health movement typically uses the term *illness* to describe severe psychiatric distress, and the usage in this chapter is consistent with that nomenclature. As noted in the introduction, the editors of this book prefer the terms *psychiatric distress* or *psychiatric struggles.*

3. If one were to locate the position of Fountain House on a continuum of services based on the source of aid in recovery—from professional to peer support—Fountain House would represent an amalgam of the two approaches, with staff assuming the expertise of social practitioners who promote mutual aid of the membership within a community working for the recovery of its members.

4. Or lately, "care management," an insurance program within a restricted network of doctors and services that promises effective care at least cost.

5. In the Unites States, the services of case management are mandated by federal law P.L. 99–660.

6. Dougherty et al. also note the crucial need for primary group supports in aiding individuals to manage such situations.

7. See Beeble & Salem, 2009; Corrigan et al., 2002, 2005; Pistrang, Barker, & Humphreys, 2008; Roberts et al., 1999; Verhaeghe, Bracke, & Bruynoghe, 2008.

8. The statement is prominently displayed at Fountain House as well as clubhouses around the world that imitate its methodology.

9. In fact, recognizing the importance of allied quality psychiatric care for people suffering from mental illness, Fountain House has always partnered with psychiatrists for assistance on clinical issues (Doyle, 2012).

Afterword

Reflections on Collecting and Telling These Life Stories

Secil Arac-Orhun, Marilyn Charles,
Michael O'Loughlin, and Montana Queler

MARILYN CHARLES

I particularly appreciate the inclusion of chapter 15, in which the collaborators who made this book possible—Fountain House members and staff, interviewers and authors—spoke about their hopes, fears, and concerns with the text, the process thus far, and the possibilities for this volume. Each of us involved in the project has their own hopes and fears, depending on precisely where we are situated in relation to the issues under discussion.

As a psychotherapist who works in a therapeutic community, and who is devoted to social issues and to behaving with as much integrity as I can muster, I was particularly interested to hear feedback regarding what I, as a therapist and an author, might be missing. In chapter 1 of this volume, I wrote about the ethical imperatives in doing research that explores the lives and experience of others. How we open up conversations in respectful ways that may illuminate certain aspects, without disrespecting or entirely disregarding others, is always a challenge. Using the metaphor of illumination, we can see that spotlighting certain areas will always leave others in relative obscurity. We can see from the very rich and probing conversation detailed in chapter 15 ways in which the authors' focus, however well-intentioned, also left other areas unexplored.

One significant theme from that conversation that I would like to take up here is that of the importance of community. Fountain House members rightfully point to the value of community as an essential component of well-being for all humans. We are, fundamentally, social beings and we need to be embedded in respectful, caring relationships with one another. From that perspective, we can locate the conversations detailed in this book in relation to the community that Fountain House has provided to those whose relational worlds had become waylaid as they struggled with symptoms of psychosis.

In the United States, there has been a breakdown in the system of community mental health that at one time provided a point of connection for those seeking services. Increasingly, however, as attention turned towards cost-efficiency and medication management, the importance of community engagement as a provision became less visible. Countering that tendency has been evidence from across the globe of the fundamental importance of community in early and ongoing intervention for those experiencing psychotic symptoms (Randall et al., 2015; Seikkula et.al., 2003).

As can be seen clearly in the chapters, the perspective of the interviewers and authors on the etiology of psychosis is both developmental and trauma-driven. Substantial research points to psychosis as a consequence of the interaction of environmental factors with individual and familial factors. Internationally, we see that most successful programs of intervention, such as the Open Dialogue Method in northern Finland, focus on building community supports for individuals experiencing psychotic symptoms. The latter method of early intervention has resulted in 75 percent of individuals experiencing a first psychotic break returning to work within two years and only 20 percent of individuals still taking medication at two-year follow-up (Seikkula et al., 2003), an important statistic given what we know about the health risks associated with antipsychotic medications (cf., Weinemann et al., 2015). Continual contact within community networks has been found to be an important factor in reducing positive and negative symptoms of psychosis and in improving social functioning and other areas of quality of life (Armijo et al., 2013).

Notably, Fountain House has provided precisely what is lacking in our culture for those struggling with psychotic symptoms: a community in which to make contact with others with similar struggles and to learn how to cope with problems and build a life in spite of them. Medical science works at removing, repairing, relieving, or otherwise moderating symptoms. Psychotropic medications, however, are not symptom-specific, and while they may alleviate distress in some cases, they also can have extremely deleterious side effects. Community interventions, at their best, help people to take stock of risks and resources and make informed decisions, while also affording the social support so essential to quality of life. Fountain House provides community, respectful engagement, and the possibility of learning life skills and applying those in daily life, thereby enlarging social networks, activities, and job possibilities.

With great respect for what Fountain House has been able to offer to individuals who have each been marginalized in particular ways, the authors in this volume have attempted to track the stories of those who so generously gave of their time. These stories point to the success of the community offered by Fountain House, but also afford us the opportunity to consider how the story might have been different if intervention had occurred at an earlier point in time. Although there is a victory in taking the present moment and making the most of it, there is also a tragedy in unfulfilled potential.

The authors come from a psychoanalytic perspective, from which vantage point we think in terms of the individual development that gets disrupted by trauma and neglect. From that perspective, without the ongoing reflective space that psychoanalysis—or other attuned, attentive relationships—can provide, we are left looking at the evolution of tragedy without being able to repair it. By opening up the missed possibilities, we hope to invite those who read this volume to recognize ways in which we each might help children in need of greater assistance and engagement to find the resources they need at as early an age as possible, so that their development might proceed more smoothly and resiliently, rather than becoming strained and waylaid.

We recognize, with gratitude, the people who have shared their lives with us in an effort to point to what Fountain House has given them, and in that process show what the type of reflective space afforded in the interviews might also offer. This, to me, is the spirit of the partnership of the project. We hope that, in bringing forward these stories in which the importance of community shines through, that we will invite people to consider how they might bring those principles into their more respectful engagement with those whose lives they touch.

SECIL ARAC-ORHUN

Fountain House Program Director Elliott Madison's suggestion to get to know the members prior to starting the interviews had not occurred to me, yet it made so much sense when he suggested it. Looking back at the whole project after its completion, I can see that it is very much in line with Fountain House's emphasis on relationships, and on the creation of shared human experience through building a working community. The horticulture unit, with daily shared tasks that required partnership and working side by side, was the ideal setting to have the members get to know who I am, and trust this stranger who was supposed to lend an ear to some of the most difficult aspects of their life stories. That is how I started my days in the horticulture unit in the heat of the summer of 2012. Jeff and I would carry the heavy water hose together to water the plants on the sidewalk outside Fountain House, or we would make rounds of the Fountain House departments to water the potted plants. Daniel and I made flower arrangements for the whole building, and we delivered them to the departments. With my goal-oriented drive, in the initial days, I remember becoming absorbed in the task at hand, yet, it took one of the staff to point out that it was not the task, per se, but the simple act of doing it together that was the point. It was the trust engendered as a result of these initial partnerships that allowed certain members to open up during our interviews, and enabled them to speak about their difficulties, and share the pride of their resilience with me. A surprising aspect was how easily the members accepted me, which speaks to the welcoming and caring atmosphere that Fountain House provides to its members. In that light, it is no wonder that Fountain House was initially protective of their members and skeptical of "clinical psychologists" who might examine or pathologize its members, or take their stories without giving back. Meanwhile, for me, with each conversation, the relationship that started while partnering on a task deepened, and each member revealed different aspects of their identities. As a result, I developed deep feelings for each member, be it for their sense of vulnerability, their resilience, or their struggles. One such person was Mary. I noted in my log at the time:

> Mary felt the need to have several weeks between each interview to feel ready for the next one. As she did not have regular individual therapy, I had a sense that the interviews were her therapy, allowing her to come to realizations about herself and her past. . . . At the end of the final interview, I remember a sense of sadness that our conversations were coming to an end, as I could tell how much she was getting out of each conversation. At the end of the third conversation, she asked me what I thought about what had happened to her, and what was my understanding of her struggles. She expressed that our conversations did not feel enough and that Fountain House should facilitate more conversations like we had. My interviews with Mary taught me how important it is to place one's life circumstances into a narrative so that one can make sense of the life events that might have contributed to his or her condition. She appeared to be very insightful and reflective, and I am troubled by the fact that she was only treated with medications, rather than offered alternative ways of coping with her traumatic experiences. More importantly, I gained an appreciation of her struggles and an understanding for the "protectiveness" of Fountain House for its members, protecting them against researchers who might come in, take away members' stories, and leave.

The conversations also allowed me to have a grasp of the resilience of the participants, and the strength they summoned against the obstacles some of the members faced. After one conversation with Courtney, I wrote, "She is such a resilient, strong woman. . . . I respected and admired the way Courtney asked for help, or tried to reach out to connect with others although she talks a lot about isolating herself." Courtney was one of the people who impacted me deeply:

As the interview ended, I felt hopeful for Courtney. First of all, she had insight-oriented therapy, and I could tell that she had internalized the therapy to a certain extent. Secondly, she had a sense of reflecting on unhelpful people in her life, including therapists, in an attempt to find more helpful ones, and her sense of resilience, along with her survival skills appeared resourceful and hopeful. Finally, I felt hopeful as I could feel that she had a strong desire to form meaningful attachments, including with me. She was very responsive to my comments and questions, which gave me a sense of hope that Courtney, a highly traumatized woman, did not lose all her hope and trust in forming attachments.

Meanwhile, the thought that perhaps the conversations touched the members in some ways made the project more fulfilling. For example, I was touched when Mary expressed her disappointment that the conversations had come to an end. I was moved, too, when Kyle gave me a set of beautiful handmade cards in which he had drawn scenes from nature. This gift spoke to his appreciation and desire to be remembered, along with providing evidence of how talented he is as an artist. After conversing with Kyle, I noted:

> Kyle raised my concerns about suicide risk, as we kept exploring the topic of "giving-up." At that moment, I did a suicide assessment, however, I was relieved that he contacted me a year later, asking me for a referral, saying "I was wondering if you may be able to refer me to any person who might NOT be a student of cognitive therapy as I feel I need some insight into my character and why I have chosen such an isolated path in life." His email gave me hope and faith in both my study and the field of psychology that had given an opportunity to explore life narrative. People can become curious about their life struggles and seek to make meaning out of their life events.

Contrary to the fears that with our research we would take from the members without giving back, when I was contacted by participants or when I heard from a staff person that the member was doing well, it meant so much to me. For example, Mary was initially nervous about the conversations we were about to have, and the questions that she might have to answer. Yet, she expressed a different opinion after we were done:

> In the end, when I asked her if she had any questions for me, she asked me what I thought about her early experiences and the way her life turned out to be . . . I gave her my understanding of it, and feared that it was not enough. . . . There was a sense of her sharing so much of her pain and suffering and I worried that whatever I said would not be enough, and that she would truly benefit from psychotherapy. . . . After the interview, I asked her how she was feeling, and she told me that the interview was not bad, she was feeling good about herself, and that talking in the interview was a "cleansing experience" for her. It was such a relief to hear that, and it makes the interviews even more

> valuable, because it feels like we are offering the members something valuable.

These conversations were quite intimate and allowed me to get a glimpse of members' lives and, after six years, I still think of them from time to time, and wonder how their lives are going. I continue to feel gratitude for the openness and generosity that allowed this project to come to fruition.

MONTANA QUELER

In hindsight, the suggestion on the part of Fountain House that we as researchers spend time immersing ourselves in the culture of the place as volunteers held a brilliant insight. Our interviews were impacted in crucial ways by this involvement. We not only had the opportunity to learn about the ways in which members related to and participated in this thriving ecosystem, they also had an opportunity to get to know us, relative outsiders who strove to make ourselves useful while also studying what it meant to be on the inside. We were learning about them, and they were learning about us. Through this mutual curiosity we built relationships, and through these relationships the interviews bloomed. The horticulture unit, where our volunteering activities were based, was perhaps a most appropriate setting for such cultivation.

Asking someone to share the intimate details of their life story is rather intrusive. There is something deeply vulnerable in such meetings for both parties, and especially so for the person being interviewed. Having spent time with some of the participants prior to the interviews, we recognized that through the interviews we were afforded access to secret windows—participants drew the curtains back for us, because we asked them to. That awareness was humbling. We also recognize that what we saw through these windows was both relationally and temporally contingent. What was being shown and how we perceived and interpreted this information was affected by personal subjectivities and the co-constructed dynamics between us, also influenced by how each person felt at that particular time on that particular day. We know that these influences render claims of objective truth about the people we interviewed impossible.

With this awareness, we approached the interviews with an appreciation of participants' humanity. One consequences of this was that we sometimes worried about the vulnerability the interviews evoked in participants. After my first interview with Faith, I wrote:

> Leaving the conversation, I felt concerned about Faith. It seemed I had reopened old wounds, and I was sad that I would be leaving her to process on her own. Her eyes were demonstrably moist as we drew to a close, and she agreed

> with my observation that much of our conversation had been difficult for her, engendering an overall uneasiness and exhaustion. After we finished Faith returned to the horticulture unit . . . the fact that she had resumed her work in the unit reassured me that she was not experiencing excessive distress, and her fairly robust support system (the Fountain House community and residence, AA fellowship which she is quite connected to, psychiatrist, and therapist) also helped me contain my anxiety that I would be leaving her to process some difficult material.

There were also moments when this kind of concern for participants emerged palpably during an interview, influencing the course the conversation took. For example, reflecting upon an interview with Dylan I noted:

> It sounded to me as though he was having these hostile hallucinations even as a child. . . . As I probed further on this subject, I began to experience a creeping sensation that we were headed into a dark place. While I felt this could lead to a richer understanding of what he had experienced, I also intuited that we might touch upon something terribly troubling for Dylan, so before proceeding I asked whether we should continue or whether he thought we should change subjects. Dylan took me up on the option to change subjects. . . . I felt protective of his need to be protected . . .

Having spent months in the horticulture unit before identifying prospective participants, some of our interactions during those months forged an unexpected background context for subsequent interviews. For example, one day on the unit Teresa enlisted my help typing a letter to her beloved "E." This elicited some mild admonishment from those around us who began to take notice. In response, Teresa clammed up about her relationship with E until outside attention seemed to subside. I had the sense that because I remained open to assisting in the letter-writing project and conveyed interest in what it was about, she felt inclined to continue elaborating on this subject during the interviews.

The personal focus inherent to the interview process also seemed to expose interpersonal longings felt by some of the people we spoke with. Many participants conveyed a yearning to be seen and loved with varying degrees of directness. After speaking at some length about her desire to reconnect with estranged family members, Eliza thanked me for taking the time to meet with her and expressed having enjoyed our time, noting, "You made me feel like a good person." Dylan, at the end of the interviews, related, "I'm just going to change my life and then see a girl and then meet her, take her on a date and then I'll marry her one day . . . the perfect girl . . . someone like you." It seemed our conversations had kindled some yearning in him to be seen and recognized. While the relationships we built with participants were relatively brief, our research took shape through the power of the bonds that formed.

MICHAEL O'LOUGHLIN

> The occasional moments of lucidity I have are becoming progressively more and more frightening. Most of the day I'm on autopilot, functioning as he wants me to. "He?" You might ask. Yeah. He. I feel as though there are two people living inside my head. The first is the "me" that has existed since my birth, the talented drummer, the Transformers fanatic, the bookworm, et cetera. The me that everyone knows and some people love. The other one is him. The self-deprecating, self-sabotaging, self-hating entity composed entirely of negativity of all types. Where all my depression/bipolar/racism/self-hatred/pessimism stems from. He's been growing and slowly taking over my consciousness since 2011. I'm currently writing this because right now, the real me has the wheel. That's where the lucidity comes from. But 99 percent of the day consists of me simply watching myself go through life. I act the same way I normally would, for the most part. He's pretty good at acting like the real me. Occasionally he slips and shows his true self, and those are the breakdowns that everyone sees, I suppose. But it's gotten to the point where I can barely tell the two of us apart. I can feel perfectly rational and present for a moment or an interaction or a conversation, but I look back after an hour and realize that wasn't me talking. Maybe I'm wrong and I don't even have the wheel right now. Sounds crazy, right? Sounds like I should be in a hospital, right? Maybe. The funny thing is, I'm not even sure I want to get better.

The material quoted here is from a spontaneous electronic communication sent to me by a young man whom I will call Doug. He is now nineteen, and I have seen Doug intermittently for therapy since he was five years old. His words are used here by kind permission, and he has reviewed and consented to this account. Doug struggled with interpersonal relations since kindergarten and he recounts a long history of bullying during childhood and adolescence. He was hospitalized a few years ago due to a fairly extreme psychic regression and an imminent desire to commit suicide. He has had significant struggles with maintaining his footing in college. He has had trouble holding fairly routine jobs, and he is currently avoiding intimate relations because of the overwhelming complexity of the interpersonal demands they entail. Doug is also an exceptionally talented musician. He lives, eats, and breathes music.

As with poet Lucy Newlyn, with whom this book opened, Doug's creative talents are a key part of his identity. On the one hand, his music is a worrisomely thin reed onto which to pin all of his hopes of life success since he will need to compete musically in a voraciously competitive business in which creative differences, commerce, greed, and a freewheeling musician lifestyle will pose extraordinary challenges. On the other hand, Doug gets up every day mainly because of the powerful creative pull of his work, and, in performing, the strongest part of what he would refer to as his original "me" is present. Doug has seen a variety of psychiatrists over the years and he is currently under the care of a capable, caring psychiatrist. He also has caring parents that are willing to extend themselves on his behalf, and he has a fairly sustained relationship with me as therapist, though it is not clear if he would attend therapy regularly without parental vigilance.

Doug's communication captures precisely the complex human dilemma this book intended to address. How are we to capture the complexity of this kind of psychic struggle, and can we develop complex understanding of the individual, familial, psychosocial, and societal variables that cause some people to have to struggle simply to *go on being*? This is the question that we fear is lost in the political debates about treatment, though it is a question that conscientious and ethical providers and treatment facilities wrestle with daily. The conundrum for such providers and facilities, as the discussion in the introduction indicated, is that in a neoliberal, capitalist healthcare system, such humanitarian concerns get squeezed in a vice by imperatives of billing, time, and bureaucratic imperatives. The cost to our society, however, of our failure to build appropriate, supportive, helpful psychosocial care is incalculable and risks producing the *wasted lives* of which Zygmunt Bauman writes so passionately in *Wasted lives* (2004).

Finally, turning again to Zygmunt Bauman, he offers an excursus on storytelling that I wish to mention briefly. Bauman states:

> Stories are like searchlights and spotlights; they brighten up parts of the stage while leaving the rest in darkness. Were they to illuminate the whole of the stage evenly, they would not really be of use. Their task, after all, is to "cure" the stage, making it ready for the viewer's intellectual and visual consumption; to create a picture one can absorb, comprehend and retain out of the anarchy of blots and stains that one can neither take in nor make sense of.
>
> Stories aid the seekers of comprehension by separating the relevant from the irrelevant, actions from their settings, the plot from its background, and the heroes or the villains at the centre of the plot from the hosts of supernumeraries and dummies. It is the mission of stories to select, and it is their nature to include through exclusion and to illuminate through casting shadows. It is a grave misunderstanding, and injustice, to blame stories for favouring one part of the stage while neglecting another. Without selection there would be no story. To say "this would be a fine story if only it did not skip this or that" is like saying "these would be fine windows for seeing through the walls if they were not framed and kept apart by the walls between them." (2004, p. 17)

Bauman's words are a reminder to us of the particularity of our vision, the selectivity of our narrative. Were time and circumstances different, we like to think we might have produced a more nuanced and situated account of the kind present for example in Annie Stopford's (in preparation) forthcoming book. Likewise, we realize that had time and opportunity permitted, we might have engaged in a more participatory action research project, or, at a minimum, created the collaborative interpretive community that was part of our initial plan. However, we are pleased to share this work and we hope it will widen the lens through which forms of severe psychic distress are viewed, and also offer a space in which the mental health professionals who toil in hospitals and other care facilities have the opportunity to step up and insist on the importance of recuperating narrative and creating spaces for psychosocial support as core elements of *care*.

Appendix

Fountain House Field Study

INTERVIEW PROTOCOL

Introductory script—First meeting

The first conversation begins with a review of the overall purposes of the research and an open invitation to the interview participant:

> Thank you for agreeing to meet with me today. I really appreciate it. Let me explain in a bit of detail what we are going to do in these conversations. Feel free to ask me any questions you have about the process.

There will be three conversations, each one lasting about one hour. In the first conversation, which we will have today, we will focus a lot on your own feelings about your life, and how your life is going for you now. In the second conversation we will ask you to talk about your childhood, your family, and memories of your past, as well as about your support system and about family and friends. In the third conversation we will ask you particularly about the different hospitals and other places you have had therapy or other treatment over the years. We are interested in how you feel you were treated, how you believe hospital staff and therapists reacted to your difficulties, and how family members reacted. We will also ask about the kinds of medications you have taken, and your feelings about whether or not medicines have helped you fell better, and we will talk to you in general about what you feel your psychiatric disability is all about. We will also ask you about your experiences at Fountain House and what you find helpful and unhelpful about being here.

Each conversation will be audiotaped and videotaped if you agree. The interview will be later typed out with your name and identifying information removed. The audiotapes and transcripts will be kept in a secure place and only available to the researchers doing this study.

We will be asking you about your feelings and emotions; about your childhood and family; and about the kinds of treatment you have received for your psychiatric difficulties. Some people may find that these questions cause them to have painful memories or to feel upset. If you think these questions might upset you, you do not have to take part in the interviews. If, you do take part and the questions are upsetting, you can stop at any time without penalty or you can say that you don't want to talk about a particular topic. OK? If we see that you are becoming upset or distressed we will stop the discussion. At the end of each conversation we will ask you how you feel and we will remind you to bring up these feelings with your staff person or Unit Leader here at Fountain House or with your regular therapist.

Before we begin I would like to go over the consent form with you and ask you to sign indicating that you give permission to have these meetings with me. OK?

Introductory script—Second and third meetings

Thank you for agreeing to meet with me again today. I really appreciate it. Do you have any questions about the process before we begin?

Let me remind you again before we start:

Each conversation will be audiotaped and videotaped if you agree. The interview will be later typed out with your name and identifying information removed. The audiotapes and transcripts will be kept in a secure place and only available to the researchers doing this study.

We will be asking you about your feelings and emotions; about your childhood and family; and about the kinds of treatment you have received for your psychiatric difficulties. Some people may find that these questions cause them to have painful memories or to feel upset. If you think these questions might upset you, you do not have to take part in the interviews. If, you do take part and the questions are upsetting, you can stop at any time without penalty or you can say that you don't want to talk about a particular topic. OK? If we see that you are becoming upset or distressed we will stop the discussion. At the end of each conversation we will ask you how you feel and we will remind you to bring up these feelings with your staff person or Unit Leader here at Fountain House or with your regular therapist.

Are you ready to start?

Life conversation—First Part

In the first conversation we are particularly interested in what Arthur Frank calls "the wounded storyteller" narrative. We are interested in when the participant first experienced psychiatric difficulties; what effect that interruption had on their life plans; what the long-term effects of the psychiatric interruption was on the participant's long-term life plans; and the participant's ability to revise the life plan and develop a new purposeful life plan subsequent to the interruption.

- If it is OK with you, I wonder if we could begin by talking about your life, beginning perhaps with why you are here at Fountain House?
- Can you tell me when you first started feeling mental distress or received a diagnosis of a psychiatric disorder? Do you know what brought it on? What did you experience? Has it been the same ever since or have your symptoms gotten better or worse?
- Looking back now, how much do you think your life has been affected by having a diagnosis? Could you, perhaps tell me what you had hoped to do with your life before you had your first episode or diagnosis?
- Do you know what you were diagnosed with back at the beginning? Has that diagnosis changed or stayed the same?
- What is your life like now? Are you satisfied or do you hope for something different?

The interviewer then follows the interview participant's lead, being particularly attentive to the participant's narration of:

- *Hopes, aspirations, disappointments, fears , anxieties, losses, disappointments, aspirations*
- *Life difficulties, including relationship dynamics, vocational successes and failures, capacity to live independently*
- *Symptoms, including distress, impairment, depression, anxiety, psychosis, and participant's understanding of these difficulties*
- *Social support systems or lack thereof*
- *Experiences of marginalization, exclusion, alienation*

Life conversation—Second Part

In the second conversation we are interested in understanding the matrix of familial, societal, and inherited factors and stressors that may have either produced the initial psychiatric crisis or contributed to the difficulty the participant had in adapting to and mastering that crisis. The second part takes up from where the first interview left off, with the emphasis this time on participant's understanding of psychosocial supports and stressors, relational successes and failures, and understanding of the origins of current and past social and psychic strains.

- I'd like to remind you again that this interview is open-ended, you can say anything about yourself that you would like.
- Could you perhaps start by telling me a bit about where you grew up and what you remember of your mom and dad?
- Are your memories of your childhood mainly happy or sad? What was the saddest or most difficult moment?
- Can you tell me about the various schools you attended and how was that experience for you? How did you do with school work?

The interviewer then follows the interview participant's lead, being particularly attentive to the participant's narration of:

- *Childhood memories of home, including caregiver/parent and sibling relationships*
- *Childhood memories of school and navigating the academic and social challenges of school*
- *Evidence for early impasses, difficulties, or suffering that might predict later psychosocial adjustment difficulties or psychological stressors and how participant negotiated these issues.*
- *Evidence of parental trauma, ancestral trauma, or cultural dislocations that might have created stressors for participant.*
- *Current quality of relationships with family members and community of origin, for example, does participant have available and use a social support system?*
- *Psychosocial stressors in current life, including social, vocational, and relational accomplishments or difficulties*
- *Aspirations and disappointments in terms of what has been and what can be achieved in the realms of family life, creativity, work, social life, leisure, and wellness.*

Life conversation—Third Part

In the third conversation we hope to understand the support structures and services that have been facilitative for the participant, as well as the participant's response to institutions and services that they found unhelpful. Here we have in mind psychiatric services, hospital in- and outpatient programs, partial hospital programs, community and government agencies, as well as the services provided by the Fountain House community. The third part takes up from where the second interview left off, with the emphasis this time on participant's understanding of the nature of the psychiatric difficulty and their feelings about the courses of treatment they have received, and their interaction with agencies, hospitals, therapeutic communities, therapeutic residences, bureaucratic agencies, social service systems, and so on. Of particular interest, in relation to the latter is their sense of the therapeutic facilitation or limitation of the various contexts which they have experienced.

- I'd like to remind you again that this interview is open-ended, you can say anything about yourself that you would like.
- Could you perhaps start by telling me about when you were hospitalized or treated for psychiatric issues?

The interviewer then follows the interview participant's lead, being particularly attentive to the participant's narration and bearing in mind the following ideas:

- *Have you been given a diagnosis or name for the psychiatric difficulties you have experienced?*
- *Has it been helpful to you or not to have been given this diagnosis/label?*
- *Do you think people react to you in a particular way if they are aware that you have a psychiatric disability or disorder?*
- *Are you taking medications now? Which ones? Are medications helpful to you now? What are the good things about your medications? What are the drawbacks or disadvantages? Do you take your medications regularly or not?*
- *If you are in therapy now or if you have been in therapy in the past, have you found/do you find therapy helpful? What kind of therapy has been most helpful for you? What kind of therapy has been least helpful for you?*
- *I would like to ask you about any hospital or outpatient clinic in which you have been treated? Can you tell me about that place/ In what ways was it helpful? What about it was not helpful to you in getting your life back on track?*
- *I would like to ask you now about your experience here at Fountain House. Why did you come here? How long ago? What are your feelings about being here? What aspects of life here are helpful to you? What do you like best about being here? What aspects of life here are not helpful to you? What do you like least about being here?*
- *What do you most wish you had in your life that you do not currently have?*
- *What is your greatest source of happiness? . . . loss?*

I would like to ask you a bit about the various symptoms you have experienced over the years or that you are currently experiencing now:

- *What are the most troublesome symptom you experience?*
- *[For each symptom] What seems to trigger it?*
- *Do you expect these symptoms are chronic, or do you expect them to go away? [If chronic] How do you feel about that? [If going away] What do you believe will help you to move past these difficulties?*
- *What do you think of labels such as "mental illness" or "disability"? Are they helpful words or not in thinking about your life?*
- *Looking back on your whole life, can you pinpoint where your psychiatric difficulties started and what made them worse?*
- *Do you ever feel stigmatized, embarrassed, or ashamed because of your psychiatric symptoms?*

Works Cited

Abraham, N., & Torok, M. (1994). *The shell and the kernel.* N. T. Rand (Ed. & Trans.). Chicago & London: University of Chicago Press.

Agamben, G. (1998). *Homo sacer: Sovereign power and bare life.* Stanford: Stanford University Press.

Amador, X. F., Strauss, D. H., Yale, S. A., Flaum, M. M., Endicott, J., & Gorman, J. M. (1993). Assessment of insight in psychosis. *The American Journal of Psychiatry, 150*(6), 873–879.

Anderson, S. B. (1998). *We are not alone: Fountain House and the development of the clubhouse culture.* New York: Fountain House, Inc.

Anthony, W. A. (1993). Recovery from mental illness: The guiding vision of the mental health service system in the 1990's. *Psychosocial Rehabilitation Journal, 16*(4), 11–23.

Apprey, M. (1993). The African-American experience: Forced migration and the transgenerational trauma. *Mind and Human Interaction, 4,* 70–75.

Aquila, R., Santos, G., Malamud, T. J., & McGrory, D. (1999). The rehabilitation alliance in practice: The clubhouse connection. *Psychiatric Rehabilitation Journal, 23*(1), 19–23.

Armijo, J., Méndez, E., Morales, R., Schilling, S., Castro, A., Alvarado, R., & Rojas, G. (2013). Efficacy of community treatments for schizophrenia and other psychotic disorders: A literature review. *Frontiers in Psychiatry, 4,* 1–10.

Atkinson, J. (2002). *Trauma trails: Recreating song lines: The transgenerational effects of trauma in indigenous Australia.* North Melbourne: Spinifex Press.

Attard, A., & Larkin, M. (2016). Art therapy for people with psychosis: A narrative review of the literature. *Lancet Psychiatry, 3,* 1067–1078.

Aulagnier, P. (2001). *The violence of interpretation: From pictogram to statement.* A. Sheridan (Trans.). London: Brunner Routledge.

Bauman, Z. (2004). *Wasted lives: Modernity and its outcasts.* New York: Polity Press.

Beard, J. H. (1978). *Beard unplugged.* Transcript of videotape. New York: Fountain House.

Beeble, M. L., & Salem, D. A. (2009). Understanding the phases of recovery from serious mental illness: The roles of referent and expert power in a mutual-help setting. *Journal of Community Psychology, 37*(2), 249–267.

Behar, R., & Gordon, D. (Eds.). (1995). *Women writing culture.* Boston, MA: Beacon Press.

Benson, P., & O'Neill, K. L. (2007). Facing risk: Levinas, ethnography, and ethics. *Anthropology of Consciousness, 18*(2), 29–55.

Bentall, R. (2003). *Madness explained: Psychosis and human nature.* London: Penguin.

Bentall, R. (2009). *Doctoring the mind: Is our current treatment of mental illness really any good?* New York: NYU Press.

Biehl, J. (2013). *Vita: Life in a zone of social abandonment.* Berkeley: University of California Press.

Bion, W. R. (1962/1988). A theory of thinking. In E. Bott Spillius (Ed.), *Melanie Klein today: Developments in theory and practice: Volume 1: Mainly theory*. London, UK: Routledge.
Bion, W. R. (1962). The psychoanalytic study of thinking. *International Journal of Pycho-Analysis, 43*, 306–310.
Bion, W. R. (1967). *Second thoughts*. London, UK: Heinemann Medical Books. [Reprinted, London, UK: Karnac, 1987.]
Bion, W. R. (1984). *Learning from experience*. London: Routledge.
Bion, W. R. (1988). A theory of thinking. In E. Spillius (Ed.), *Melanie Klein today, Vol. I: Mainly theory*. London: Routledge.
Birchwood, M., Meaden, A., Trower, P., Gilbert, P., & Plaistow, J. (2000). The power and omnipotence of voices: Subordination and entrapment by voices and significant others. *Psychological Medicine, 30*, 337–344.
Black, K. (2004). *Mothering without a map: The search for the good mother within*. New York: Penguin.
Bollas, C. (2013). *Catch them before they fall: The psychoanalysis of breakdown*. London & New York: Routledge.
Bollas, C. (2016). *When the sun bursts: The enigma of schizophrenia*. New Haven: Yale University Press.
Breggin, P. R. (1991). *Toxic psychiatry: Why therapy, empathy, and love must replace the drugs, electroshock, and biochemical theories of the "new psychiatry."* New York: St. Martin's Press.
Britzman, D. (1995). Beyond innocent readings: Educational ethnography as a crisis of representation. In W. Pink & G. Noblit (Eds.), *Continuity and contradiction: The future of the sociology of education*. New York: Hampton Press.
Burstow, B. (2015). *Psychiatry and the business of madness: An ethical and epistemological accounting*. London: Palgrave.
Bustamante, L., Cerqueira, R., Leclerc, E., & Brietzke, E. (2017). Stress, trauma, and post-traumatic stress disorder in migrants: A comprehensive review. *Brasileira Psiquiatria, 40*(2), 220–225.
Carolan, M., Onaga, E., Pernice-Duca, F., & Jimenez, T. (2011). A place to be: The role of clubhouses in facilitating social support. *Psychiatric Rehabilitation Journal, 35*(2), 125–132.
Castañeda, Q. E. (2006). Ethnography in the forest: An analysis of ethics in the morals of anthropology. *Cultural Anthropology, 21*(1), 121–145.
Chamberlin, J., Rogers, E. S., & Edison, M. L. (1996). Self-help programs: A description of their characteristics and their members. *Psychiatric Rehabilitation Journal, 19*(3), 33–42.
Chambers, I. (1996). Signs of silencing, lines of listening. In I. Chambers & L. Curti (Eds.), *The post-colonial question*. New York and London: Routledge.
Charles, M. (2000). The intergenerational transmission of unresolved mourning: Personal, familial and cultural factors. *Samiksa: Journal of the Indian Psychoanalytical Society, 54*, 65–80.
Charles, M. (2009). Psychosis and the social link: Fighting chronicity through human connections. *Bulletin of the Michigan Psychoanalytic Council, 5*, 33–44.
Charles, M. (2013). Bullying and social exclusion: Links to severe psychopathology. In M. O'Loughlin (Ed.), *Psychodynamic perspectives on working with children, families, and schools* (pp. 207–226). New York: Jason Aronson.
Charles, M. (2014). *Working with trauma: Lessons from Bion and Lacan*. Lanham, MD: Jason Aronson.
Charles, M. (2014a). Trauma, childhood, and emotional resilience. In N. Tracey (Ed.), *Transgenerational trauma and the aboriginal preschool child: healing through intervention.* (pp. 109–131). Lanham, MD: Rowman & Littlefield.
Charles, M. (2014b). The intergenerational transmission of trauma: Effects on identity development. In N. Tracey (Ed.), *Transgenerational trauma and the aboriginal preschool child: Healing through intervention* (pp. 133–152). Lanham, MD: Rowman & Littlefield.

Charles, M. (2014c). Trauma, fragmentation, memory and identity. In M. O'Loughlin & M. Charles (Eds.), *Fragments of trauma and the social production of suffering.* (pp. 25–44). Lanham, MD: Rowman & Littlefield.

Charles, M., & O'Loughlin, M. (2012). The complex subject of psychosis. Special Issue: Psychosis, M. Charles, Guest Editor. *Psychoanalysis, Culture, and Society, 17*(4), 410–421.

Charmaz, K. (1983). Loss of self: A fundamental form of suffering in the chronically ill. *Sociology of Heath and Illness*, *5*(2), 168–195.

Clay, S. (2005). *On our own together: Peer programs for people with mental illness.* Nashville: Vanderbilt University Press.

Clifft, M. A. (1986). Writing about psychiatric patients: Guidelines for disguising case material. *Bulletin of the Menninger Clinic, 50(*6), 1–11.

Comaroff, J., & Comaroff, J. (2003). Ethnography on an awkward scale: Postcolonial anthropology and the violence of abstraction. *Ethnography, 4(*20), 147–179.

Cooper, D. (1967). *Psychiatry and anti-psychiatry.* London: Tavistock Publications.

Corin, E. (1992). Positive withdrawal and the quest for meaning: The reconstruction of experience among schizophrenics. *Psychiatry, 55(3)*, 266–278.

Corin, E., & Lauzon, G. (1992). From symptoms to phenomena: The articulation of experience in schizophrenia. *Journal of Phenomenological Psychology, 25,* 3–50.

Corin, E. (1998). The thickness of being: Intentional worlds, strategies of identity, and experience among schizophrenics. *Psychiatry*, *61*, 133–145.

Corrigan, P. W., Calabrese, J. D., Diwan, S. E., Keogh, C. B., Kock, L., & Mussery, C. (2002). Some recovery processes in mutual-help groups for persons with mental illness. I: Qualitative analysis of program materials and testimonies. *Community Mental Health Journal, 30*(4), 287–301.

Corrigan, P. W., Slopen, N. A .M., Garcia, G., Phelan, S., Keogh, C. B., & Kock, L. (2005). Some recovery processes in mutual-help groups for persons with mental illness; II: Qualitative analysis participant interviews. *Community Mental Health Journal, 41*(6), 721–735.

Cosgrove, L., & Krimsky, S. (2012). A comparison of *DSM*-IV and *DSM*-5 panel members' financial associations with industry: A pernicious problem persists. *PLoS Med 9(3): e1001190*. https://doi.org/10.1371/journal.pmed.1001190.

Cosgrove, L., & Wheeler, E. (2013). Industry's colonization of psychiatry: Ethical and practical implications of financial conflicts of interest in the DSM-5. *Feminism & Psychology, 23*(1), 93–106.

David, A. S. (1990). Insight and psychosis. *British Journal of Psychiatry, 156(6),* 798–808.

Davoine, F., & Gaudillière, J.-M. (2004). *Psychoanalysis and trauma: history beyond trauma: Whereof one cannot speak, thereof one cannot stay silent*, S. Fairfield (Trans.). New York: Other Press.

Dorman, D. (2003). *Dante's cure: A journey out of madness.* New York: Other Press.

Dougherty, S. J., Campana, K. A., Kontos, R. A., Lockhart, R., & Shaw, D. (1996). Supported education: A qualitative study of the student experience. *Psychiatric Rehabilitation Journal, 19*(3), 59–70.

Doyle, A. (2012). Fountain House and community psychiatry. In W. E. Sowers, J. M. Ranz, and J. M. Feldman (Eds.). *Handbook of community psychiatry* (pp. 369–378). New York: Springer.

Doyle, A., Lanoil, J., & Dudek, K. (2013). *Fountain House: Creating community in mental health practice*. New York: Columbia University Press.

Dykeman, C. (1993). Encountering the face of the other: The implications of the work of Emmanuel Levinas for research in education. *Journal of Thought, 28*(3/4), 5–15.

Epstein, M. (1995). *Thoughts without a thinker: Psychotherapy from a Buddhist perspective*. New York: Basic Books.

Epstein, M. (1998). *Going to pieces without falling apart.* New York: Random House.

Estroff, S. (1981). *Making it crazy: An ethnography of psychiatric clients in an American community.* Berkeley: University of California Press.

Estroff, S. (2004). Subject/subjectivities in dispute: The poetics, politics, and performance of first-person narratives of people with schizophrenia. In J. Hunter Jenkins & R. Barrett

(Eds.), *Schizophrenia, culture, subjectivity* (pp. 282–302). Cambridge, England: Cambridge University Press.
Fabian, J. (2012). Cultural anthropology and the question of knowledge. *Journal of the Royal Anthropological Institute, 18*, 439–453.
Fairbairn, W. R. (1954). *An object-relations theory of the personality*. New York: Basic Books.
Fassin, D., & Rechtman, R. (2009). *The empire of trauma: An inquiry into the conditions of victimhood*. Princeton, NJ: Princeton University Press.
Ferenczi, S. (1988). Confusion of the tongues between adults and the child—The language of tenderness and of passion. *Contemporary Psychoanalysis, 24*(2), 196–206. doi:10.1080/00107530.1988.10746234.
Fine, M. (1994). Working the hyphens: Reinventing self and other in qualitative research. In N. K. Denzin & Y. S. Lincoln (Eds.), *Handbook of qualitative research.* Thousand Oaks: Sage Publications.
Fink, B. (2014). *Against understanding: Commentary and critique in a Lacanian key*. New York & London: Routledge.
Fonagy, P., & Target, M. (2000a). The place of psychodynamic theory in developmental psychopathology. *Development and Psychopathology, 12*(3), 407–425. doi:10.1017/S0954579400003084.
Fonagy, P., & Target, M. (2000b). Playing with reality: III. The persistence of dual psychic reality in borderline patients. *International Journal of Psycho-Analysis, 81*(5), 853–873.
Foster, R. P. (2001). When immigration is trauma: Guidelines for the individual and family clinician. *American Journal of Orthopsychiatry, 71*, 153–170.
Fowler, J. C., & Perry, J. C. (2005). Clinical tasks of the dynamic interview. *Psychiatry, 68*(4), 316–336.
Frank, A. W. (1995). *The wounded storyteller: Body, illness, and ethics*. Chicago: University of Chicago Press.
Fraser, S. (1987). *My father's house: A memoir of incest and healing*. New York: Harper & Row.
Fricker, M. (2007). *Epistemic injustice: Power and the ethics of knowing.* Oxford: Oxford University Press.
Fromm-Reichmann, F. (1954). Psychotherapy of schizophrenia. *The American Journal of Psychiatry, 111*(6), 410–419.
Fromm-Reichmann, F. (1959). Loneliness. *Contemporary Psychoanalysis, 26*, 305–329.
Garcia-Coll, C., & Marks, A. K. (Eds.). (2012). *The immigrant paradox among children and adolescents: Is becoming an American a developmental risk?* Washington, DC: American Psychological Association. doi: 10.1037/13094-000.
Garland, C. (1998). (Ed.). *Understanding trauma: A psychoanalytical approach.* London: Karnac.
Gartner, R. (2001). *Betrayed as boys. Psychodynamic treatment of sexually abused men*. New York: Guilford Press.
Gartner, R. (2017). *Healing sexually betrayed men and boys: Treatment for sexual abuse, assault, and trauma*. New York & London: Routledge.
Georgiana, C. (2013). Cultural identity and diaspora. *Philobiblon, XVIII(1)*, 161–174.
Gilchrist, P., Holmes, C., Lee, A., Moore, N., & Ravenscroft, N. (2015). Co-designing non-hierarchical community arts research: the collaborative stories spiral. *Qualitative Research Journal*, 15(4), 459–471. https://doi.org/10.1108/QRJ-06-2015-0036.
Giorgi, A. (1970). *Psychology as a human science*. New York: Harper & Row.
Giorgi, A. (2009). *The descriptive phenomenological method in psychology: A modified Husserlian approach.* Pittsburgh: Duquesne University Press.
Goffman, E. (1961). *Asylums: Essays on the social situation of mental patients and other inmates*. London: Penguin Books.
Greenberg, J. (1986). *I never promised you a rose garden.* London: Penguin.
Grinberg, L., & Grinberg, R. (1989 & 2004). *Psychoanalytic perspectives on migration and exile.* N. Festinger (Trans). New Haven: Yale University Press.
Grob, G. N. (1994). *The mad among us: A history of the care of America's mentally ill.* New York: The Free Press.

Grotstein, J. (1995). Orphans of the "Real": I. Some modern and post-modern perspectives on the neurobiological and psychosocial dimensions of psychosis and primitive mental disorders. *Bulletin of the Menninger Clinic, 59*(3), 287–311.

Guillemin, M., & Gillam, L. (2004). Ethics, reflexivity, and "ethically important moments" in research. *Qualitative Inquiry, 10*(2), 261–280.

Hammersley, P., Burston, P., & Read, J. (2004). Learning to listen: Childhood trauma and adult psychosis. *Mental Health Practice, 7*(6), 18–21. doi: 10.7748/mhp2004.03.7.6.18.c1794.

Haslam, N. (2000). Psychiatric categories as natural kinds: Essentialist thinking about mental disorder. *Social research, 67*(4), 1031–1058.

Healy, D. (1993). *Psychiatric drugs explained.* London: Mosby.

Healy, D. (2012). *Pharmageddon.* Berkeley: University of California Press.

Healy, D. (2019). Drug trial secrets: How drug companies and medical experts dupe you and your doctor. Toronto: Lorimer.

Herman, J. L. (1997). *Trauma and recovery: The aftermath of violence from domestic abuse to political terror*. New York: Basic Books.

Hofstadter, R. (1944). *Social Darwinism in American thought, 1860–1915*. Philadelphia: University of Pennsylvania Press.

Hogan, M. F. (1994). *Recovery: The new force in mental health.* Ohio: Department of Mental Health.

Hook, D. (2018). *Six moments in Lacan.* London and New York: Routledge.

Hunter Jenkins, J., & Barrett, R. J. (2004). *Schizophrenia, culture and subjectivity: The edge of experience.* Cambridge: Cambridge University Press.

Jackson, M. (2005). *Existential anthropology: Events, exigencies, and effects*. New York & Oxford: Berghahn Books.

Khanna, R. (2003). *Dark continents: Psychoanalysis and colonialism*. Durham: Duke University Press.

Kirmayer, L. J., Corin, E., & Jarvis, G. E. (2004). Inside knowledge: Cultural constructions of insight in psychosis. In X. Amador and A. David (Eds.), *Insight and psychosis: Awareness of illness in schizophrenia and related disorders* (pp. 197–229). Oxford: Oxford University Press.

Klein, E. (2006). In the community: Aftercare for seriously mentally ill persons from their own perspectives. In J. Rosenberg & S. Rosenberg (Eds.), *Community mental health: Challenges for the 21st century* (pp. 35–46). New York: Routledge.

Klein, M. (1946). Notes on some schizoid mechanisms. *International Journal of Psychoanalysis, 27*, 99–110.

Kleinman, A., Ramphele, M., & Reynolds, P. (2000). *Violence and subjectivity.* Berkeley: University of California Press.

Kohut, H. (1977). *The restoration of the self.* New York: International Universities.

Kohut, H. (1984). *How does analysis cure?* A. Goldberg & P. E. Stepansky, (Eds.). Chicago: University of Chicago Press.

Kohut, H., & Wolf, E. S. (1978). The Disorders of the self and their treatment: An outline. *International Journal of Psycho-Analysis, 59*, 413–425.

Kristeva, J. (1982). *Powers of horror: An essay on abjection.* L. S. Roudiez (Trans.). New York: Columbia University Press.

Krugman, S. (1987). Trauma in the family: Perspectives on the intergenerational transmission of violence. In B. A. van der Kolk (Ed.), *Psychological trauma* (pp. 127–151). Washington, DC: American Psychiatric Press.

Lacan, J. (1977). Of the subject who is supposed to know, of the first dyad and of the good. In *The four fundamental concepts of psycho-analysis*, A. Sheridan (Trans.), (pp. 230–243). New York: W. W. Norton.

Lacan, J. (1978). The function and field of speech and language in psychoanalysis. In *Écrits: A selection*, A. Sheridan (Trans), (pp. 30–113). New York: W. W. Norton.

Lacan, J. (2002). *Écrits: A selection* (A. Sheridan, Trans.). New York: W. W. Norton & Co.

Lacan, J. (2006). *Écrits: The first complete edition in English.* B. Fink (Trans.). New York: W. W. Norton.

Laing, R. D. (1969). *The divided self: An existential study in sanity and madness*. London: Penguin.

Lamb, H. R. (1994). A century and a half of psychiatric rehabilitation in the United States. *Hospital and Community Psychiatry, 45(10)*, 1015–1020.

Laplanche, D. (1997). The theory of seduction and the problem of the other. *International Journal of Psycho-Analysis, 78*, 653–666.

Lehman, A. F., Kreyenbuhl, J., Buchanan, R. W., Dickerson, F. B., Dixon, L. B., Goldberg, R., Green-Paden, L. D., Tenhula, W. N., Boerescu, D., Tek, C., Sandson, N., & Steinwachs, D. M. (2004). The schizophrenia patient outcomes research team (PORT). *Schizophrenia Bulletin, 30*(2), 193–217.

Levinas, E. (1987). Meaning and sense. In *Collected philosophical papers*, A. Lingus (Trans.), (pp. 75–107). Dordrecht: Martinus Nijhoff.

Levinas, E. (1998). *Otherwise than being: Or beyond essence,* A. Lingus (Trans.). Pittsburgh: Duquesne University Press.

Levinas, E. (1999). Philosophy and transcendence. In: *Alterity and transcendence*, M. B. Smith (Trans.), (pp. 3–38). New York: Columbia University Press.

Lewin, R. (1992). *Complexity—Life at the edge of chaos*. New York: Macmillan.

Liotti, G. (1999). Disorganization of attachment as a model for understanding dissociative psychopathology. In J. Solomon & C. George (Eds.), *Attachment disorganization* (pp. 291–317). New York & London: Guilford Press.

Liotti, G. (2004). Trauma, dissociation, and disorganized attachment: Three strands of a single braid. *Psychotherapy: Theory, Research, Practice, Training, 41*, 472–486.

Lyons-Ruth, K. (2008). Contributions of the mother-infant relationship to dissociative, borderline, and conduct symptoms in young adulthood. *Infant Mental Health Journal, 29*, 203–218.

Lysaker, P. H., Erickson, M., Ringer, J., Buck, K. D., Semerari, A., Carcione, A., & DiMaggio, G. (2011). Metacognition in schizophrenia: The relationship of mastery to coping, insight, self-esteem, social anxiety, and various facets of neurocognition. *British Journal of Clinical Psychology, 50*, 412–424.

Lysaker, P. H., Gumley, A., & Dimaggio, G. (2011). Metacognitive disturbances in persons with severe mental illness: Theory, correlates with psychopathology and models of psychotherapy. *Psychology and Psychotherapy: Theory, Research and Practice, 84*, 1–8.

Lysaker, P. H., Roe, D., & Yanos, P. T. (2007). Toward understanding the insight paradox: Internalized stigma moderates the association between insight and social functioning, hope, and self-esteem among people with schizophrenia spectrum disorders. *Schizophrenia Bulletin, 33*(1), 192–199.

Main, M., & Hesse, E. (1990). Parent's unresolved traumatic experiences are related to infant disorganized/disoriented attachment status: Is frightened and/or frightening parental behavior the linking mechanism? In M. Greenberg, D. Cicchetti, & E. M. Cummings (Eds.), *Attachment in the preschool years: Theory, research, and intervention* (pp. 161–182). Chicago: University of Chicago Press.

Malatesta, C. Z., & Haviland, J. M. (1985). Signs, symbols, and socialization. In M. Lewis & C. Saarni (Eds.), *The Socialization of emotion* (pp. 89–115). New York: Plenum Press.

Mancini, M. A. (2006). Consumer-providers' theories about recovery from serious psychiatric disabilities. In J. Rosenberg & S. Rosenberg (Eds.), *Community mental health: Challenges for the 21st century* (pp. 15–24). New York, Routledge.

Mandiberg, J. M. (2010). Another way: Enclave communities for people with mental illness. *American Journal of Orthopsychiatry, 80*(2), 167–173.

Mandiberg, J. M. (2012). The failure of social inclusion: An alternative approach through community development. *Psychiatric Services, 63*(5), 458–460.

Martin Baró, I. (1996). *Writings for a liberation psychology.* Cambridge: Harvard University Press.

McKay, C. E., Yates, B. T., & Johnson, M. (2006). Costs of clubhouses: An intentional perspective. *Mental Health Services Research and Administration and Policy in Mental Health, 343*(1*)*, 62–72.

McWilliams, N. (2011). *Psychoanalytic diagnosis, second edition: Understanding personality structure in the clinical process.* New York: Guilford Publications.

Mendelson, M. D. (1997). Aspects of self-esteem in life and in analysis, with reflections on its functions and rightful place. *Contemporary Psychoanalysis, 33*, 481–497.

Millar, M., Canavan, J., & Byrne, A. (2004). Developing inclusive research methodologies: Testing the voice centred relational method of qualitative data analysis in a collaborative research project on early school leaving. *Political Science and Sociology*, NUI, Galway; Child & Family Research and Policy Unit, WHB/ NUI Galway. https://aran.library.nuigalway.ie/xmlui/handle/10379/234.

Moncrieff, J. (2013). *The bitterest pills: The troubling story of antipsychotic drugs*. London: Palgrave.

Morgan, A. (2010). Schizophrenia, reification and deadened life. *History of the Human Sciences, 23*(5), 176–193.

Mowbray, C., Chamberlain, P., Jennings, M., & Reed, C. (1988). Consumer-run mental health services: Results from five demonstration projects. *Community Mental Health Journal, 24*(2), 151–156.

Muller, R. (2008). *Doing psychiatry wrong: A critical and prescriptive look at a faltering profession*. New York & London: Routledge.

Murray, M. (2016). *Jacques Lacan: A critical introduction*. London: Pluto Press.

Myin-Germeys, I., & van Os, J. (2007). Stress-reactivity in psychosis: Evidence for an affective pathway to psychosis. *Clinical Psychology Review, 27*, 409–424.

Newlyn, L. (2018). *Diary of a bipolar explorer*. Oxford: Signal.

Ødegaard, Ø. (1932). Emigration and insanity. *Acta Psychiatra Neurologica*, 1–206.

O'Loughlin, M. (2002). Is a socially responsible and critical psychology of difference possible? *Race, Gender & Class Journal, 9*(4), 175–192.

O'Loughlin, M. (2007a). Bearing witness to troubled memory. *Psychoanalytic Review, 94*(2), 191–212.

O'Loughlin, M. (2007b). On losses that are not easily mourned. In L. Bohm, R. Curtis, & B. Willock (Eds.), *Psychoanalysts' reflections on deaths and endings: Finality, transformations, new beginnings* (pp. 103–120). New York: Routledge.

O'Loughlin, M., & Johnson, R. (Eds.). (2010). *Imagining children otherwise: Theoretical and critical perspectives on childhood subjectivity*. New York: Peter Lang Publishing.

O'Loughlin, M. (2012). Countering the rush to medication: Psychodynamic, intergenerational, and cultural considerations in understanding children's distress. In U.S. Nayar (Ed.), *International handbook on mental health of children and adolescents: Culture, policy & practices* (pp. 275–288). Delhi, India: Sage.

O'Loughlin, M. (2013). Reclaiming genealogy, memory and history: The psychodynamic potential for reparative therapy in contemporary South Africa. In C. Smith, G. Lobban, & M. O'Loughlin (Eds.), *Psychodynamic psychotherapy in contemporary South Africa: Contexts, theories, practices* (pp. 242–272). Johannesburg, SA: Wits University Press.

. O'Loughlin, M. (2016, June). Unconscious dominions: The limits of psychoanalysis and the impossibility of the migrant's dilemma. Presented at *Psychosocial Studies Conference*, University of West of England, Bristol, U.K.

O'Loughlin, M. (2017). [Podcast]. Exploring narrative approaches to psychological distress. https://www.madinamerica.com/2017/09/michael-oloughlin-exploring-narrative-approaches-psychological-distress/.

O'Loughlin, M. (2018a). Book Review: *Psychoanalysis, the NHS, and mental health work today,* A. Vaspe (Ed.), *Psychoanalysis, Culture & Society, 23(4)*, 459–462.

O'Loughlin, M. (Ed.). (2018b). Introduction: Bearing witness to South Africa's moral trauma. In L. Muofhe & P. Phaswana, *And we forgave them: Life stories from apartheid South Africa* [M. O'Loughlin, Ed.] (pp. 1–18). Pretoria: UNISA Press.

O'Loughlin, M. (2018c, February). Rethinking psychosis and its treatment: Psychodynamic and psychosocial considerations. Presented at Grand Rounds Summa Healthcare, Akron, OH.

O'Loughlin, M., & Charles, M. (2012). Psychiatric survivors, psychiatric treatments, and societal prejudice: An inquiry into the experience of a marginal group. In G. Cannella & S.

Steinberg (Eds.), *Critical qualitative research reader* (pp. 500–511). New York: Peter Lang Publishing.

O'Loughlin, M., & Charles., M. (Eds). (2015). *Fragments of trauma and the social production of suffering.* Lanham, MD: Rowman & Littlefield.

O'Loughlin, M., Charles, M., Crosby, J., Arac, S., & Queler, M. (2014). Field note: Closing the gap: Narrating the prose of severe psychic suffering. *Psychoanalysis Culture & Society, 19*(1), 98–106.

O'Loughlin, M., & Queler., M. (2019). Faith: A woman interrupted. In M. E. Brown & M. Charles (Eds), *Women and the psychosocial construction of madness.* Lanham, MD: Lexington Books.

Pandolfo, S. (2008). The knot of the soul: Postcolonial conundrums, madness and the imagination. In M. Good, S. Hyde, S. Pinto, & B. Good (Eds.), *Postcolonial disorders: Ethnographic studies in subjectivity* (pp. 329–358). Berkeley: University of California Press.

Parks, J., Svendsen, D., Singer, P., & Foti, M. E. (2006). *Morbidity and mortality in people with serious mental illness*. Alexandria: National Association of State Mental Health Program Director (NASMHPD) Medical Directors Council.

Patai, D. (1991). U.S. academics and third world women: Is ethical research possible? In S. B. Gluck & D. Patai (Eds.), *Women's words: The practice of oral history* (pp. 137–154). London: Routledge, Chapman & Hall.

Patai, D. (1987). Ethical problems of personal narrative: Or who should eat the last piece of cake? *International Journal of Oral History, 8*, 5–27.

Peciccia, M., & DiBenedetto, G. (1998). The integration of sensorial channels through progressive mirror drawing in the psychotherapy of schizophrenic patients with disturbances in verbal language. *Journal of the American Academy of Psychoanalysis* [Special Section: Contemporary Psychoanalysis in Italy], *26,* 109–122. Retrieved from https://doi.org/10.1521/jaap.1.1998.26.1.109.

Penney, D., & Stastny, P. (2009). *The lives they left behind: Suitcases from a state hospital attic.* New York: Bellevue Literary Press.

Phillips, A. (2007). *Winnicott.* London: Penguin.

Pistrang, N., Barker, C., & Humphreys, K. (2008). Mutual help groups for mental health problems: A review of effectiveness studies. *American Journal of Community Psychology, 42,* 110–121.

President's New Freedom Commission on Mental Health. (2003). *Achieving the promise: Transforming mental health care in America.* Rockville: DHHS Publication No. SMA-03-3832.

Putnam, R. D. (2000). *Bowling alone: The collapse and revival of American community*. New York: Simon & Schuster.

Randall, J. R., Vokey, S., Loewen, H., Martens, P. J., Brownell, M., Katz, A., Nickel, N. C., Burland, E., & Chateau, D. (2015). A systematic review of the effect of early interventions for psychosis on the usage of inpatient services. *Schizophrenia Bulletin, 41*(6):1379–1386.

Rapp, C. A., & Goscha, R. J. (2006). *The strengths model: Case management with people with psychiatric disabilities* (2nd ed.). New York: Oxford University Press.

Read, J., Goodman, L., Morrison, P., Ross, C., & Aderhold, V. (2004). Childhood trauma, loss and stress. In J. Read, L. Mosher, & R. Bentall (Eds.), *Models of madness: Psychological, social and biological approaches to schizophrenia* (pp. 223–252). London & New York: Routledge.

Read, J., & Gumley, A. (2008). Can attachment theory help explain the relationship between childhood adversity and psychosis? *Attachment: New Directions in Psychotherapy and Relational Psychoanalysis, 2*, 1–35.

Read, J., & Ross, C. A. (2003). Psychological trauma and psychosis: Another reason why people diagnosed schizophrenic must be offered psychological therapies. *Journal of the American Academy of Psychoanalysis and Dynamic Psychiatry 31*(1), 247–268.

Read, J., van Os, J., Morrison, A. P., & Ross, C. A. (2005). Childhood trauma, psychosis and schizophrenia: A literature review with theoretical and clinical implications. *Acta Psychiatrica Scandinavica, 112*, 330–350.

Ready, T. (2016). *Music in therapeutic practice: Using rhythm to bridge communication barriers*. Lanham, MD: Rowman & Littlefield.
Ritsher, J. B., & Phelan, J. C. (2004). Internalized stigma predicts erosion of morale among psychiatric patients. *Psychiatry Research, 129*, 257–265.
Roberts, L. J., Salem, D., Rappaport, J., Toro, P. A., Luke, D. A., & Seidman, E. (1999). Giving and receiving help: Interpersonal transactions in mutual-help meetings and psychosocial adjustment of members. *American Journal of Community Psychology, 27*(6), 841–868.
Rose, N. (2003, November/December). Neurochemical selves. *Society,* 46–59.
Rose, S. M. (1992). *Case management & social work practice*. White Plains, NY: Longman.
Rosenhan, D. L. (1973). On being sane in insane places. *Science, 179*, 250–258.
Saks, E. (2008). *The center cannot hold: My journey through madness*. New York: Hyperion.
Sarason, S. B. (1974). *The psychological sense of community: Prospects for a community psychology*. San Francisco: Jossey-Bass.
Sass, L. A., & Parnas, J. (2003). Schizophrenia, consciousness, and the self. *Schizophrenia Bulletin, 29*(3), 427–444.
Sass, L. A. (2017). *Madness and modernism: Insanity in the light of modern art, literature and thought*. Oxford: Oxford University Press.
Sass, L. A. (2007). "Schizophrenic person" or "person with schizophrenia"? An essay on the illness and the self. *Theory & Psychology*, *17*(3), 395–420.
Scheper-Hughes, N. (1995). The primacy of the ethical: Propositions for a militant anthropology. *Current Anthropology, 36*(3), 409–420.
Scheper-Hughes, N. (2003). A genealogy of genocide. *Modern Psychoanalysis, 28,* 167–197.
Scheper-Hughes, N. & Lock, M. M. (1986). Speaking "truth" to illness: Metaphors, reification, and a pedagogy for patients. *Medical Anthropology Quarterly*. 17(5): 137–140.
Schielke, H. J., Fishman, J. L., Osatuke, K., & Stiles, W. B. (2009). Creative consensus on interpretations of qualitative data: The Ward Method. *Psychotherapy Research, 19*, 558–565.
Seikkula, J. (2001). Open dialogue in psychosis II: A comparison of good and poor outcome cases. *Journal of Constructivist Psychology*, *14*, 267–284.
Seikkula, J., Alakare, B., Aalotonen, J., Holma, J., Rasinkangas, A., & Lehtinen, V. (2003). Open dialogue approach: Treatment principles and preliminary results of a two-year follow-up on first episode schizophrenia. *Ethical Human Sciences & Services*, *5*(3):163–182.
Seikkula, J., & Olson, M. (2003). The open dialogue approach to acute psychosis. *Family Process, 43,* 403–418.
Smith, J. A. (2011). Evaluating the contribution of interpretative phenomenological analysis. *Health Psychology Review, 5*(1), 9–27.
Smith, J. A., Flowers, P., & Larkin, M. (2009). *Interpretative phenomenological analysis: Theory method and research*. London: Sage.
Smith, J. A., & Osborn, M. (2003). Interpretative phenomenological analysis. In J. A. Smith (Ed.), *Qualitative psychology: A practical guide to research methods* (pp. 53–80). London: Sage.
Solomon, P. (2004). Peer support/peer provided services underlying processes, benefits, and critical ingredients. *Psychiatric Rehabilitation Journal, 34*(4), 392–401.
Sontag, S. (1978). *Illness as metaphor*. New York: Farrar, Straus, and Giroux.
Soros, E. (2015). Eyes! Birds! Walnuts! Pennies! In L. Tanslely & M. Maftei (Eds.), *Writing creative non-fiction: Determining the form* (pp. 155–166). Canterbury: Gylphi Press.
Sowbel, L. R., & Starnes, W. (2006). Pursuing hope and recovery: An integrated approach to psychiatric rehabilitation. In J. Rosenberg & S. Rosenberg (Eds.), *Community mental health: Challenges for the 21st century* (pp. 25–34). New York: Routledge.
Stauffer, J. (2015). *Ethical loneliness: The injustice of not being heard*. New York: Columbia University Press.
Stopford, A. (In preparation). *Violence, segregation, and resistance: A psychosocial study of trauma and economic injustice in four American locations*. Lanham, MD: Lexington Books.
Styron, W. (1990). *Darkness visible: A memoir of madness*. New York: Random House.
Sullivan, H. S. (1929). Research in schizophrenia. *American Journal of Psychiatry, 86*, 553–567.

Sullivan, H. S. (1956). *Clinical studies in psychiatry*. New York: Norton & Company, Inc.
Szasz, T. (1961). *The myth of mental illness: Foundations of a personal theory of life*. New York: Harper & Row.
Szasz, T. (2008). *Psychiatry: The science of lies*. Syracuse: Syracuse University Press.
Tangney, J. P., Wagner, P., & Gramzow, R. (1992). Proneness to shame, proneness to guilt, and psychopathology. *Journal of Abnormal Psychology,* 101, 460–478.
Taussig, M. T. (1980). Reification and the consciousness of the patient. *Social Science & Medicine*, 148, 3–13.
Tranulis, C., Corin, E., & Kirmayer, L. J. (2008). Insight and psychosis: Comparing the perspectives of patient, entourage and clinician. *International Journal of Social Psychiatry, 54*(3), 225–241.
Trout, D. L. (1980). The role of social isolation in suicide. *Suicide and Life-Threatening Behavior, 10*(1), 10–23.
Vallath, S., Luhrmann, T., Bunders, J., Ravikant, L., & Gopikumar, V. (2018). Reliving, replaying lived experiences through auditory verbal hallucinations: Implications on theories of management. *Frontiers in Psychiatry*, https://www.frontiersin.org/articles/10.3389/fpsyt.2018.00528/full.
Van Haute, P. (2002). *Against adaptation: Lacan's subversion of the subject*. New York: Random House.
Vanheule, S. (2014). *The subject of psychosis: A Lacanian perspective*. Basingstoke, Hampshire: Palgrave Macmillan.
Varese, F., Smeets, F., Drukker, M., Lieverse, R., Lataster, T., Viechtbauer, W., Read, J., van Os, J., & Bentall, R. P. (2012). Childhood adversities increase the risk of psychosis: A meta-analysis of patient-control, prospective- and cross-sectional cohort studies. *Schizophrenia Bulletin, 38*(4), 661–671.
Vaspe, A. (Ed.). (2017). *Psychoanalysis, the NHS, and mental health work today*. London: Karnac.
Verhaeghe, P., Bracke, P., & Bruynooghe, K. (2008). Stigmatization and self-esteem of persons in recovery from mental illness: The role of peer support. *International Journal of Social Psychiatry, 54*(3), 206–218.
Vermeylen, S., & Clark, G. (2017). An alternative ethics for research: Levinas and the unheard voices and unseen faces. *International Journal of Social Research Methodology, 20*(5), 499–512.
Waegemakers Schiff, J., Colman, H., & Miner, D. (2008). Voluntary participation in rehabilitation: Lessons learned from a clubhouse environment. *Canadian Journal of Community Mental Health, 27*(1), 65–78.
Watkins, M., & Shulman, H. (2010). *Toward psychologies of liberation.* London: Palgrave Macmillan.
Watters, E. (2010). *Crazy like us: The globalization of the American psyche*. New York: Free Press.
Weinemann, S., Aderhold, V., Haegele, C., & Heinz, A. (2015). Brain atrophy and antipsychotic medication—A systematic review. *European Psychiatry—Supplement, 30*(1), 64. https://doi.org/10.1016/S0924-9338(15)30055-9.
Welch, S. (2000). *A feminist ethic of risk.* Minneapolis: Fortress Press.
Wertz, F. J. (2011). The qualitative revolution and psychology: Science, politics, and ethics. *The Humanistic Psychologist,* 39, 77–104.
Whitaker, R. (2010). *Anatomy of an epidemic: Magic bullets, psychiatric drugs and the astonishing rise of mental illness in America.* New York: Crown.
Whitaker, R. (2001). *Mad in America: Bad science, bad medicine, and the enduring mistreatment of the mentally ill.* New York: Basic Books.
Whitley, R., & Drake, R. E. (2010). Recovery: A dimensional approach. *Psychiatric Services, 61*(12), 1248–1250.
Winnicott, D. W. (1958). The capacity to be alone. In D. W. Winnicott (Ed.), *The maturational processes and the facilitating environment* (pp. 29–36). London: Karnac Books.
Winnicott, D. W. (1960). The theory of the parent-child relationship. *International Journal of Psychoanalysis, 41*, 585–595.

Winnicott, D. W. (1971/1982). *Playing and reality*. New York: Routledge.
Winnicott, D. W. (1974). Fear of breakdown. *International Review of Psychoanalysis, 1*, 103–107.
Winnicott, D. W. (1982). *The maturational processes and the facilitating environment*. London: The Hogarth Press.
Zubin, J., & Spring, B. (1977). Vulnerability: A new view of schizophrenia. *Journal of Abnormal Psychology, 86*, 103–126.

Index

About the Contributors

Michael O'Loughlin, is professor in the College of Education and Health Sciences and in Derner School of Psychology at Adelphi University. He is co-editor of the journal *Psychoanalysis, Culture & Society*. He published *The Subject of Childhood* in 2009 and edited *Imagining Children Otherwise: Theoretical and Critical Perspectives on Childhood Subjectivity* with Richard Johnson in 2010. He is co-editor with Cora Smith and Glenys Lobban of *Psychodynamic Psychotherapy in Contemporary South Africa: Contexts, Theories, and Applications* (2013), and in 2013 he also edited two books on children's emotions: *The Uses of Psychoanalysis in Working with Children's Emotional Lives* and *Psychodynamic Perspectives on Working with Children, Families, and Schools*. He edited *The Ethics of Remembering and the Consequences of Forgetting: Essays on Trauma, History, and Memory*, in 2015, as well as a companion volume, co-edited with Marilyn Charles, *Fragments of Trauma and the Social Production of Suffering*. In 2018 he edited and wrote the introduction to Lillian Muofhe and Ndanganeni Phaswana's book, *And We Forgave Them: Stories from the Struggle Against Apartheid in Venda, South Africa.* He also edits a book series, *Psychoanalytic Studies: Clinical, Social, and Cultural Contexts*, and he is co-editor with Awad Ibrahim, Gabrielle Ivinson, and Marek Tesar of a second book series, *Critical Childhood & Youth Studies: Clinical, Educational, Social and Cultural Inquiry*, both with Lexington Books. He has a private practice for psychotherapy and psychoanalysis on Long Island, New York. Website: michaelloughlinphd.com.

Secil Arac-Orhun is a licensed clinical psychologist, currently working at Lenox Hill Hospital in the Inpatient Psychiatry Department, in New York. She completed a PhD in Clinical Psychology at Adelphi University's Derner

Institute, where she researched narrative experiences of individuals struggling with psychiatric difficulties. She completed her predoctoral psychology internship and postdoctoral training at Lenox Hill Hospital in New York City. She holds a masters degrees in Psychology from New York University, and a masters degree in Political Science from Fordham University. Secil was born and raised in Turkey and is currently living in New York with her husband and son.

Marilyn Charles is a psychologist and psychoanalyst at the Austen Riggs Center in Stockbridge, Massachusetts, and is affiliated with Harvard University, The University of Monterrey, the Boston Graduate School of Psychoanalysis, and the Chicago Center for Psychoanalysis. As co-chair of the Association for the Psychoanalysis of Culture and Society (APCS) and past president of Division 39 (Psychoanalysis) of the APA, she is engaged in mentoring and promoting community involvement, psychoanalytic training, outreach, and research initiatives. Interests include creativity, psychosis, resilience, and the intergenerational transmission of trauma. Books include: *Patterns: Building Blocks of Experience*, *Constructing Realities: Transformations through Myth and Metaphor*, *Learning from Experience: A Guidebook for Clinicians*, *Working with Trauma: Lessons from Bion and Lacan, Psychoanalysis and Literature: The Stories We Live, Introduction to Contemporary Psychoanalysis: Defining Terms and Building Bridges,* and *Fragments of Trauma and the Social Production of Suffering* (with Michael O'Loughlin). Forthcoming: *Women & Psychosis: Multidisciplinary Perspectives* and *Women and the Psychosocial Construction of Madness* (with Marie Brown), also *The Importance of Play in Early Childhood Education: Psychoanalytic, Attachment and Developmental Perspectives* (with Jill Bellinson).

Alan Doyle EdD, was the Director of Education at Fountain House, New York, where he developed an international training institute for a community approach to psychiatric recovery that originated at Fountain House and has since been replicated worldwide. Previously he was the assistant director for a regional vocational school on Long Island, New York, providing occupational training to adults and high school students and literacy education to immigrants. While there he also created an alternative high school for disaffected teenagers. He has served as the liaison of the Massachusetts State Education Commissioner to the state's congressional delegation in Washington, DC, and was a teacher of Latin in the Great Neck Public Schools and Regis High School in New York. He holds a Doctorate in educational planning and social policy from Harvard University Graduate School of Education. He is the co-author of *Fountain House: Creating Community in Mental Health Practice* published by Columbia University Press (2013). He is currently retired and living in New York City.

Kenneth Dudek is a recognized leader in the mental health field. He has led Fountain House and the international development of clubhouses since 1992. He has directed development of groundbreaking programs that address the housing, employment, educational, and health needs of people living with mental illness. During his tenure, Fountain House has been honored by many organizations—including receiving the world's largest and most prestigious, Conrad N. Hilton Humanitarian Prize—and widely praised by leading scholars, psychiatrists, government officials, and others working in the mental health field. Prior to joining Fountain House, Dudek was director of community support at the Massachusetts Department of Mental Health, where he created twenty-five model clubhouses and many other community-based mental health programs. Because of Fountain House's outstanding track record, Dudek is frequently quoted by media, invited to serve on key advisory committees, and asked to speak throughout the world. He appeared in and co-produced the award-winning documentary, "West 47th Street," as well as two short films on mental illness and stigma, "A Family Matter" and "Lance's Story." Dudek is a co-author of the book *Fountain House: Creating Community in Mental Health Practice*.

Elliott Madison has worked alongside people managing severe mental illness for over twenty-five years. Elliott is the program director at Fountain House, where he has worked for over eighteen years. He first became involved in working with people suffering from mental illness doing his anthropological fieldwork among Romani people in Eastern Europe. For the past few years he has trained staff and others on Social Practice, the therapeutic model used at Fountain House.

Veronica Ozog is currently a PhD candidate in Clinical Psychology at the Derner School of Psychology at Adelphi University. She holds a Bachelor's Degree in Psychology from Monmouth University and Masters Degrees in Clinical Psychology from Teachers College, Columbia University as well as from the Derner School of Psychology at Adelphi University. She has worked with marginalized populations including those experiencing psychosis, incarcerated males, foster system youth, and asylum seekers. Veronica's (in-progress) dissertation is entitled, "A Qualitative Inquiry into the Psychosocial Experiences of Persons Hospitalized for Severe Psychic Distress," for which she is interviewing individuals currently hospitalized in an inpatient psychiatric facility about their lived experiences.

Mario Pinot is a longtime member of the Fountain House community.

Montana Queler, PhD, LMHC is a psychologist and licensed mental health counselor. Her work has been devoted to developing an approach to healing that honors suffering and engages in narrative discourse through which new, transformative potential can emerge. Montana earned a Master's degree in Psychological Counseling at Columbia University Teachers College and a Doctoral degree in Clinical Psychology at The Derner Institute of Advanced Psychological Studies at Adelphi University. She has worked in a variety of settings including community mental health, urban hospitals, and college counseling. She has a private practice in New York City.

Andrew Schonebaum has worked at Fountain House for nearly twenty-five years as a social practitioner, as supervisor, and now as CFO. He has a background in sociology and social work. He initially came to the field of mental health through his work with the deaf community.

Erin Soros is a postdoctoral fellow in the University of Toronto's Department of Applied Psychology, where she is a nonIndigenous contributor to a project on Indigenous mental health. She has published fiction and nonfiction in international anthologies and journals, including *Short Fiction*, *The Iowa Review*, *The Indiana Review*, *Exile Literary Quarterly*, *Geist*, *Prism*, *West Coast Line*, *Fiddlehead*, and *enRoute*, and her stories have been produced for the CBC and BBC as winners of the CBC Literary Award and the Commonwealth Award for the Short Story. Her academic articles weaving psychoanalysis, philosophy, and autobiographical narrative have appeared in such journals as differences: *A Journal of Feminist Cultural Studies*, *The Journal of Intercultural Studies*, *The Journal of Curriculum Theorizing*, and *The Canadian Journal of Women and the Law*. New work has appeared in *Literatures of Madness*, published by Palgrave Macmillan, and in *Women and the Psychosocial Construction of Madness*, published by Lexington Press. Soros has been a visiting writer at four universities, most recently at St. John's College at the University of Cambridge, which funded travel to learn from Inuvialuit oral history in Canada's Western Arctic. In 2019–2020 she will hold a position as a postdoctoral fellow with the Society of Humanities at Cornell University, where she is researching psychosis and psychic energy as understood within psychoanalysis.

www.ingramcontent.com/pod-product-compliance
Ingram Content Group UK Ltd.
Pitfield, Milton Keynes, MK11 3LW, UK
UKHW041128071026
15587UKWH00009B/288